S0-BZV-995

CONSTRUCTIVE PSYCHOTHERAPY

CONSTRUCTIVE *Psychotherapy*

A Practical Guide

MICHAEL J. MAHONEY

Foreword by C. R. Snyder

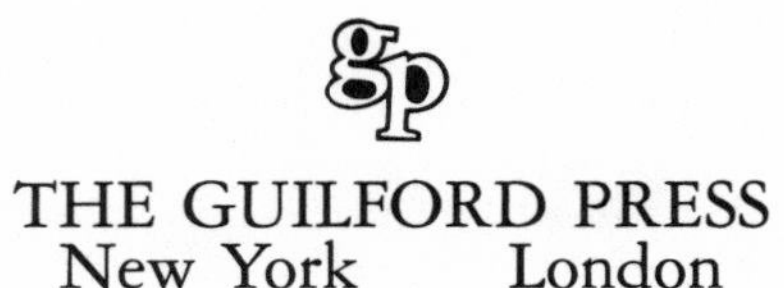

THE GUILFORD PRESS
New York London

A Division of Guilford Publications, Inc.
72 Spring Street, New York, NY 10012
www.guilford.com

Printed in the United States of America

This book is printed on acid-free paper.

Last digit is print number: 9 8 7 6 5 4 3 2 1

Library of Congress Cataloging-in-Publication Data

Mahoney, Michael J.
Constructive psychotherapy: a practical guide / Michael J. Mahoney.
p. cm.
Includes bibliographical references and index.
ISBN 1-57230-902-4
1. Psychotherapy. 2. Personal construct therapy. 3. Constructivism (Psychology). 4. Eclectic psychotherapy. I. Title.
RC480.5.M315 2003
616.89′ 14—dc21

2003007876

To
the Wump
and
da Mo

Grazie, ragazzi.

About the Author

Michael J. Mahoney, PhD, is Distinguished Consulting Faculty at Saybrook Graduate School and Research Center (San Francisco), Distinguished Professor at the Institute for Post-Rationalist Psychology and Psychotherapy (Rome), and Professor of Psychology at the University of North Texas (Denton). Honored as a Fellow by the American Association for the Advancement of Science, the American Psychological Association, and the World Academy of Art and Science, he serves as Executive Editor of the journal *Constructivism in the Human Sciences*.

FOREWORD

"On the Wings of Words . . . "

Reading this book, I was reminded of a comment that my youngest son made many years ago. He was about 5 years old, and he and I were watching a young bird attempt its first flight from the nest. After watching this little drama for some time, my son said, "There's lots of flappin', but not much flyin'." I have the same assessment of most new books that I read in psychology these days. Michael Mahoney's latest volume, however, is the exception. His ideas and heartfelt writing literally take off and make my mind soar with possibilities. Somehow, Mahoney can reach places in my soul that go untouched by other psychologists. The places on which he lays his writer's hands are deeply human; they are reached only by a scholar with quintessential scientific insights and limitless humility.

This volume is Mahoney's magnum opus. I say this with some degree of history, in that I have read most everything that this man has written. When evaluating psychologists, I think of the positive end of the continuum that goes from those who do good work to those whose ideas set the agenda for others and those whose research and words are cited widely—and then there is the "Mahoney category" that entails all the virtues, yet transcends normal terms of description. To rekindle my son's early metaphor about flight, Mahoney's ideas ascend—with grace and sway resulting from simple and convincing logic. There is an ease and exhilaration in Mahoney's writing that, for me, comes from the pleasures of having learned very sophisticated notions that heretofore have escaped my own more limited powers of thought. Indeed, perhaps the highest praise I can give this book is that it takes me places I could not go on my own.

Since the retirement of one of my mentors, Hans Strupp, whom I saw as the most insightful scholar *and* eloquent writer about the psychotherapy process, Michael Mahoney has ascended to the point where, in my estimation, he now is the alpha psychotherapy scholar and writer.

Mahoney composes with the active voice of a sports writer, yet there is a grace and precision to his words that makes me think that, if needed, he could vividly describe shades of black. This is the best written psychology book that I, the son of an English teacher, have read. I base this opinion on the fact that Mahoney lucidly describes the most complex of human processes—psychotherapy.

Unlike some brilliant scholars who become increasingly impressed with their own insights, Mahoney is the antithesis of such arrogance. Indeed, "humble" captures his stance toward himself and his subject matter. For all of the insights (and there are many) that he delivers about the constructivist approach to psychotherapy, Mahoney's conclusions are presented in a form that is more akin to child-like wonder than smug satisfaction. Throughout the chapters of this latest book, Mahoney continually reminded me of the amazement and respect that he holds for the power of psychotherapy, *along with its participants*. And, in many instances, Mahoney describes how he laughed and cried with his clients. For Mahoney, psychotherapy clearly is conducted *with* and not *to* people.

We humans are a stubborn sort. We like things the way they have been in the past. We almost treat the maintenance of the status quo as if it were the most important principle of our lives. Related to this point, Mahoney's volume helped me to unravel a long-held conundrum of mine—how at times we humans passionately desire change, yet such change must happen in concert with this powerful need to remain the same. In this regard, Mahoney easily could have titled his latest book *The Dance of Change* rather than *Constructive Psychotherapy*. There are two reasons, however, why this would not be a good idea. First, it would confuse Mahoney's book with Harriet Lerner's string of best-selling *Dance of* ___________ (fill in the blank) volumes. Second, and more importantly, the essence of Mahoney's message is that we constantly are "constructing" ourselves, and it is such regeneration that drives the change process. *In fact, we must change even to maintain the status quo*. Consider Mahoney's observation that, every 7 years, the human body recomposes itself physically. Psychologically, therefore, the answer to my earlier conundrum is that change is part of maintaining an evolving equilibrium.

If you are a therapist and are wondering if "constructive psychotherapy" is some form of New Age treatment that is unrelated to what you do in helping people, the answer is "no" on both counts. What Mahoney offers is applicable to every psychotherapist, and you probably will be able to translate his ideas to your work effortlessly. For me, his ideas served as epiphanies for my previous helping activities and vague insights about how people struggle to change.

Mahoney's book provided vivid support for my previously held view that we humans are the link between the ape and civilized people. So too do I believe that this very journey will be informed by science and humanity. In the pages of *Constructive Psychotherapy,* Michael Mahoney offers a compassionate companion for this marvelous journey. As such, this book and its author are visionaries in the very best sense; that is, instead of instructing us, Mahoney walks *with* us and shares the wonderment of the unfolding journey.

C. R. SNYDER, PHD
Wright Distinguished Professor of Clinical Psychology
University of Kansas, Lawrence

PREFACE

This is a book about the practical side of human change processes. Its central question is, What can one do to help? Many theories and thousands of research studies aim at answering that question. In this book, I do not compare the theories or tabulate every piece of evidence. I respectfully take them into account, but I do not try to review them exhaustively. My goal here is to summarize what I have learned in more than 30 years of research, teaching, training, and practice.

What I have learned is that human change is a complex and dynamic process. There are, indeed, basic principles at work. Those principles reflect both the complexities and the simplicities of the mysteries of change. I offer here a brief summary of those principles as I now understand them. The particulars of any given life are unique, of course, and I emphasize this. We must respect such uniqueness in offering professional life counsel.

Psychology and psychotherapy have become heavily categorical. The profession seems to both breathe and breed classification. Classification is a useful tool, of course. It helps us to organize and communicate our experience. But tools can sometimes become tyrants. Abraham Maslow called it the law of the hammer: We start to find ourselves pounding everything. When we fall into the habit of experiencing and describing our clients as nothing but their diagnoses, we have lost control of a very powerful tool. More important, we have lost a precious sense of our clients' uniqueness as flesh-and-blood, trial-and-error persons. I here write about flesh and spirit, errors and unexpected epiphanies.

This book addresses the personal side of psychotherapy—what it feels like to change. Change is often a distressing experience. So is its absence. People may feel frustrated by how hard it is to change. They may also feel overwhelmed by how suddenly and sweepingly their life is changing. Sometimes these feelings exist in the same person simultaneously. A constructive therapist—a therapist who appreciates the complexities of human change—helps her clients to honor such puzzling experiences. Such a therapist respects the courage required by everyday life. Personal problems and life crises require even more than everyday courage. They also demand resourcefulness, relatedness, persistence, and patience.

I emphasize the term "constructive" throughout this book. A constructive therapist experiences his clients as intentional agents in their own lives. As people ask me what constructivism is, I find that my responses continue to develop. This, I believe, is consistent with the philosophy that it represents. Constructivism is a view of humans as active, meaning-making individuals who are afloat on webs of relationships while they are moving along streams of life that relentlessly require new directions and connections. Whether they realize it or not, most clients are constructivists. They construct meanings, and they live their lives from an invisible web of meanings they have woven thus far. A large part of what therapists and clients do together in constructive psychotherapy is to weave new possibilities for experiencing. This is much easier said than done. My emphasis in this book is on the doing.

Much in these pages also reflects the personal side of being a psychotherapist. Therapists are not—and should not be—emotionally neutral technicians. We are human, to be sure, and we continue to become even more human as a consequence of our work. Clients are not the only ones who change. We therapists are deeply changed by the many lives we are privileged to serve. We are forced to develop in ways that we could never have anticipated—just like our clients. And we serve our clients well when we show them our own humanity and integrity in the face of the unexpected. We teach our clients most powerfully by risking learning in front of them. We learn, we hope, and we serve. As will be apparent toward the end of this book, much of what we learn is about the sacred nests of our connections. Let me, therefore, acknowledge some of the many connections that have served both this writing and my life.

This book was written in many places and with the help of countless others. My indebtedness to libraries, publishers, and other authors is vast. Also vast is my gratitude to the many people who have shared the gift of inspired inquiry with me. Teachers have repeatedly touched my life, from early on until yesterday. Thank you all, and particularly Mrs. Graves (first grade), Mr. Brust (sixth grade), Mrs. Lambert (principal), Miss Busch (sophomore English), Mr. Baker (wrestling), Miss Senffner (geometry), Mrs. Fike (junior English), and Mrs. Stewart (junior college psychology). Thank you, Milton Erickson, for giving me permission to trust my intuitions about my path. Thank you, Dave Rimm, Jerry Davison, and Dave Rosenhan, for your generous encouragement in my early ventures. And thank you so much, Al Bandura, for your personal modeling of scholarship and science with such generous helpings of wit, wisdom, and engaged social responsibility.

Students and friends have contributed to the joys of my teaching and learning. I wish I could list them all here, for they are alive inside me even when they are long gone or far away. Some have helped me with aspects of this book, often by co-creating a gentle atmosphere of nurturance. Thank you, Marla Arvay, Gualberto Buela Casal, Antonio Caridi, Isabel Caro, Randy Cox, Don and Mitzi Eades, Margo Edmunds, Diana Fosha, Sophie Freud, Don Granvold, Andy Giffney, Les Greenberg, Rich Herrington, Michael Hoyt, Marie Hoskins, Irma and Antti Karila, Mairi Keenleyside, Walter and Lula Kerr, Ed and Diane Lewis, Bert Moore, Cris Nabuco, Karina and Anil Raina, Mario Reda, Tammie Ronen, Michael Rosenbaum, Mukesh Saraiya, Laurie Schwegler, Joyce Stein, Ruth Stimer, Newt Trail, Scott Warren, and Barry Wolfe.

My life has been blessed with a body that enjoys movement, play, and physical challenge. I am grateful to my playmates, competitors, and coaches in baseball, basketball, track and field, wrestling, cycling, and Olympic weightlifting. It seems too good to be true that I have been able to combine my work with my love of sports. For their trust and support, I thank the United States Olympic Committee and the many athletes, coaches, and trainers I have been privileged to know and serve. Olympic weightlifting has played a central role in my sporting life, and I nod a bright-eyed "namaste" to all my gravity-challenging friends. We lift much more than weights. Special salutes are sent to Joe Amendolaro, Howard Cohen, Mark Cohen, Derrick Crass, Walter Imahara, Tommy Kono, Paul Lambert, Russ Leabch, Anne Lehman, Joe McCoy, Chuck Meiole, Harvey Newton, Jim Pumphrey, Dennis Reno, Jan Schlegel, Tim Smith, and Bob Sweeney. Thanks also to Jeff Schuckers, Mike McDaniel, and the entire Elite Fitness staff.

Mind and body are integral themes in my life. So is spirit.

Many years ago, I was spiritually adopted by two good Samaritans who soon became dear friends. Frances Vaughan and Roger Walsh took me under their loving wings and lifted my gaze toward heartful wisdom. They also introduced me to Ken Wilber. With their collective support, I discovered whole communities of gentle, compassionate, and developing beings who continue to shape and inspire my own pilgrimage. Some of our journeys together have been sponsored by the Esalen Institute, Fetzer Institute, Integral Institute, Institute of Noetic Sciences, and the Transnational Network for the Study of Physical, Psychological, and Spiritual Well-Being. I bow in gratefulness to Angeles Arrien, Richard Baker Roshi, Joseph Goldstein, Elmer and Alyce Green, Stan and Christina Grof, Michael and Sandra Harner, Brugh Joy, Jon Kabat-Zinn, Stan Krippner, Father Thomas Keating, Bob Kegan, Jack Kornfield, George Leonard, Michael Murphy, Mark Nepo, Kate Olson, Brendan O'Regan, Kaisa Puhakka, Ram Dass,

Sharon Salzberg, Zindel Segal, Brother David Steindl-Rast, Charlie Tart, Gordon Wheeler, and Gary Zukav.

If the heart has a first language, it is music. Music has been my companion through many adventures and more than a few long, lonely nights. The forms and the artists have expanded over my lifetime, but music itself has been changeless. I offer special thanks to my mother, who hummed and sang from my cradle to her grave. With grateful tears and taps of my being, I also salute Buddy Holly, Chuck Berry, Kris Kristofferson, Harry Chapin, John Denver, Tom T. Hall, and Cris Williamson.

Deep and enduring friendships are among the most precious blessings of a human life. I have been generously blessed. Through copious personal example, Neil Agnew has put my eccentricities in epistemic perspective. Giampiero Arciero continues to teach me what true loving friendship can be. Until his sudden death in 1999, Vittorio Guidano was a soul companion. Andre Marquis gently reminds me that to shine *is* the way of the heart. Holly Van Horn has been a precious "always there" ever since fourth grade. And the three Pats of my life keep me laughing, even when we hurt. Thank you, my dear ones.

Penultimately, I thank my clients. In their courage and their honesty, they have stretched me much further than I thought humanly possible. For many years now, most of my clients have been therapists themselves. They have taught me, again and again, that this profession we share is itself a privilege. Bearing authentic witness to private lives and offering wise counsel on life's mysteries is a responsibility that dances with reverence.

Finally, I thank my two best friends, who happen to be my children. Sean and Maureen have filled my life with welcome worries and boundless laughter. I am most grateful for the gifts of their being. Such gifts are beyond the reach of words.

This book, however, is full of words. Please forgive my excesses. I hope that some my words may serve as a small gift from me to all who wonder about what to say, what to do, and how to be while being helpful. May you grow sweeter as you serve, and may the dance that you dance be full of heart.

MICHAEL J. MAHONEY

CONTENTS

1 CONSTRUCTIVISM 1
A Brief Introduction
Human Change Processes 1
The Essence of Constructivism 3
Principles and Personal Revolutions 9

2 CONSTRUCTIVE PSYCHOTHERAPY 13
An Overview of Practice
Compassionate Relationship as the Heart of Psychotherapy 14
Collaboration and Action 19
Affirmation and Hope 21
Balancing Skills and Cycles of Experiencing 24
Summary 28

3 CONSTRUCTIVE ASSESSMENT 38
Measurement and Diagnostics 38
Constructive Themes in Assessment 42
Problems, Patterns, and Processes 44
Core Ordering Processes 48
Attunement 52

4 BASIC CENTERING TECHNIQUES 57
Breathing Exercises 59
Body Balance Exercises 62
Relaxing into Center 66
Finding Stability in Relationships, Places, and Patterns 69

5 PROBLEM SOLVING 73
Basic Behavioral and Cognitive Techniques
Problem Solving 74
The Essence of Behavioral Methods 76
Cognitive Restructuring 81
When Problem Solving Doesn't Work 85

6 PATTERN WORK 88
Personal Journaling and Bibliotherapy 90
Life-Review Exercises 95
Narrative Reconstruction 100
Coming Home to Process 104

7 BASIC PROCESS WORK 108
Meditation and Embodiment
Meditation 110
Embodiment Exercises 113

8 DRAMA, FANTASY, DREAM WORK, AND STREAM OF CONSCIOUSNESS 130
Role Playing "As If" 131
Fantasy and Dream Work 135
Stream of Consciousness 140

9 SELF-RELATIONSHIP AND SPIRITUAL SKILLS 152
Mirror Time 154
Spiritual Skills and Personal Development 161
A Postscript on Techniques 168

10 THE EXPERIENCE OF CHANGE 170
Static Cling: A Compassionate Look at People Who Don't Change 172
Core Change: Personal Revolutions 177
Emotionality and Change 180
Courage and Creativity 181
Transition and Termination 187

11 BEING HUMAN AND A THERAPIST 193
Vicarious Suffering: The Wounds of Helping 195
The Person and Personal Life of the Therapist 197
A Therapist's Personal Life 199
Therapist Self-Care 205
Personal and Spiritual Development 206
The Challenges of Practicing Constructively 207

Appendices

A Constructivism: History and Current Relevance 211

B Consent Form 226

C Personal Experience Report 230

D Breathing Exercises 242

E Body Balance Exercises 244

F Relaxation 247

G Mindfulness Meditation 249

H Mirror Time 251

I Kindly Self-Control 253

J Self-Comforting Exercise 254

K Spiritual Skills Exercises 256

L Human Change Processes: A Synopsis 257

M Recommendations for Therapist Self-Care 260

N Recommendations for Constructive Practice 262

References 265

Index 295

CHAPTER 1

CONSTRUCTIVISM

A Brief Introduction

What are the laws or principles of change? How and why do *we* change? What can we do to anticipate and direct change? Such questions are fundamental to all teaching, and they are central to the practice of psychotherapy. They are also at the heart of this book. I have sought to understand human change processes all of my life. I am, of course, still seeking and learning, but I also appreciate the significance of recent developments in our ways of thinking about human experience and adaptation. Relative to what was known only 10 or 20 years ago, our scientific understanding of human development has made substantial leaps. Some of these advances have been humbling and others are truly inspiring.

HUMAN CHANGE PROCESSES

Three questions are fundamental to the profession of psychotherapy: Can humans change? Can people help one another change? Are some forms of helping better than others? The questions seem simple. Their answers are more complicated than one might expect, and good answers lead to further questions.

Can we change? Yes, but it is rarely easy, simple, or pleasant. We are, in fact, capable of more change than most scientists and therapists had imagined. We are an incredibly resilient and creative life form, and we are capable of surviving and adapting to circumstances that stretch the imagination. But human change is more complex and difficult than many specialists had once thought. We do not change our lives as easily as we change our clothes. We cannot simply choose a new personality or a new sense of ourselves and implement such a change in a few weeks of casual practice. Changing our habitual patterns of being is a formidable challenge, and it is now clear that there are good reasons for this. This does not mean that we are incapable of such changes. Nor does it rule out sudden leaps in our ways of being. It does mean, however, that we are wise to appreciate the self-protective conservatism of change processes. We resist change even more passionately than we seek it. We are sometimes desperate in our quests for different ways of being, yet we gravitate toward old and familiar patterns. Change is a risky and sometimes lonely adventure.

Can we help one another change? Most definitely. In fact, most change takes place in contexts of human relatedness. We are fundamentally relational beings. Our relationships with one another are crucial to our survival and adaptation. We live in and from the bonds of belonging. A child's development is influenced by his or her parents. Parents are also changed by their children. We are changed, for better and for worse, by our families and friends, our teachers and students. We are changed by the drunk driver and the good Samaritan. We affect one another, and we create intricate webs of influence that merit our reflection and respect. Some relationships entrap us in patterns that prevent or complicate our change. And some relationships provide us with precious opportunities to develop.

Are some forms of helping more effective than others? Yes, and we now know some of their characteristics. Our understanding of human change processes has harvested valuable lessons from clinical practice, careful scientific research, and studies of the wisdom embedded in multicultural spiritual traditions. More effective forms of helping tend to be more sensitive to our personal needs, our developmental history, our styles of learning, our cycles of experiencing, the changing circumstances of our lives, and our relationships, communities, and cultures. Effective forms of helping are also more creative, more affirming, and more likely to respect our capacities for development. They reflect a perspective that has gained increasing visibility. That perspective is called "constructivism." Constructivism offers considerable promise in guiding our efforts to serve the lives and development of other human beings professionally. This book is an attempt to convey that promise in as clear and practical a manner as possible.

My goal in this book is to translate a multidisciplinary understanding of human development into guidelines for the practice of psychotherapy. Although I offer resources and suggestions for further reading, I do not survey or summarize the existing literature. Indeed, I have struggled to resist temptations to be encyclopedic. The "big picture" is a seductive one for me, but it also exacts a price that few readers are willing to pay. Fortunately, there are valuable research reviews and extensive literature surveys available.[1] My focus here is on weaving a coherent fabric of conceptualization for practice. An inherent theme in my work as a weaver is one of integration. The major conceptual traditions in psychotherapy—behavioral, biological, cognitive, existential–humanistic, psychodynamic, systems, and transpersonal—have each contributed valuable insights and exercises to what is called "constructive" psychotherapy. Constructivism also embraces contributions from anthropology, biological science, cognitive neuroscience, philosophy, sociology, and a range of spiritual wisdom traditions. It is an approach that bridges and balances many calcified contrasts, particularly those between mind and body, head and heart, self and society, and science and spirituality. Constructivism offers a positive and promising way of conceptualizing human experience as a complex, lifelong experiment. We are neither prisoners of our pasts nor free to choose any future. We are, however, vigilant protectors of what we hold close to our hearts—our view of reality, our sense of ourselves, our values, and our sense of control. When we are asked to change these, as we often are in our development, the challenge to change may feel overwhelming. I believe that constructivism offers a promising choice in ways of thinking about and dealing with human change processes. It is, in my opinion, the best conceptual system we now have that integrates multidisciplinary knowledge about human development.

THE ESSENCE OF CONSTRUCTIVISM

Constructivism is expressed in a range of perspectives on human experiencing. The range is so wide and their legacy so deep that describing them could easily require many volumes. Here, I only touch on major themes and influences. More elaborate technical information on the history and contemporary voice of constructivism is presented in Appendix A. For information on journals, conferences, and training, the Society for Constructivism in the Human Sciences is a valuable resource.[2]

Constructivism is neither new nor narrow. In Asian philosophy, it was anticipated in the teachings of Lao Tzu (6th century BC) and Buddha (560–477 BC). The Tao (literally, the "path" or "way") outlines an ancient wisdom tradition that recognizes the fluidity of life and its essential embrace of seemingly opposite elements (the "yin" and "yang"). Buddhism also acknowledges the changing (impermanent) nature of our lives, particularly our inner lives. Prince Siddhartha (more commonly called "the" Buddha) realized that we play a large role in the construction of our worlds by means of our thoughts, fantasies, and all manner of imaginings. Constructivism earned its name from its emphasis on acts of construction. The verb "to construct" means to organize or create order. As we shall see, order is essential to perception and fundamental to meaning. But in English, the word "structure" tends to have connotations of a static thing, such as a building, that does not change. The sense of permanence here is contrasted with the dynamic emphasis of ongoing reorganization emphasized by constructivism.

In Western Culture core aspects of constructivism were expressed by the presocratic philosopher Heraclitus (540–475 BC). He argued that everything that is must also be becoming. Centuries later, this would be called process philosophy. It was Heraclitus who immortalized the statement that one cannot step into the same river twice. It is not just the water that is moving or the river that is changing. The person is also changed by the experience. We are neither spectators nor pawns in our lives. As Cris Williamson has put it in musical verse, we are both the changer and the changed.[3] This is a valuable insight with practical clinical implications. No matter how small our voice may seem, it is part of the cosmic choir. Every life and every act within a life makes a difference.

The three writers most often credited as the formal originators of constructivism are Vico, Kant, and Vaihinger. Recent studies suggest that Schopenhauer may also deserve some of that credit. Giambattista Vico (1668–1744) of Naples wrote poetically on philosophy, history, and the human construction of human experience. Vico's contributions have become the focus of entire fields of scholarship.[4] Immanuel Kant (1724–1804) portrayed the mind as an active organ of self-organization. Kant argued that rather than being a passive recipient of experience, we construct our knowledge by means of categories. We perceive and feel and think in channels, and there may be much that exists beyond the channels to which we are attuned. Arthur Schopenhauer (1788–1860) respected these insights of Kant, and he went on to elaborate a theory of will and representation that is still being studied by modern scholars.[5] Hans Vaihinger (1852–1933) was also inspired by Kant's work, particularly the part that emphasized our human tendency to carry on our activities "as if" some things were the case. Vaihinger's *Philosophy of As If* explored the functional values of mental fictions.[6] His work would influence later constructivists such as Alfred Adler and George Kelly.

Major 20th-century constructivists included Alfred Adler, Albert Bandura, Gregory Bateson, Jerome Bruner, James Bugental, Mary Whiton Caulkins, Viktor Frankl, Kenneth Gergen, Vittorio Guidano, Hermann Haken, Sandra Harding, Friedrich Hayek, William James, Evelinn Fox Keller, George Kelly, Karin Knorr-Cetina, Humberto Maturana, Jean Piaget, Joseph Rychlak, Esther Thelen, Francisco Varela, and Paul Watzlawick. Fortunately, some of these pioneers are still constructing. Across the diversity of their interests and emphases, however, there are shared themes. I believe these themes capture the organic essence of constructivism.

The five basic themes of constructivism are (1) active agency, (2) order, (3) self, (4) social–symbolic relatedness, and (5) lifespan development. Let me state them succinctly and then briefly elaborate. Constructivism maintains the following:

1. Human experiencing involves continuous *active agency.*
2. Much human activity is devoted to *ordering processes*—the organizational patterning of experience; these ordering processes are fundamentally emotional, tacit, and categorical (they depend on contrasts), and they are the essence of meaning making.
3. The organization of personal activity is fundamentally self-referent or recursive, making the body a fulcrum of experiencing and encouraging a deep phenomenological sense of *selfhood* or *personal identity.*
4. Self-organizing capacities and creations of meaning are strongly influenced by *social–symbolic processes*; persons exist in living webs of relationships, many of which are mediated by language and symbol systems.
5. Each human life reflects principles of *dynamic dialectical development*; complex flows among essential tensions (contrasts) are reflected in patterns and cycles of experiencing that can lead to episodes of disorder (disorganization) and, under some circumstances, the reorganization (transformation) of core patterns of activity, including meaning making and both self- and social relationships.

Together, then, these themes suggest that a constructive view of human experience is one that emphasizes *meaningful action by a developing self in relationship*. The five themes are expressed very tersely here, of course. They are reviewed again in Chapter 2, in which the focus is on clinical practice. For the moment, I elaborate only briefly.

Activity

Like existential philosophy, constructivism says that we humans are active participants in our own lives. We choose, and our choices make important differences in our lives and in the lives of all with whom we are connected. We are often reactive, to be sure. Constructivism does not deny our capacity for unreflective reflex and conditioning. But our efforts to survive are also fundamentally proactive. We anticipate. We lean into life. We fall forward into our being. And just like the skydiver in free fall or the wind surfer, sailor, or skier, our posture in that process influences its form and direction. We are moving in the midst of forces far greater than ourselves, yet we have voice and choice within those forces. We may not be able to command the stars or the winds, but we can learn to read them better and to set our sails and our actions in ways that serve our movement. And, lest all of this sound a bit ambitious or audacious, we can also learn the sacred arts of stillness and acceptance in the never-ending dance of effort and surrender.

The central point of this first theme is that humans are not passive pawns in the game of life. We are agents that act on and in the world: hence, the emphasis on self-efficacy (Bandura) and acts of knowing

(Bruner). Freud and Skinner, who were both determinists, argued that humans are no more than machines being driven by internal (psychic) or external (environmental) forces. In constructivism, the individual is an active agent in the process of experiencing. Paying attention is an act of agency (James). Like the processes of "natural selection" that contributed to our biological evolution, we are each engaged in acts of selection at every moment (Bateson).

Order

The second principle of constructivism acknowledges that we need order. We organize our worlds and we respond to the order within them (Hayek). We develop patterns and create meanings (Haken, Frankl), and we do most of this without being aware of what we are doing. We are creatures of habit, to be sure, and well might we wonder whether it is we who possess our habits or our habits that possess us. Almost as quickly as we learn a new skill, we become mindless of it. It goes underground, so to speak, and enters into the root structure of our life patterning. And this applies not only to our physical actions but also to our patterns of thinking and feeling. This explains a large part of the difficulty in our change projects. We long to change, yet there is a powerful momentum to the ways we have come to be. This is why the most important changes in our lives may require ruptures and repairs to the very fabric of our lives.

Our emotions develop as powerful biological forces in our self-organization (Guidano). Emotions serve critical roles in directing our attention, shaping our perceptions, organizing our memory, and motivating our active engagement with the learning that life relentlessly requires of us. We feel our way. Constructivism views emotions as central to human experiencing. Feeling is not bad or dangerous or unhealthy. On the contrary, not feeling or fighting against what we are feeling is a more formidable threat to our health and well-being. Our relationships with our feelings are often at least as important as the feelings themselves. This point has important implications for our understanding of what it means to be human, and what we can do in constructive psychotherapy (Bugental).

Self

We organize our worlds by first organizing ourselves (Piaget). Biological self-regulation emerges from bodily experiences. Early in life we struggle to separate ourselves from our caregivers—to individuate into a coherent and differentiated identity. The body and its boundaries become an axis for the organization of experience (Bateson). Like our relationships with our emotions, our relationships with our bodies may become complicated and painful. So, too, at more abstract levels of self-relationship. All psychotherapy is, in a sense, a psychotherapy of the self (Guidano)—an act of assistance in self-organization.

The uniqueness of each self-organizing life is emphasized in constructivism. Terms emphasize individual being (Adler), recursive self-construction (Maturana, Varela), and the personal nature of the order created (Kelly). The unique perspective of the experiencing agent is honored. Moreover, what people experience is integrally related to how they have learned to create an orderly reference point—a metaphorical center. The "who" that is experiencing is one of the more elusive phenomena in consciousness. The self is a process, not an entity (Caulkins, James). And the self is not separated or isolated. Another way to say this might be that the self is a fluid coherence of perspective from which we experience. But the sense of self emerges and changes primarily in relationship to others.

Social–Symbolic Relatedness

Much of the order that we seek and the meaning that we create emerges out of what we feel with one another. We are born in relationship, and it is in relationship that we most extensively live and learn (Bandura). Our languages lack words to convey adequately our social and symbolic embeddedness. Throughout psychology and philosophy, there are creative gestures at capturing the elusive ever-presence of "alterity," "intersubjectivity," and "interbeing."[7] A simplifying analogy would be a fish trying to describe water. Plato was making much the same point in his allegory of the cave. The forms that make up our personal experience are themselves shaped by forces we can hardly claim to imagine, let alone know. The words that you are now reading are more than symbols on a page. What they invoke in your experience depends on a vast network of relationships (Gergen, Rychlak, Watzlawick). Some words and concepts will be more familiar than others. The less familiar ones may give you occasional pause, and you may unconsciously interpret them in terms of what is more familiar. What is familiar and comfortable depends of your personal history, the vocabulary and concepts closest to you, and so on. These are, in turn, reflections of your vast connections with people and ideas (past and present).

The active organization of a self takes place not only "in" a body but also simultaneously "with" and "through" social bonds and systems of symbols (Harding, Keller, Knorr-Cetina). We humans are fundamentally social creatures, and there is no meaningful way of separating our sociality from our symbolic capacities. We may talk about living "in" our heads because we spend so much time thinking, but the form and structure of our thinking is itself relational. One of our favorite ways of organizing our own experience and relating to one another is through stories (Bruner). In other words, a large part of our meaning making is experienced and expressed as narrative (story): our stories, our selves. Stories may teach and sooth. They can also challenge and inspire. Much of what I share in this book is in story form.

Lifespan Development

In its emphasis on the lifelong dynamics of our development, constructivism speaks to the cycles and spirals of experiencing. Like Sisyphus in Greek mythology, we live our lives seeking to achieve a balance that can never quite be perfectly mastered. Some of us get nearer to that balance more often than others, but everyone falls occasionally and eventually. Small falls teach us important lessons about paying attention, learning what is risky, holding on, and recovering control. Big falls overwhelm us. If we are lucky, we hit something soft and are caught in the loving embrace of family and friends. But even in the best of circumstances some falls may feel endless and fatal—what existentialists and mystics have called "the void" and "the dark night of the soul." Whatever the precipitating event, in these there is a felt loss of everything—of meaning, of life order, of control, of identity, and of hope. This kind of hard fall may feel like an agonizing death—a loss not only of all balance but also of wholeness and health. It is, in fact, a metaphorical form of death and a disintegration (a literal loss of integration) of the active life order that preceded it. Often experienced as a living hell, it is something that career psychotherapists witness more often than they might wish.

Constructivism emphasizes developmental processes (Piaget, Thelen). Sometimes we develop via "baby steps" of gradual change. Other times, life demands a large leap. Changes outside of us and inside us may suddenly emerge. When these changes are large, we may undergo a personal revolution. In the face of overwhelming challenges, it is common to do two seemingly opposite things: rigidify and disorganize. We resist the challenge to change. At the same time, however, if the challenge persists or increases, we show signs of variability. Our usual patterns of order begin to disintegrate. This is particularly evident in cycles of energy, moods, sleep, attention, appetite, and digestion. Our formerly "normal" life begins to deviate from its own norms. Such variability and disorganization—literal "disorder"—are natural expressions of a life that is trying to reorganize itself. The shift from an old order to a new one is seldom easy or painless. But it can be "naturalized" and facilitated by a therapist who appreciates the developmental dynamics of self-organizing systems.

A constructive approach to psychotherapy does not deny the struggles of life or the pain of losing meaning or balance. It does not promise quick and easy solutions to tragedies and lifelong struggles. What constructive therapy does offer is compassion and hope borne of an understanding and trust in the powerful wisdom of life processes reorganizing themselves. It offers practical suggestions for coping and incorporates techniques that have been extensively evaluated. More importantly, however, constructive therapy offers an authentic human relationship in which clients are encouraged to experience in their own way, to explore what has happened and is happening in their lives, and to experiment with possibilities for living more fully. Beyond the safety, nurturance, and wisdom offered in the helping relationship, constructivism offers a widely embracing conceptualization of life and development. Patterns of distress and dysfunction are not viewed as diseases. They may be excruciatingly painful and persistent, of course, but they are not seen as something that is biologically or morally "wrong" with the person. There are, of course, biological structures and processes that shape any individual's experiencing. Neuroscientists pursuing the constructivist tradition are among those at the leading edge of our rapidly expanding knowledge of how bodies and brains organize and reorganize themselves.[8] Their findings emphasize the five themes—that is, that biochemically and neurologically, humans are ever-active organizers whose biological patternings develop and change in ways that reflect an extensive network of dynamic relationships. When the many factors influencing any given life moment are taken into account (genetic constraints and activations, cultural and developmental history, current health, skills development, and life circumstances), each human being can be seen as doing and feeling what is "natural" for him or her. They are still responsible for their actions, and an important part of that responsibility is engagement in future development.

Constructive therapy affirms and encourages a hopeful engagement with the mysteries and complexities of each developing life and the connectedness of all lives. It addresses the painful limitations of some personal beliefs, the gain and loss of meanings as life unfolds, and the chaos that often accompanies major life changes. What happens when the order of a life is challenged? What happens when a personal paradigm no longer holds the world together? What are the structures and processes of personal revolutions? On the practical level, what can both client and therapist do to facilitate the kinds of changes that best serve quality of life and wise paths of development? My responses to these questions form the heart of this book.

PRINCIPLES AND PERSONAL REVOLUTIONS

Before turning to the practical aspects of constructive psychotherapy, the complexity of human change processes merits appreciation. Human development rarely follows a simple, linear path. It is more often a zigzag course, with frequent sticking points, repetitive circles, occasional regressions, and a few startling leaps and falls. The particulars may seem dizzying in their diversity, yet there are patterns. Patterns suggest principles. Understanding the principles of human development is essential to the task of psychotherapy. The quest for such principles has been an intense one. Theories of personality and psychopathology have proliferated. Such theories have tried to describe the order and disorder in human lives. With few exceptions, the common assumption has been that order is healthy, normal, and desirable. Disorder has been used as a synonym for disease and dysfunction. The implicit goal of psychotherapy has been to help the disordered individual return to order. But our conceptions of order and disorder are now in the midst of a revolution. Chaos theory, dynamic systems theory, and the sciences of complexity have encouraged new ways of thinking about life and its challenges.[9] Without belaboring the technicalities, I amplify and illustrate that encouragement in this book.

What happens when old ways of being fail to satisfy the demands of new challenges in life? In the harshest of scenarios, that being dies. Fortunately, most human failures do not result in death. We are a flexible life form. We find ways to continue. We try something different, explore alternatives, turn the challenges into opportunities. When circumstances permit, our determination and flexibility allow us to find a better way of being. Our success is more than a matter of our cleverness, however. Our viability reflects the fundamental processes that have characterized the development of life on this planet. Biological evolution has been demonstrating this clever persistence and flexibility for a long time.[10] Change and exchange are the essence of life as we know it. This is one of the central emphases of constructivism. Order is not the opposite of disorder. They are complementary processes. Relative stabilities can be described, but we should be careful not to think of stability or structure as the opposite of process. Consider the apparently stable structure of our bodies. The human body recomposes itself every 7 years. The organic materials that make up our bodies are regularly recycled (at different rates for different tissues). Because the new material (protein, mineral, etc.) is introduced slowly and takes up the positions and functions of the old material, we experience a continuity of structure despite the high rate of exchange via processes.

This same kind of continuity and change applies to our psychological lives. There are processes that are crucial to our psychological existence. Structured continuities are often described in terms of traits, "true" or "real" selves, personality, and character types. Psychology is full of typologies. Constructivism is full of challenges that are not simply protests against typologies.

Constructivism suggests that it is typical for humans to typify. As Kant put it, we are categorical creatures. Schopenhauer wryly noted that there are two kinds of people in the world: those who believe that there are two kinds of people in the world, and those who do not. This observation deserves more than casual reflection. Our penchant for dichotomy and simplification continues to plague our conceptualizations of human development.[11] Problems arise most often when our categories are inadequate to our experiencing. This is when we most need a revolution in our thinking and being. Indeed, as I demonstrate, periods of disorganization and fluctuations in our experiencing are a natural and necessary part of development. Such episodes may not be pleasant, but they often reflect promise and possibility in our processes of being.

I can speak to the phenomena and phenomenology of personal revolutions at several levels. I have been privileged to participate in quite a few revolutions. Some have been with my clients. Others have been with scientific researchers. And still others have been with psychotherapists themselves. Revolutions are often revelations to those involved. I have experienced several myself, personally and professionally. In my quest to understand and help people who are changing, I have changed myself. I am not the same person I was when I began practicing psychotherapy more than 30 years ago. I have been deeply touched by the many lives in which I have participated. I have wept and laughed and yelled—sometimes with clients, often in my private reflections on their lives.

The demands of being a therapist are formidable. Psychotherapy is a difficult profession. We practice a privilege, and we often pay a high personal price. One does not serve such an intimate and responsible role without being changed in the process. One does not bear close witness to the human heart without getting bloody. Broken hearts and lost souls fill our appointment books. If we let them (and I believe we should), they do get to us. They touch the core of our being. Sometimes it is too much to bear. Dozens of lives simultaneously circle around our counsel, each placing its own demands on our wisdom and strength. Even the wise and the strong have their needs and their follies. Therapists need therapy, too. I did not appreciate that fact when I was a beginning therapist. I now emphasize it to my students and colleagues. Clients are not the only ones who change. We therapists are changed by what we do. We also teach in large part by learning. We teach our clients to risk aliveness by taking such risks with them. We teach them to change by being open to change ourselves.

I have learned valuable lessons from my clients. I have also learned from being a client myself. I have been comforted, counseled, and encouraged by colleagues. And I have served as a therapist for many therapists. It has been an honor to serve those who are serving others. My clients, therapists and otherwise, continue to teach me what we all need to learn—that life can be brutally hard and simply beautiful, that we are stronger than we know (or might wish), and that the human heart shines most brilliantly when it is engaged and shared.

In these pages, I share much of who I am and how I try to be in my role as a therapist. I relate intimate stories. Some tell of people struggling to endure and develop in the face of life's relentless challenges. Other stories illustrate the inevitable surprises of therapeutic work. I describe some of my mistakes and discoveries—these two being often related. My life has been enriched by the privilege of practicing and teaching psychotherapy. Its demands are formidable. It is likely to be even more demanding—and more important—in the future. Life is complex, and it is becoming more complex all the time. Being a psychotherapist is an exponentially complex life path. It is a principled attempt to serve the development of lives in process. Drawing upon wisdom and knowledge that embrace a diversity of disciplines and traditions, constructivism offers an integrative approach to professional helping. Let us now turn to what that means for psychotherapy.

NOTES

1. Anderson (1990, 1995, 1997, 2003); Brower and Nurius (1993); Carlsen (1988); Caro (1993, 1994, 1997); Franklin and Nurius (1998); Gergen (1994, 1999); Goldberger, Tarule, Clinchy, and Belenky (1996); Hoffman (1998); Hoyt (1998); Mahoney (1991, 1995a, 1995b, 2000a); Martin (1994); Neimeyer (1995b); Neimeyer and Mahoney (1995); Neimeyer and Raskin (2000); Polkinghorne (1988); Raskin and Bridges (2002); Ronen (1997, 1999, 2001); Rosen and Kuehlwein (1996); Sexton and Griffin (1997); Walker, Costigan, Viney, and Warren (1996).
2. Constructivism, Box 311280, Denton, TX 76203; *www.constructivism123.com*.
3. Williamson (1975).
4. Berlin (1976); Mancuso (2001); Mazzotta (1999); Pompa (1975); Verene (1981).
5. Magee (1983, 1997); Schopenhauer (1932).
6. Vaihinger (1911/1924).
7. Anderson (1997); Arciero (1999); Bretherton (1995); Caputi (1988); Caputo (1987); Cushman (1995); Foucault (1965, 1970); Gergen (1991, 1994); Hargens (2001); Hoffman (1998); Palmer (1969); Sampson (1993); Stern (1985); Thompson (2001); Varela and Shear (1999); Velmans (2000).
8. Cytowic (1998); Damasio (1995, 1999); Freeman (1995); Gallese (1995); Núñez and Freeman (1999).
9. Arciero, Gaetano, Maselli, and Gentili (2003); Beck and Cowan (1996); Chamberlain and Bütz (1998); Combs (1996); Gleick (1987); Haken (1996); Hayek (1964); Kauffman (1993, 1995); Kelso (1995); Krippner (1994); Mahoney (1991); Mahoney and Marquis (2002); Mahoney and Moes (1997); Masterpasqua and Perna (1997); Pagels (1988); Palombo (2000); Pattee (1973); Prigogine (1980); Prigogine and Stengers (1984); Robertson and Combs (1995); Schiepek, Eckert, and Weihrauch (2003); Weimer (1982, 1987); Wilber (1999).
10. Capra (1996); Margulis (1998); Margulis and Sagan (1995); Thompson (1996).
11. Bateson and Martin (2000); Goldberger et al. (1996); Keller (1983, 1985); Koestler (1978); Lowen (1982); Oyama (2000); Smith (1988); Wilber (1998).

CHAPTER 2

CONSTRUCTIVE PSYCHOTHERAPY

An Overview of Practice

What is constructive psychotherapy? I had a close encounter with this question at a recent meeting of mental health professionals. I was on an elevator with half a dozen people in a large hotel, all of us caught in the silence of our commute. The elevator stopped at several floors and people shuffled in and out, quietly making room for each other. At one stop, a woman entered and quickly scanned the name badges of the occupants. When she saw mine, she said, "Aren't you giving a talk on constructive psychotherapy this afternoon?" I said, "Yes." "Well," she said, "I can't come to your talk . . . can you give me a one-sentence definition of constructive psychotherapy?" At this point, the elevator stopped and she stepped between the doors to exit, holding them open while she waited for my response. I felt speechlessly "on the spot" and self-conscious about the fact that we were delaying the other passengers. Then some Irish elf within me spoke up and said, "In one sentence, constructive psychotherapy is the opposite of destructive psychotherapy." We all smiled and the elevator doors closed. I had never quite thought about it in that way before that moment. On reflection, I don't think it was a bad rendition, on the spur of the moment.

Her question and my response reminded me of Schopenhauer's aphorism on there being two kinds of people in the world (those who believe there *are* two kinds of people in the world and those who do not.) More than being a cute play on words, this saying captures the heart of the constructivist insight—that we organize our experiences primarily by means of classifications and categorizations. Without being aware of our tendency, we tend to think in terms of kinds. Try to describe anything—a person, an object, an experience, or whatever—and you will quickly find yourself thinking in terms of what it is like and what it is not. In my spontaneous attempt to describe constructive psychotherapy to that woman on the elevator, I unconsciously reacted by invoking its opposite.

There is, in fact, a "positive spin" to constructive philosophy and its applications in psychotherapy. Constructivism emphasizes possibility and therefore hope, and it offers a refreshingly humanizing conceptualization of disorder and development. In this sense, at least, constructivism is an important part of the recent movement toward developing a more "positive psychology."[1] Constructivism is a philosophy of participation: It encourages individuals and communities to be actively involved in their own unfolding.

This chapter is an overview of how I approach constructive practice. As noted in Chapter 1, there are many different expressions of constructive psychotherapy. Some reflect a legacy from cognitive-behavioral traditions, and others are nested in existential–humanistic or psychoanalytic approaches. In what follows, I refer to constructivism and constructive practice in a general sense that is meant to embrace the legitimacy of this diversity. My generalizations are not intended to homogenize that diversity or to suggest that there is only one way of viewing constructive practice. Constructive psychotherapy includes a diversity of techniques. It is not defined by specific techniques so much as by the individualization and developmental pacing of different techniques. More importantly, a constructive approach to psychotherapy recognizes the importance of human relationship in well-being and development. To avoid repetitive qualifications, let me emphasize from the outset that I am describing a personal and ever-evolving view of practicing a developmental philosophy called constructivism. Table 2.1 presents a summary of the five basic themes of constructivism as they relate to human experience and development. Table 2.2 offers an overview of constructive practice in terms of its emphases on human relationships, a rationale for understanding change, and the role of rituals or structured exercises in facilitating change.[2] These conjectures are elaborated in subsequent chapters. Finally, Table 2.3 offers a flexible structure for conceptualizing sessions in constructive practice. As is evident in that table, compassionate human presence is a central emphasis.

COMPASSIONATE RELATIONSHIP AS THE HEART OF PSYCHOTHERAPY

There is probably more written about human relationships than almost any other dimension of human experience, and this is clearly the case in the domain of psychotherapy.[3] Mountains of volumes and thousands of studies have accumulated, and still we struggle with translating all of this into clear and practical guidelines for how to be with another human being. It is such a basic and sacred ability, yet it still mystifies researchers. I am reminded here of a story told by John O'Donahue[4] about a young anthropologist who had traveled to the rain forests of South America. The anthropologist wanted to interview and study shamans (tribal healers), and he learned of an elder shaman who was considered the most gifted of the group. The anthropologist asked one of the junior shamans to approach the elder and ask if he would be willing to be interviewed. The young shaman went into the forest to convey the message respectfully. He returned some time later with a response. The old man said that he would consider an interview, but first he would have to spend time with the young man. The anthropologist agreed and was told to follow the messenger. They walked for several miles, until they came to where the tiny gray-haired healer sat under a towering tree. The old shaman motioned for his would-be interrogator to sit across from him. The young man sat down respectfully, ready to respond to questions such as "What is your name?", "Where do you come from?", "Why are you here?", "What do you want from me?" But instead, the old man sat there and simply looked at him. Several minutes passed and the anthropologist felt so uncomfortable that he began to say something. The shaman motioned for him to remain silent. It was torture for the young man, who sat there under the direct and relentless gaze of a very wise and perceptive spiritual healer. After more than 2 hours of this, a welcome sense of peacefulness began to fill the young man, and he later said that he had never felt so "known" by anyone before. The old man then began talking.

I shall not attempt to capture in words the essence of the therapeutic relationship and the art of being humanly *present* to another person. I will, however, reiterate the foundational importance of human relatedness in constructive practice. The client–therapist relationship provides a special context for vital experiments in living. For many clients, that relationship also becomes a transformational crucible in which they can risk exploring new ways of relating to themselves. Finally, even when it lasts for only one or a few sessions, the therapeutic relationship can become a lifelong source of compassion and encouragement that exerts an influence not only on the client but also on the people whose lives are touched by that client. One clear and crystalline moment of understanding and caring can ripple across endless lives and generations. Unfortunately, the same is true for moments of judgment and cruelty.

After the first session, each meeting with a client is itself a form of reunion. Just as no two clients are ever alike, no two sessions are identical. Part of what makes them different is more than the passage of time and the changing contents of their current focus. Sessions are made different by each participant's presence to the other and to themselves. "Presence" is a very difficult thing (or process) to define. Most psychotherapy experts agree that presence, like empathy, is very important, but they differ quite a bit on its definition and measurement.[5] Most of us can recall moments when we were embarrassingly not present in a conversation with clients or friends. "Our lights were on," so to speak, "but we were not home." We may have been looking directly into their eyes and even nodding our head in apparent understanding, but our consciousness was somewhere else. People who know us well or are attuned to the subtleties of our presence may call us on such lapses: "Are you with me?", "Where are you?", "Hello in there . . . " More often, they are polite and say nothing. I believe that we psychotherapists develop unusual abilities to look like we are present and paying attention when we are not.

The therapist should be as present as possible and invite a genuine contact with the client as another human being. It is crucial not only to beginning the session but also to fostering the continuing human relationship that is the essence of the practice. Sometimes, on the way to greet a client, I intentionally slow the pace of my walk, take a deep breath, and recite the simple phrase "Be here now" silently to myself. [6] When a client enters my visual field, I am usually unaware of my facial expression. On the outside, I am focusing on his eyes, and face, and movement toward me. On the inside, I am focusing on my intention to be there in that moment with him, and to be there for him in the time that we have scheduled together.

In the beginning of my relationship with clients, I try to be attuned to what they are seeking and their level of comfort in being with me. In general, I find that they are more comfortable with me when I am comfortable with myself. Opening is a process that is facilitated by relaxation, and I often concentrate on relaxing my breathing and my voice. If I sense that they want or need to talk, I invite them to do so with questions that are familiar to all practitioners (e.g., "What brings you here?", "Can you tell me a little bit about what is going on with you?", "How might I help?"). I try not to rush toward judgments based on first impressions but, at the same time, I make a mental note of how they approach being in conversation with me. I do not push for private or emotional material in the early stages of our getting to know one another, and I try to develop a sense of their rhythm of expressing themselves. If they appear to be tense or to feel awkward, I may reflect something like "I realize that this may be difficult for you, and I want to respect your feelings as we continue."

In the first session, I often ask whether they have been in therapy before. This is often an ice breaker in that it leads toward two possible paths of conversation. If this is their first experience of professional counseling, then we can discuss some of their assumptions and possible concerns. Any new experience is likely to feel strange at first, and I acknowledge this. If clients have been in therapy before, they may have had experiences that they may or may not want to repeat. In either case, their response to the question provides a point from which we can navigate toward topics of current concern to them. Some clients, of course, do not need help in getting started. They may launch into a long or detailed list of personal problems, or they may express strong emotions from the *outset*. Whether they communicate reluctantly, quietly, loudly, or demandingly, I try to express respect for what they are feeling and compassion for their dilemma.

I believe compassion is the heart of constructive psychotherapy. Compassion is more crucial than the transmission of scientific information or even the sharing of wise counsel. The latter are important, to be sure, but they are not the heart. Caring is at the heart of all helping.[7] How that caring is expressed is a matter of controversy in the psychotherapies spawned by Western civilization. Still, such caring is an essential component of constructive counseling. Evidence for its importance is pervasive in the literatures of human development and psychotherapy. It reflects the essence of our social embeddedness and our symbolic capacities to imagine and honor what someone else may be feeling. But, I gladly confess, the evidence most compelling to me has not come from rigorous experiments and elaborate clinical trials. It has come from clients. One of the clearest examples for me came from a woman named Linda.

I had been invited to give a talk at a professional conference, and my topic was supposed to include the most important components of effective therapy. I had another week before I left for the conference, and I was busy getting things in order. In between my sessions with clients, I had been making notes to myself in preparation for my talk. The group that I was to address comprised primarily psychotherapy researchers, and I was understandably inclined to use technical and scientific terms in my presentation. I had a yellow note pad on my desk filled with ideas for my talk.

That was when Linda arrived for her weekly session. She was a large and imposing figure. We had been working together for months on her long-standing issues of self-esteem. Even though Linda presented a rugged exterior to her employees and business associates, she felt inauthentic because of some core feelings of inadequacy that had haunted her since childhood. I greeted her at the office door and invited her in. As she was moving toward her chair, I offered to get her a soda or glass of water from the refrigerator down the hall. She requested a soda. When I returned seconds later with our drinks, Linda was still standing. She was halfway to her chair, lingering at the side of my desk and staring down at my scribbled notes on "The Essential Ingredients in Effective Psychotherapy." I closed the door behind me, and Linda, purse still on her shoulder, put her hand on my note pad and said, "Where's the caring?"

"What?" I was not prepared for her question. Walking over to my desk, I saw what had prompted it.

"Where's the caring?" she repeated.

I managed an awkward smile and an "Ummm . . . " as I handed Linda a soda. She accepted it, dropped her purse to the floor, and sat down.

"You may have done some of those other things," she continued (and we both glanced toward my note pad), "but the most important thing you have done for me has been to care."

I was tempted to look away from her direct gaze and to cushion the force of her sudden gesture of appreciation. But I was aware of my awkwardness and discomfort, and I sensed that it was an important moment for both of us. For Linda, it was a rare disclosure of feeling and an affirmation of the importance of our relationship. For me, it was a welcome reminder of practical relevance. In preparing my talk for the researchers, I had begun to drift into the technical language of theory and the laboratory—and I had begun to lose the relevance of the "real thing" in the consulting room. Linda's honesty and courage helped to bring me back to the fact that our relationship—and, in her words, my "caring"—had been an essential aid to her development.

"Thank you," I said, as I pulled out my pen and wrote "CARING" at the top of the list. We smiled at each other and moved on with our work.

As strongly as I believe that compassion lies at the heart of psychotherapy, I am quick to admit that our theories and scientific research in this domain are barely rudimentary. The same is true of our training programs. With rare exceptions (e.g., in Buddhist and humanistic approaches), compassion has not been an explicit emphasis in the training of mental health practitioners. At its etymological root, compassion literally means "with feeling" or "feeling with." The optimal "emotional distance" between therapists and clients has been one of the longest running debates among theorists of psychotherapy. Should the therapist assume a posture of maximal detachment? How should the therapist respond to a client's requests for emotional engagement? There is no single accepted answer to such questions. But the perseverance of such questions should alert us to the fact that our capacities and willingness to relate to our clients is a central aspect of all forms of psychotherapy.[8] My personal opinion is that compassion and caring, which are related to comforting and encouragement, account for a sizable portion of what we contribute to our clients' lives.

Other constructive therapists might well respond with a range of opinions to questions about the ideal emotional posture of the therapist or the most appropriate therapeutic distance. Less variable, I believe, would be their acknowledgment that human relatedness lies at the center of all human experience and, therefore, of constructive psychotherapy. Across time and space and many bridges of symbols, every individual is connected with every other—past, present, and future. This fact has a richness of importance that I can only superficially address within the confines of this chapter, but it is one whose further appreciation and exploration will, I believe, powerfully shape the experiences of our planetary inheritors. It will also shape the future of psychotherapy.

COLLABORATION AND ACTION

Compassion and caring are central to a constructive helping relationship. The same is true of collaboration and action. The essence of collaboration is an egalitarian (nonauthoritarian) contract that distributes the responsibilities for change. The client is the primary agent of change. She is the resident expert on herself and what she is experiencing. Besides being the primary actor and monitor of what is happening in her life, she is the one who bears the burdens and blessings of her choices. As therapists, we can offer our reflections and advice on courses of action. But our clients are the ones who live in and on the front lines of their own lives. They are the ones who pay the prices and reap the benefits of their own actions (and failures to act). They and their life companions endure or enjoy the consequences of their choices.

Collaboration is a critically important aspect of constructive psychotherapy. Clients are not viewed as objects, but as agents. Psychotherapy is not something that is done *to* them, but *by* them. It is a change process in which they are the central character, the primary benefactor, and a potential victim. What they choose to do is critical to their development. They are the ones who make the difference in their own lives. They are the ones who must live out the consequences of their choices. There are always choices, whether we want them or not. We do not have total control or absolute knowledge, of course. We cannot perfectly know what will result from our actions. But we must and do choose, even when we struggle to avoid choosing. Not choosing is a choice. We have no choice but to be always in the process of choosing.

The importance of action—of engaged practice ("praxis")—will be apparent in many later chapters on therapeutic techniques and the experience of change. I place a high priority on what my clients are actually doing in their lives. Their actions are more important than their intentions. Change is an active process, and exerting an influence on its direction often requires attention to subtle details. I rely heavily on homework assignments that are to be tried and repeated in clients' daily lives. There are times, of course, when clients may be trying too hard. They may have developed patterns of "learned restlessness," and they might benefit from being told "Don't just do something, sit there."[9] There are subtleties to the practical balance of effort and surrender. Not all action is effortful, and surrender is often anything but effortless.

Collaboration literally means "working together." Laboring together is an essential aspect of constructive psychotherapy. The work of changing—indeed, the work of living—cannot be done on one's behalf by another person. As one of my clients put it most poignantly, "No one else can live for you or die for you." Life is your own project, and it is always a uniquely personal undertaking. No one else has been or ever will be *you*—in your circumstances, with your background, facing this moment and its options. A constructive therapeutic collaboration recognizes and respects this fact. The demands of living are somewhat different for each of us. We can learn important lessons from those who have gone before us and from scientific inquiries into the processes of adaptation. But, ultimately, each of us faces a unique configuration of challenges and a very personal responsibility for the choices we make in moving onward with our lives. We have only partial information, limited understanding, and imperfect control. Yet the physical world and our social communities hold us responsible. Such is our shared existential predicament.

Two essential dimensions of collaboration are dialogue and coordination. These are therefore central aspects of constructive psychotherapy. Dialogue, as used here, is more than the exchange of words. Indeed, it is more than a simple exchange process. Physicist David Bohm devoted much time and energy to issues of dialogue and the development of human consciousness.[10] He came to believe that much that masquerades as genuine dialogue is a talking around things, the avoidance of difficulties, or negotiations toward compromise. In the constructive sense, dialogue is an open and emergent process in which the participants are mutually enriched (and often surprised) by what they share with one another (and what they learn, in the process, about themselves). Verbal dialogue becomes more than an exchange of words. And nonverbal copresence becomes a precious experience of coordination and experiential validation. In its more intimate and elegant forms, psychotherapy becomes a process of "interbeing"—an open-ended exploration of possibilities of being. Traditional theories of communication have yet to accommodate this aspect of an emerging relationship of creative change. Be this as it may, it is a familiar phenomenon to those who practice it daily. The working together—the talking together in an open-ended form of teleonomy[11]—is a common aspect of constructive psychotherapy.

The importance of coordination in constructive psychotherapy lies in its emphasis on the resonance between the efforts of therapist and client in co-ordering their activities in the service of the client's adaptation and development. If there is not some semblance of synchrony in this process, there will be difficulties. However, if the process runs too smoothly, the effects may be less than optimal. This is an observation being made with increasing frequency by specialists in development and psychotherapy process.[12] Examples include the recent work of Daniel Stern and colleagues on what they term "hot" or "now" moments when the interaction between therapist and client leads to a surprise that catches them both off guard. It can take any form in terms of content, but it is always emotionally charged. There is a momentary loss of balance by both beings, and the challenge is in how it is handled. It can be ignored, but it rarely goes by unnoticed. The therapist can revert to a ritualized response (e.g., a reflection, an interpretation, or a distancing that is communicated in various ways). Under ideal circumstances, such surprises become opportunities for a genuine "moment of meeting." In such moments, there is mutual authenticity and a jointly emergent response that deepens the relationship and reflects its capacity to encounter future unexpected events. Psychotherapy then becomes an actively intimate and emotional dance between its participants. There are inevitable missteps, painful moments of feeling stepped on, and occasional periods of beautiful attunement. Coordination and a commitment to refining that coordination are important to both the therapeutic relationship and to therapeutic process.

AFFIRMATION AND HOPE

Along with compassion and collaborative action, affirmation is central to constructive psychotherapy. It is a basic dimension of the therapeutic relationship and an important component in the client's perseverance and change. The therapist is often a primary or sole source of encouragement in a client's life, and I have frequently been impressed with what a few words and good wishes have meant to my clients. To say that the constructive therapist encourages or affirms clients does not mean that such a therapist is a professional cheerleader or an unwavering and enthusiastic promoter of whatever the client is doing. What it does mean, however, is that the constructive therapist respects the importance of working with clients in a manner that capitalizes on their current strengths, while addressing the consequences and problems associated with their past choices and activity patterns.

The term "affirmation" is a derivative of a much earlier word referring to the process of strengthening. To affirm someone is essentially to offer them strength or to compliment their strength. But what happens when that person's ways of being are dysfunctional or damaging? And how does affirmation differ from what behaviorists have called "reinforcement"? Let me begin with the latter and then return to the former. In my opinion, affirmation is not simply reinforcement—a head nod or an "Mm-hmm," or even a verbalized "Well done" that is given contingent on the client's having said or done something that the therapist considers positive, appropriate, or progressive. Nor is affirmation simply a statement of the fact that "You're OK, whatever you are doing." Affirmation is a style of relating that is fundamentally encouraging and responsibly hopeful. This style of relating is not mechanical or calculating: It does not select certain dimensions of experiencing and then praise only them. Nor is it indiscriminately positive about everything a client has done, is doing, or hopes to do.

An affirmative therapeutic style is one that embraces the client as active agent—a unique, self-organizing, and self-protective life force. An important part of our task as psychotherapists is to serve clients in ways that strengthen their best and encourage even better ways of experiencing (where "better" is individually defined but generally attuned to their well-being, their development, and their responsible participation in the collective community of their family, friends, and society).

How do we do this? We do much of it, I believe, by inviting and supporting the kind of relationship thus far described in this chapter: a relationship that is safe, compassionate, respectful, and trusting. But we can also do it more directly. We can dare to make human-to-human contact and actually communicate our caring, our compassion, and our encouragement. An example is offered by a client who had suffered through many years of intense depression. It took several weeks to get her started on homework and a personal journal. Even then, she was slow to engage. It therefore felt sudden to me to have her leave a session by handing me a brown envelope without a comment. Inside was a copy of her most recent journal entry, which described a reaction to a recent moment in our work together:

> So there I was, telling him things I could not even admit to myself. I don't know even now if they were all exactly true, but it was scary just to say them. And he *listened*. It was more than just hearing. I could tell that he had heard a lot from other people. I imagined that he had lived a lot himself. And still he was interested in me. In ME! He wanted to hear what I had to say, and I could tell that he hurt *with* me when I hurt.
>
> And today he did something that I never expected. I had been crying—oh, more like whining and weeping—on and off for a while. He was silent, but I could tell he was with me. Then he called me by my name and asked me to look into his eyes. I didn't want to. I felt so foolish. He called my name again and I lifted my head and looked at him. There were tears in *his* eyes! And he said, "JoAnn, I wish I could say something to make it hurt less." I don't remember if I said anything or just sat there frozen, staring into those two soft eyes. "I wish I could talk (or did he say "take"?) your pain away, but I can't. All I can say is that I am sorry that you are hurting, and I admire your strength." When he said that, I sort of startled, and blew my nose. "Strength! I'm not strong!" I must have looked down, because he reached toward my chin and just made a motion with his hand to lift my gaze again—he didn't even touch me, but I got the message and I looked at him again. "You *are* strong," he said, "even though you may not feel that or know that right now." And I just stared at him in disbelief.
>
> I left there in a daze, half wanting to argue and half wondering what had just happened. I felt angry with him for giving me a shot of hope. But why angry? He wasn't feeling sorry for me. And it wasn't like he was for-

> giving me for all my mistakes. It was like he was saying that I was one helluva person to have survived all that pain and still kept my bearings. He really respected me, problems and all.

This excerpt from her diary conveys more, I think, than I can put into technical words. For me, at least, it captures something essential about the affirmative spirit of constructive psychotherapy.

Affirmation is often paired with suggestions for explorations or homework exercises. I deal with these at more length later. I believe that homework is often valued by clients, if only because it provides tentative suggestions for things they might do to feel a greater sense of agency in their lives. Depending on clients' current individual needs, homework may be intended to create stability in their lives or to destabilize and restructure the patterns that they have developed.

The constructive practitioner has faith in possibilities. Things could be different than they are. They could get worse, but they could also get better. And the meanings of "good" and "bad" are open to interpretation. From some perspective, bad things often present good opportunities. A flat tire may contribute to a "bad day" at one level, but it may also have fringe benefits (e.g., it didn't cause a fatal accident, it forced a challenge, it slowed life down, perhaps serving as a reminder of many things that are going well without being appreciated, etc.). Each person is an active participant in making meaning of life and enacting that meaning in his or her engagement with self and others, and the world at large. At least in this sense, the constructive therapist is a devoted practitioner of "positive psychology" and a faithful guardian of hope.[13] He or she believes and teaches that life is a precious gift. As it is said so beautifully in Spanish, "La vida vale la pena" [Life is worth the pain]. Jerome Frank wisely saw that a central function of all forms of psychotherapy is the restoration and protection of hope on the part of the client. And, as I have said elsewhere, hope is not something that automatically and endlessly renews itself:

> Contrary to Alexander Pope's famous assurance, hope does *not* spring "eternal in the human breast." Rather, it must be vigilantly nurtured through an active—enactive—faith in the possibilities and preciousness of human life in process. If nothing else, our vast literatures and laboratories have taught us that the meaning of life does not lie comfortably nestled within any single theory, model, or scripture. The lesson, it seems, is that such meaning must be endlessly and individually re-created in our lived-life struggles and triumphs.[14]

Hope and engagement with life are not processes we can assume are always operative in a client. One of the primary and most demanding responsibilities of psychotherapy involves our socially sanctioned role as protectors or promoters of hope.

BALANCING SKILLS AND CYCLES OF EXPERIENCING

Psychotherapy is a special form of human relationship that serves the immediate and long-term developmental needs of the client. Ideally, that relationship becomes a safe and secure source of compassionate counsel and encouragement. In the context of that relationship, a client should feel free to feel, to reflect, and to ask for and receive help. As therapists, our primary responsibilities are to respectfully listen and witness or honor our clients' presentations of themselves and their experiences. With sensitive attunement to their current needs and capacities, we offer comfort, reassurance, and encouragement. At appropriate times, we may challenge our clients to change—to consider different ways of viewing themselves, to risk feelings that may be uncomfortable or frightening, and to experiment with new ways of living. How do we do this? We do it, I believe, by skillfully and flexibly balancing our interactions with them to suit their unique and unfolding requirements for help. I conceptualize such balancing in terms of two basic and interrelated dimensions. Both are simplifications, but I find them helpful in organizing my own way of being therapeutic. One dimension is created by the contrasts of opening and closing. The other is created by the contrasts of comforting and challenging.

Opening and Closing

Imagine that there are two kinds of processes in the world: opening and closing. "To open" generally means to expand or enlarge. It also can mean to begin or to create. When it has been preceded by barriers or blockage, opening involves a process of freeing the flow or movement of restrained processes. "To close" generally means to constrict or narrow. Closing something can also refer to finishing it, as in closing a book. To close also means to stop or to shut, as well as to secure or to cover. It is not coincidental that these verbs serve as powerful metaphors that are related to multiple bodily actions and processes. They are both associated with a vertical dimension: we open "up" but we close "down."[15]

It may be useful to think about life as cycles of openings and closings. This metaphor may be expressed in experiences ranging from a moment to a lifetime. Each therapy session is a dynamic exchange in which the client is opening and closing to possible experiences. This is, of course, a natural expression of dynamic self-organization and attempts to maintain or regain a sense of order in one's life. A significant part of the therapist's role, in my opinion, involves an ongoing attunement with each client's processes of multidimensional expansion and contraction. A person in extreme contraction is literally cut off from some kinds of exchange with his world. A person in extreme dilation (expansion) may risk giving and receiving at rates that exceed what her system can currently accommodate.

Processes of learning and development require a delicate, dynamic balance that protects the coherence of the person's core ordering processes, while allowing for encounters with manageable novelties. *Change requires new experience* and, therefore, at least episodic openness to such experience. But the living system is fundamentally conservative: Its first priority is to protect itself and its life support systems. This is especially true when it is exploring new territory. It is also true in the context of both pleasure and pain. Thus, even after rewarding or satisfying excursions into new experience patterns, it is common for the system to pull back, to contract, to close itself off for a while. This is readily apparent in most therapeutic sessions, where close attention to subtle cues will often reflect the client's dance toward and then away from significant themes and potential experiences. I believe each client expresses her own tempo and style of opening and closing. It is her habitual manner of moving through her life, and her style is often amplified in the personally charged moments of a therapeutic hour.

Neither opening nor closing is inherently good or bad. Both are required in the dynamic maintenance of a living system. To assign a value judgment to one of them would be to overlook their necessary reciprocity in life support. It would be like saying inhalation is better or worse than exhalation in our breathing. But the metaphorical opening and closing I am talking about is much more complex than our respiration, our digestion, or any of the other processes that are essential to our being.[16] One cannot assign a meaningful overall score to our experiential openness or closure. This is not only because it keeps changing, but also because we may be simultaneously open and closed at different levels—and there are, of course, many "degrees" in between. A physical illustration of this might be in terms of all the organs and parts of our bodies that dilate and contract: pupils, pores, sinuses, arteries, lungs, heart, digestive tract, and so on. They have complex and variable rhythms that cannot be captured in a single summary number. Isn't it possible—indeed, likely—that our consciousness also reflects rhythmic cycles? The idea is complex, to be sure, but that is how we are: Life is complex, and so is psychotherapy.

Imagine that this complex coordination of expansion and contraction processes is illustrated in the contrasts between thinking and feeling. Although this separation is an artificial one that colludes in the mind–body dualism of classical rationalism,[17] it is such a familiar one that most of us can easily relate to it.[18] We can recognize the difference between being mostly in our heads and totally "out of our minds" and into our bodies. We know when we are intellectualizing about a problem versus experiencing it in parts of our body. Indeed, there are ample reports that suggest that shuttling back and forth along the dimensions of conceptualization and experiencing is a common developmental process, both inside and outside psychotherapy.[19] Vittorio Guidano described it as the dance between experiencing and explaining. In later work with Giampiero Arciero, this dialectical process was refined to address the complexities of maintaining and restoring emotional coherence.[20] We seem to make risky excursions into existential *dasein*, which means "being there" and involves being present to what Milan Kundera termed "the unbearable lightness of being," and then we pull back from our absorption in bodily experience and bracket it with words and concepts (descriptions, commentaries, interpretations, analyses, explanations).

A client who is coming mostly out of his head (i.e., at the conceptualizing end of this dimension) might be showing signs of opening by asking questions, exploring meanings, and playing with ideas or possibilities. Signs of closing at a conceptual level could take the form of firm declarations of answers, rigid categorizations, or inabilities to understand. A client who is opening at the experiential level might be showing signs of emotional or behavioral exploration, risking or experimenting in an embodied manner. Experiential closing is often signaled by a return to "Let's just talk about it," but it can also take the forms of emotional or behavioral perseveration (stereotypy), numbing, and—in the extreme—loss of consciousness.

Whether we think of it as oscillations along the dimensions of thinking and feeling or along any number of other dimensions, it is important that we recognize that our clients are always moving to the rhythms of their own self-organizational processes. Instead of being motionless in their chairs, our clients are doing anything but sitting still. They are expanding and contracting in multiple ways at every moment. We are, too. And neither of us can be totally aware of our own cycling. It is, in fact, when our habitual rhythms are disrupted that we are likely to glimpse them.

Comforting and Challenging

In our role as professional helper, we accept special responsibilities. These include our being sensitively attuned to cycles of experiencing in our clients, in ourselves, and in the unfolding moments of our interactions. We are professional mentors trying to teach life skills.[21] We do our best to keep our own balance while we delicately adjust our actions to the student's immediate and imminent needs. I believe we do this by organizing our actions along a dimension that might be called "comforting and challenging."

Comforting is something with which most of us are quite familiar. We know what it feels like to want comforting, and most of us have been fortunate enough to have felt genuinely comforted by people in our lives. Seeking comfort, being comforted, and learning to comfort ourselves may help us in comforting others. We hug or hold someone, or we listen with compassion, inviting him to lean on us in a metaphorical sense. A good friend in the role of a caregiver is someone who is "there" for us, silently or otherwise, in a difficult time, witnessing our pain and reducing the loneliness of our struggle. If psychotherapy can be thought of as something like a "one-way friendship,"[22] then it is the therapist who is always in the caregiving role and always a potential source of comfort.

We often think of challenges as taking place at the edges of ability and possibility. But there are two kinds of challenges: aggressive and progressive. They can have very different felt meanings depending on their emotional tone, their context, and the quality of the relationship from which they issue. An aggressive challenge is issued in anger, and it may imply dominance or convey doubt about the capacities of the other. This is the kind of challenge encountered in confrontations (e.g., on the battlefield, on the playground, or in power struggles). It often takes the form of an insult or a dare, and aggressive challenges often lead to destructive actions.

The other kind of challenge is an invitation to stretch, and it is in this sense that it can be called "progressive." Such a challenge issues from a caring relationship and conveys a message of faith in the ability of the other. It encourages a stretching forward toward new capacities and is an essential aspect of dynamic development.

> The loving mother teaches her child to walk alone. She is far enough from him so that she cannot actually support him, but she holds out her arms to him. She imitates his movements, and if he totters, she swiftly bends as if to seize him, so that the child might believe that he is not walking alone. . . . And yet, she does more. Her face beckons like a reward, an encouragement. Thus, the child walks alone with his eyes fixed on his mother's face, *not* on the difficulties in his way. He supports himself by the arms that do not hold him and constantly strives towards the refuge in his mother's embrace, little suspecting that in the very same moment that he is emphasizing his need of her, he is proving that he can do without her, because he is walking alone.[23]

Just as a parent or teacher will often challenge children or students to stretch themselves and their skills, a constructive therapist does likewise with clients. In so doing, the therapist is helping clients to learn and refine capacities that will ultimately reduce their need for therapy.

A client caught in the grip of a severe contraction of anxiety or depression often wants to be comforted. For some clients, the comfort and compassion afforded by the helping relationship constitute its most valuable component. Some clients do not change during the course of therapy. This does not mean that their therapy failed. The provision of safe harbor for the heart is no small achievement. But many clients also want to be coaxed toward again taking risks. In this progressive sense of the term, challenge is an invitation to explore or experiment—to look for or try something different. Because novelty—a different or unfamiliar experience—is essential to change, challenge lies at the heart of teaching and many forms of helping. The form, focus, and timing of challenges must be attuned to the person's current skills and systemic balance, of course. This is part of what can be so demanding about parenting, teaching, and psychotherapy. This is, so to speak, the challenge of challenging. An inappropriate challenge—an excessive one—can present a barrier to learning and cause the individual to feel overwhelmed. An inadequate challenge—one that does not ask the person to risk new frontiers—may not only waste time and energy but it may also collude in maintaining old and dysfunctional ways of being.

Bear in mind that I have created an artificial contrast for the sake of simplifying a practical point. I do not believe caring, compassion, and comfort are incompatible with progressive developmental challenge. Comfort and challenge need not be a disjunction in helping style. Both are essential to optimal therapy. The necessity of comfort and security is clear in research on both early and lifespan emotional development. And challenge is also an integral part. Life keeps coming at you. Indeed, it is the capacity of challenges to overwhelm persons that often motivates their search for professional help. Within psychotherapy, challenges initiated by the therapist should come only when safety and caring are already trusted. Such challenges should emerge out of a collaborative dance. Authoritarian demands dictated by the therapist are not recommended. The client who is challenged prematurely or excessively is often done more harm than the client who is never challenged at all. As one of my teachers put it, bad therapy is often worse than no therapy at all. Challenge should emerge out of the dynamics of the therapeutic relationship, with mutual consent that new opportunities for experiencing are possible in the overall balance of the client's personal system. The client always retains the right to say, "This is too much; this is too fast." Although some therapists will pressure clients about such objections,[24] my experiences have taught me to trust the client's sense of pacing in personal development. If I err, I prefer to err in the direction of challenging too little rather than too much. When clients show signs of withdrawing, I respect that. I also encourage them to witness their process of closing down and to honor its intent, which is self-protection.

SUMMARY

Constructive psychotherapy involves compassionate relationship, collaborative action, affirmations of hope, and balancing the cycles of experiencing. Each of these honors phenomenology—the uniquely constructed reality in and from which each person exists. Coming to know that person and his or her phenomenology is the essence of constructive assessment, to which I turn next. Because my emphasis in this book is on illustrations of how to practice constructively, I have condensed much of the conceptual scaffolding into Tables 2.1 and 2.2, and Appendix L. In teaching constructive psychotherapy I have also learned that students appreciate concrete visual aids that can help to convey how concepts may be translated into actions within the therapeutic encounter (Table 2.3).Constructive psychotherapy involves a sensitive coordination of comforting and challenging in response to each client's cycles of opening and closing to experiences. This is the essence of Johann Herbart's (1776–1841) "respiratory philosophy of education," which inspired Jean Piaget to develop his theory of "equilibration" (dynamic balance) in psychological development. Constructive therapy is literally an ongoing gesture of sensitive attunement with the client's current sense of balance (emotionally, conceptually, and otherwise).

The metaphor of balance figures prominently in my presentation of a constructive approach to psychotherapy. I often begin consultation with assessments and exercises that emphasize a client's abilities to find and return to a sense of calm center (e.g., relaxation, physical balance, breathing meditation) (Chapters 3 and 4, Appendices D–F). For some clients, this will be a significant part of our work together. Learning to find their balance may be a formidable challenge. Skills in centering are essential to a sense of coherence, safety, and personal competence. Such skills become an important part of establishing and utilizing an internal "base camp" from which clients can energize, orient, and organize their continuing efforts to develop.

As clients become skilled in finding and expanding a sense of balance in their lives, we move on to more advanced exercises in exploratory behaviors and experimentation with new patterns of experiencing (Chapters 5–9, Appendices G–K). Such explorations and experiments inevitably lead to further losses of balance. Centering skills therefore remain at the heart of coping with new challenges. The processes of development have their own dynamics, and these are experienced and expressed uniquely by each living system. A principled order unfolds, however, and it often reflects an expanding center and refinements in the skills that connect the center with the edges. This is where disorder and order dance the dialectic, and it will be the focus of some final chapters on the process of change in complex systems such as our selves (Chapter 10). Witnessing and fostering engagement with life is a privilege that places formidable demands on the person who is a therapist. I therefore conclude this volume with reflections on the burdens and blessings of professional helping, with special emphasis on the importance of therapist self-care (Chapter 11). My message is simple: Our work is complex. That complexity begins with meeting and trying to understand another human being. Let us begin there.

NOTES

1. Bandura (1997); Rosenbaum (1990, 1998); Snyder (1999); Snyder and Lopez (2001).
2. I have borrowed the "three R's" (relationship, rationale, rituals) idea from Jerome Frank's (1973) insightful analysis of helping processes.
3. Ainsworth (1979); Atkinson and Zucker (1997); Bailey, Wood, and Nava (1992); Baringholtz (1998); Bohart and Greenberg (1997); Bowlby (1969, 1973, 1979, 1980, 1988); Bretherton (1995); Buber (1958); Cassidy and Shaver (1999); Fogel (1993); Fromm (1956); Gergen (1994); Kahn (1991); Kernberg (1975, 1976, 1995); Kohut (1971, 1977); Levine and Levine (1997); Mahler (1968); Mahler, Pine, and Bergman (1975); May (1969); Mayeroff (1971); Mitchell (1988, 1997); Mitchell and Black (1995); Rogers (1957, 1961, 1980); Simpson and Rholes (1999); Solomon and George (1999); Sroufe (1979); Stern (1985); Taylor (1995); Watkins (1986); Wheeler (2000); Zimmerman and McCandless (1998).
4. O'Donahue (1997, 1998).
5. Bohart and Greeberg (1997).
6. These and similar simple phrases can be powerful incantations to the mindfulness optimal in helping: Epstein (1995); Ram Dass (1971); Ram Dass and Gorman (1985).
7. Bugental (1978, 1987); Fogel (1993); Fromm (1956); Kornfield (1993, 2000); Mayeroff (1971); Ram Dass and Gorman (1985); Taylor (1995).
8. Fogel (1993); Leitner (1995); Schwartz (1993).
9. Boorstein (1996); Fogle (1978).
10. Bohm (1985, 1996).
11. Teleonomy is usually contrasted with teleology. Teleology involves movement toward a specified destination (e.g., going home, reaching a specific future point, etc.). In other words, teleology refers to a directionality that is defined by a specific destination. Teleonomy, on the other hand, refers to an emergent directionality that is apparent only historically. In teleonomy, the direction emerges from ever-emerging choice points. Its pattern of self-organization becomes apparent only after considerable complexities of action in the face of options. The classical example of teleology is that of following a map: pursuing a course of action aimed specifically at a concrete and singular choice of destination. Teleonomy, on the other hand, is best illustrated in biological evolution and human personality development, where there are patterns that become clear in retrospect, but which were not apparent in the early stages of development.
12. Brent (1978); Dell (1982a, 1982b); Dell and Goolishian (1981); Hayes (1996); Kohut (1971, 1977); Lyddon (1993); Mahoney (1991); McAdams (1994); Miller and C'de Baca (1994, 2001); Orlinsky, Grawe, and Parks (1994); Orlinsky and Howard (1975); Pervin (1994); Rice and Greenberg (1984); Robertson and Combs (1995); Safran and Muran (2000); Schiepek, Eckert, and Weihrauch (2003); Sluzki (1992, 1998); Thelen and Smith (1994); Van Geert (1998, 2000); Woodcock and Davis (1978).
13. Snyder (1999); Snyder and Lopez (2001); Snyder, McDermott, Cook, and Rapoff (1997).

14. Mahoney (1991, p. 374).
15. Johnson (1987); Lakoff (1987); Lakoff and Johnson (1980, 1999).
16. Kokoszka (1999).
17. Lakoff and Johnson (1999); Mahoney (1991).
18. Epstein (1973, 1993); Haviland and Kahlbaugh (1993); James (1890); Lewis and Haviland (1993); Magai and McFadden (1995).
19. Angus (1996); Angus and Hardtke (1994); Caro (1993, 1994, 1997); de Rivera and Sarbin (1998); Gonçalves (1994, 1995); Gonçalves, Korman, and Angus (2000); Greenberg and Pascual-Leone (1995); Guidano (1987, 1991).
20. Arciero (1999); Arciero & Guidano (2000).
21. Bruner (1979, 1986, 1990, 2002); Daloz (1999); Glazer (1999); Palmer (1998).
22. I am indebted to Sophie Freud (personal communication) for this suggestion.
23. Kierkegaard (1938, p. 85).
24. Davis and Hollon (1999); Dowd (1999); Eagle (1999); Prochaska and Prochaska (1999); Reid (1999); Wachtel (1982, 1999).

TABLE 2.1. Constructive Themes in Human Experience and Development

Activity

- Human beings are active participants in shaping their own experiences. We are agents of choice.[a] Our actions and activities reflect our choices, and our choices influence who and how we are. We are unaware of most of our choices.
- Much of our activity is anticipatory. With important exceptions, we tend to anticipate what we remember, that is, we expect our future to resemble our past.
- Attention is a powerful form of activity and frequently an important focus in therapy. Many clients are helped by learning attentional skills. To be optimally useful, insight must be paired with action. Practice is a high priority.

Order

- We actively seek order in the face of constant challenges to our order-seeking.
- Human activity is primarily focused on the creation and maintenance of a viable order or organization in life. We seek and create meanings.
- Meanings are relationships that connect particulars. Loss or lack of meaning is experienced as chaos. The network or matrix of our personal meanings make up our "personal realities." Although we share much with each other, we each live in and from uniquely personal realities. Major changes in psychological experiencing involve changes in meanings and, therefore, in personal realities.
- Biologically, emotional processes, which are intimately related to attention, are powerful organizers of our experiencing. Emotions are evaluative appraisals and preparations for action. Emotions are natural expressions of our biological nature—our quests for order (viable meanings) and our reactions to the lack, loss, or change of order in our lives.
- Challenges to our order are essential for all learning and development. Novelty or new experiences are crucial.
- We live seeking a dynamic balance—seeking to achieve or regain a sense of equilibrium amid the ever-unfolding challenges to our ordering processes.
- Professional counseling is often sought as an attempt to change or regain a sense of order, meaning, or balance in life. Many clients benefit from developing a healthy relationship to the power and presence of emotions. Emotional experiencing and expression are often as important as emotional control.

Identity

- The creation and change of order hinges on contrasts. Change is experienced relative to what remains the same.
- A primitive and powerful contrast in most humans is that between self and not-self. The emergence of a sense of self appears to be crucial to healthy human development.
- The body and its sensations are fundamental to experiencing selfhood or personal identity. The body serves as a center of operations. Center and centering are important metaphors in psychological life.

(continued)

TABLE 2.1. ***(continued)***

- Sense of self and sense of reality are intimately related. Challenges to the sense of self are often experienced as life threatening. The self is paradoxical in being simultaneously changing and unchanging (historically continuous).
- Relationships with self are critical to life quality. These include self-concept, body image, self-esteem, and capacities for self-reflection and self-comfort.
- The sense of self can become dysfunctional when it is fragmented and its capacities for balance and coherence are insufficiently developed. Difficulties also occur when an individual identifies with a problem or rigidly resists the changing aspects of life. Foreclosure on the complexity or flexibility of the self can lead to painful patterns of felt isolation, unworthiness, or insufficiency.
- Sense of self and relationships with self most often develop and change in the context of strong emotional relationships with others. Counseling can provide a secure base for examining and changing self- and interpersonal relationships.

Social–symbolic processes

- Self-organization is fundamentally shaped by social bonds and symbolic processes (e.g., imagery, language). We live in and from relationships (past, present, and potential). Symbols and symbolic processes connect us and help us to organize our experiencing. Words and symbols reflect powerful processes of organization and communication.
- The quest for order and meaning is often expressed in narrative form (i.e., in the form of an unfolding story). Narrative sharing—storytelling, story creation, story revision—is a powerful form of human bonding and a common element in professional counseling.
- Religious and spiritual beliefs, communities, and traditions are often powerful sources of support and guidance. Counseling can encourage quests for meaning via shared communities and enduring traditions.
- Changes in personal experience and activity patterns are often accelerated by changes in relationships. Changes in patterns of thinking may be a valuable component of counseling.
- Human consciousness involves capacities to transcend time and space (e.g., to remember and anticipate). Living primarily in the present is often a challenge. Counseling can encourage the development of balanced skills in being present, as well as planning.

Dynamic dialectical development

- Equilibration (balance) reflects our attempts to deal with the contrasts (dialectics) between old and new patterns.
- Resistance to change expresses a healthy tendency to protect against changing too much, too quickly.
- Cycles or waves of opening and closing (expansion and contraction) are common experiences in development.
- When a challenge to our ordering capacities is overwhelming, severe contraction is a natural response.
- Disorganization is a natural and necessary component of reorganization in life-ordering processes.

(continued)

TABLE 2.1. ***(continued)***

- The new life order that may emerge from waves of disorganization is usually more complex and differentiated than its predecessor.
- There are two kinds of change: gradual and abrupt (quantum). Most human lives reflect both. Counseling can encourage patience, hope, and persistence in the face of both change and its felt absence. Particularly valuable skills involve centering (finding and regaining balance) and exploratory decentering (risking excursions into new possibilities for experiencing).

[a]The issue of will and determinism permeates the literatures of psychology and philosophy: Baltes and Staudinger (2000); Bandura (1997); Barrett (1958, 1967); Bartley (1984); Bateson (1972, 1979); Durant (1926); Durant & Durant (1935–1975); Fischer (1987); Hunt (1995); James (1890, 1902); Kaufmann (1974); Kovel (1991); Lewis (1997); Magee (1983, 1997); May (1969); Russell (1945); Schwartz (2000); Sperry (1988); Wundt (1912). Personally, I believe in "costly will" rather than the free variety: Our agency has a price.

TABLE 2.2. Basic Principles of Constructive Practice

Professional psychotherapy involves a special form of human *relationship*, a *rationale* that makes sense of the client's experience and possible courses of constructive action, and the active practice of *rituals* aimed at changing experience patterns. The *processes of change* are principled, but they are also complex, individualized, and nonlinear.

Relationship

- The helping relationship is a *co-created human bond* between the individual(s) seeking counsel and the individual(s) offering to serve.
- A constructive helping relationship is characterized by a nonauthoritarian *collaborative style* in which the persons involved work together and share a joint responsibility for the process and results of their endeavors.
- *Compassion, caring, and empathy* on the part of the therapist are critical ingredients in the quality of the helping relationship.
- The therapeutic relationship provides a *secure base*—a consistently safe and confidential interpersonal context—in which and from which the client can both explore and experiment with new ways of experiencing.
- The *client* is the primary agent of change.
- The *person and personal characteristics of the therapist* are important ingredients in the helping relationship and in the therapeutic enterprise. Of particular significance are his or her continuing personal development, authenticity, tolerance for ambiguity, patience, comfort with emotionality, and faith in the possibilities of human development.
- The constructive therapist focuses on the *client's strengths, resources, and capacities* to change in personally meaningful ways.
- The constructive therapist is a consistent and trustworthy source of *affirmation, encouragement, and hope.*

(continued)

TABLE 2.2. *(continued)*

Rationale

- *Life is change*, and *change is stressful.*
- People organize their lives into patterns of activity that are meaningful and that have been functional for them. These patterns become *uniquely personal realities* and styles of living. Personal realities are generally *tacit* and *anticipatory*; they operate without our awareness, and they assume that the future will resemble the past.
- When life challenges are not successfully resolved by old and familiar methods of coping, people are likely to *experience disorder and disorganization* in many dimensions of their life.
- Disorder and disorganization are often accompanied by *strong negative emotions* and a sense of confusion.
- *Emotions are not dangerous*. Emotions are powerful patterns of organizing our experience as preparations for action and ways of communicating with self and others.
- *Emotions are natural expressions* of people's attempts to protect or regain a sense of meaning, order, and control in their lives.
- Although it may be distressing, disorder can create variations or changes in old patterns of experiencing; this *variability is necessary for the emergence of new forms of adapting.*
- *Chronic distress and dysfunction* often reflect reductions in variability as a result of habitual patterns of activity (including thinking and feeling). Such patterns may have been functional (adaptive) in earlier life circumstances, but they have become costly and counterproductive. In this sense, many chronic "disorders" are excessively orderly. They are rigid or rutted processes that reduce possibilities for novel or enriching experience.
- People can facilitate their own change by *actively experimenting* with new ways of being and by *selectively practicing* (strengthening) new patterns that serve them well.
- As well as being the primary agent of change, the client is always the *resident expert on self* and his or her own experience.
- The primary purpose of psychotherapy is to provide compassionate encouragement and professional counsel as individuals work to *reorganize themselves and their lives.*
- *Personal reorganization* often involves multiple attempts to *emotionally rethink* (revise) one's *life story* while *redirecting* one's *attention* and everyday *activity.*
- The primary responsibilities of the therapist are to *honor* the *phenomenology* (felt experience) of the client, *to offer appropriate comfort* and reassurance, to respectfully *assess personal realities and activities*, *to challenge old patterns* of coping that are unsuccessful or dysfunctional, to be sensitively *attuned to* the client's *pace of change*, and *to encourage* responsible and self-caring *experiments in new ways* of perceiving, acting, thinking, and feeling. For many clients, these experiments involve more viable narratives (stories) about themselves, their characteristics, and their capacities.
- The primary responsibilities of clients are to remain as *engaged* as possible *in their own development* and to be both *patient with their process* and *persistent in their participation.*

(continued)

TABLE 2.2. ***(continued)***

Rituals

- Rituals (techniques, exercises, and homework assignments) are *structured experiments* in experiencing.
- Rituals are an important expression of people's *intention to change* and their *active participation* in that pursuit. As such, rituals are *trial-and-error* endeavors.
- Rituals often reflect *symbolic meanings* regarding past events, present experiences, and future directions of development. These meanings may be more important than the actual content or form of the ritual itself.
- Many rituals are aimed at *developing skills* (e.g., attention or awareness, communication, conceptualization, emotional regulation, experiential risk taking, impulse control, perspective taking, and self-relationship—especially self-comforting).
- Some of the most common rituals in psychotherapy reflect *basic contrasts in* the *processes* of living (beginning or ending, opening or closing, centering or edging, accelerating or decelerating, effort or surrender, giving or receiving, etc.).
- Many therapeutic techniques involve *creative reconstructions* of clients' life stories (narratives) in a manner that *modifies the meaning(s) of their past* and changes clients' *self-characterizations*, their sense of *agency*, and their sense of alternative *possibilities and hope*.
- *Personalized rituals*—experiments created for or by an individual—may be particularly helpful in the exploration of new action patterns.
- *Careful observation*, especially self-observation, of the experience and effects of a ritual can provide important information on its utility in facilitating change processes and can help to strengthen new patterns of adjustment.
- Rituals or exercises involving *supportive groups or significant others* can be particularly powerful in influencing developmental pace and direction.
- The *regular practice* of rituals can add a sense of *order and commitment* to the change process.

Processes of change

- Changes in patterns of experiencing are usually *nonlinear*, reflecting mixtures of mostly *slow, small steps*; frequent *returns to earlier patterns*; and occasionally *large, sudden leaps*.
- Although change processes reflect orderly principles, the *particulars can never be perfectly predicted* for a given individual (e.g., how long it will take, the consequences and repercussions of a particular course of action, the degree of difficulty or effort required).
- The reorganization of life patterns often occurs in *waves or oscillations* of success and failure, progress and regress, and *expansion and contraction*.
- Small initial changes may be *amplified* into large and enduring ones.
- Changes in any area of functioning can affect all other areas; change is systemic or *holistic*.
- Reluctance or *resistance to change* is common, natural, and most intense when core ordering processes are involved; such resistance is an expression of *self-protection*.

(continued)

TABLE 2.2. ***(continued)***

- *Old and new patterns* of coping *compete for dominance* and control within the individual; change is often experienced as *an internal struggle or conflict.*
- Even when new patterns are well-practiced and apparently stabilized, *old patterns* of activity *are never completely eliminated*; old patterns are most likely to reappear in contexts of fatigue, prolonged stress, and novel challenges.
- Psychological development is often reflected in *shifts of attention*, *changes in perceptions* and *personal meanings*, changes in *interpersonal relationships*, improved *capacities to rebound* from setbacks (to "regain balance"), and changes in *self-relationships.*
- Among the more common and important changes in self-relationships that occur during and after psychotherapy are *increased self-awareness*, *increased comfort with emotional experience* and its expression, greater *openness to experience*, greater *self-acceptance* or *improved self-esteem*, increased capacities to *self-comfort* and to receive and give *affection*, a greater *sense of personal agency* or *empowerment*, and a sense of more *hopeful or grateful engagement with life.*

TABLE 2.3. A Flexible Session Structure

1. Human presence in first contact
2. Assess current attention and establish immediate agenda
3. Practice attunement in balancing client's cycles of experiencing

    Comforting * * * * * * Challenging

    Opening
*
*
*
*
*
Closing

4. Practice exercises or techniques
5. Invite processing and reflections
6. Offer affirmations, suggestions, and possibly homework
7. Separate with presence and good will

CHAPTER 3

CONSTRUCTIVE ASSESSMENT

Just as constructive therapy is not something done "to" a client, constructive assessment is not something separate from constructive therapy. Each meeting is an opportunity for both client and therapist to examine and creatively experiment with their experience of the other and how their being together, even briefly, is reflected in self-experiences. Recall that constructivism views the creation and experience of meaning as central to human life. We actively organize our lives into meaningful realities. The fundamental dimension of meaning is relationship. The meanings assumed by and assigned to things in our lives depend on their relationships with other things. The individual letters in these words, for example, contribute to different meanings, depending on how they are arranged and related. The words assume different meanings in relationship to sentences, paragraphs, and themes. Their meaning does not reside "in" them so much as in their relationships. Their relationships may change. This is why I place such emphasis on the relationship between therapist and client in constructive practice. A therapeutic relationship should be a coming together of human beings in such a way that the person being served can learn valuable lessons about his or her patterns and possibilities.

MEASUREMENT AND DIAGNOSTICS

In the realm of assessment, a commentary is warranted on the issues of measurement and diagnostics. Measurement is often equated with numbers. Pythagoras (570–500 BC) believed numbers to be the essence of being.

Rationalism and rationality derive from the concept of a "ratio" scale (which requires an absolute zero as a reference point and equal intervals of distinction). Numbers are still the name of the game in science's claims to authority. "Quantophilia" is the assumption that reality and quantification are synonymous. We should remember that numbers are constructions of category and sequence. They offer valuable (but not infallible) means for thinking about patterns.[1] In more ways than one, the scientific revolution has been a synergy of mathematical and experiential possibilities. We are wise to honor the contributions of both.

But the limitations of numbers to capture important qualities is readily apparent when it comes to the measurement of meaning, particularly personal meaning. Quantifiable measures of persons are plentiful, but meaningful measures are elusive. This becomes a particularly important issue in the realm of psychological measurement and assessment. Assessment has been traditionally viewed as something performed before a treatment is rendered. Indeed, it has become standard practice in some helping professions for the assessment and diagnostics to be performed by specialists who are relatively disconnected from the treatment process. An "intake" or "evaluation" may be performed by one professional as part of a sequence in which other professionals assume the responsibility of actual treatment. In the approach I am practicing, however, assessment and intervention are interwoven into the fabric of a developing human relationship. Other than beginning with informed consent and collecting basic information at the outset, however, I exercise considerable freedom about whether and when I use particular assessment methods with individual clients.

In much contemporary practice of psychotherapy, it is assumed that the therapist possesses an errorless "psychic dipstick" for measuring levels of clients' functioning. In the lingo of the profession, the client is evaluated, tested, and perhaps profiled. The tested individual may undergo an assessment "battery." More often than not, the assessment results in a diagnosis or classification that purports to capture clients' personalities, their problem(s), and possible risks associated with people like them. Only recently has attention been given to developing and utilizing psychological instruments that focus on the strengths, creativity, and resourcefulness of the person.[2]

Because my focus in this book is on practice, I do not dwell on the theoretical controversy, empirical limitations, and ethical complexities that abound in the realm of psychological assessment. The existing literature on this topic is vast, and its implications are hardly reassuring for proponents of traditional assessment and diagnosis.[3] I believe it is practically important, however, to emphasize some of the differences between conventional and constructive uses of psychological measures. There is a certain irony in the historical fact that psychological measurements were originally developed to document individual differences, yet have come to be used in ways that diminish those differences. Sir Francis Galton, the talented cousin of Charles Darwin, pioneered the measurement of human differences.[4] In the century since his work on "anthropometry," thousands of instruments have been designed for measuring 10s of thousands of variables thought to be meaningful to our understanding of human experience. Besides their reliability and validity, the meaningfulness of those measures is a topic of continuing debate.

Constructivists have participated in those debates and often have challenged the assumptions, functions, and effects of many psychological measures. It is important to note that the issue is not simply "number bashing"; constructivists do not deny the impressive power of mathematics as a symbolic tool. Rather, constructivists have emphasized that personal meanings—the orderly patterns by which we organize our life activities—are not easily or adequately captured in simple summary numbers. Moreover, constructivists have emphasized that mathematical and categorical representations of a person take on significant meanings (e.g., for the client, therapist, and third-party payers). Some of those meanings can become potential obstacles to the change process. When a person is assigned a summary score (e.g., estimating her intelligence) or given a rigid diagnostic label, it is common to assume that her score or diagnosis is a capsule summary of who she is or what she is capable of becoming. George Kelly cautioned about a tendency toward "hardening of the categories," and this hardening often takes place despite repeated cautioning. A person who has accepted a psychological "type casting" must often face formidable obstacles if he desires to change his styles of experiencing. A person who has come to identify with his problems, for example, faces more daunting challenges in changing those problems than does someone for whom such problems represent less central features of the self. This is one of the dimensions I listen for in my ongoing assessment of a client: How does he classify or categorize himself? I also listen for hints of implicit models of personality. Does he believe his personality can change? Is personality different from personal identity or one's fundamental self? These are not just abstract questions deserving philosophical reflection. They are questions that are critical to every person who is seeking to understand and redirect his or her life. Not surprisingly, such questions can be found at the forefront of research on consciousness itself and lifespan human development.[5]

My remarks here and elsewhere are not intended to damn psychological tests or to deny some of the functions that can be served by an adequately individualized and dynamic classification system. We should realize, however, that classification and categorization have come to assume formidable powers in our profession. Research funding and the approval of drugs by the U.S. Food and Drug Administration now require specific diagnoses drawn from the current versions of the *Diagnostic and Statistical Manual of Mental Disorders* or the *International Classification of Diseases*.

These classification systems continue to be elaborated, and their lingo enters everyday conversation. Different diagnoses and drugs go through cycles of popular use. Importantly, the constructs beneath the labels become less flexible. Patterns of human activity become entombed as categorical imperatives. Assessment and diagnosis become focused exclusively on problems, deficiencies, and dysfunctions, most of which are talked about as if they were permanent entities inside the client. Some clients welcome a diagnosis, of course. If their problem is due to their disorder, it may seem less mysterious, they may feel less lonely, and they may use their diagnosis to explain their ways of being. A diagnostic label also conveys the message that a professional is confident that he or she has identified the problem. In many medicinal cultures, diagnosis is the first step toward treatment. But most treatments for psychological problems are still highly experimental, and those with good scientific evidence are generally nonspecific. In other words, our most effective therapies—including psychotropic medications—tend to work well with a wide range of dysfunctions. Diagnoses appear to be serving functions other than specifying the best form of treatment. My concern is that, through the proliferation and continuing entrenchment of a pathology-centered diagnostic system, our personal and collective tendencies toward categories are being exploited in ways that do not optimally serve our clients or our professional focus.

A client's description of her current concerns or presenting problem is obviously important, and I am interested in her assumptions about causes and possible solutions. As research and clinical experiences have amply documented, the client's theory of change is often at least as important as the theory believed by the therapist.[6] Our theories of change (our clients' and our own) are largely tacit. Even though it may be helpful to make attempts to describe such theories, our words are not likely to capture the powerful abstract processes by which we organize our active experiencing.

When I reflect on the mistakes I am aware of having made as a therapist, I am often struck by the obvious clues I ignored. For example, a woman named Martha, who consulted me after having been dissatisfied with several previous therapists, was unhappy in her marriage and dissatisfied with her work, and she reported a range of struggles in her daily functioning (anxiety, depression, irritability, indigestion, and poor sleep). Repeated medical tests had revealed nothing, and she reported that her previous therapists simply did not understand her.

At the time, I was still practicing a rudimentary form of cognitive-behavioral therapy, and my questions to her were focused primarily on self-statements and goal setting. In our first two sessions, she asked me if I thought she might be an alcoholic. Both times I inquired about how much she drank, how frequently, for what effect, and in what contexts. Both times she reported that she consistently consumed one or two beers every evening after her husband went to bed. She said she had never exceeded this amount, had never been intoxicated (privately or publicly), and that she drank to relax and get sleepy. I presumed she was pathologizing her modest indulgences, and I reassured her that small amounts of soft liquor could be included in a healthy program of stress management. She asked my opinion of Alcoholics Anonymous (AA) and I voiced a cautious acknowledgment of its benefits for some people.[7] By the middle of our third session, I had a strong sense of not understanding or serving her very well, and I expressed this. She agreed that we did not seem to be making progress, and she accepted the name and phone number of a colleague who I felt might better serve her. A year later, I had an opportunity to speak confidentially with that colleague, and I inquired about her progress. He said she was doing very well. I was curious about how he had helped her. He said, "Well, she asked my permission to join AA and I encouraged her to do so." She had apparently become a regular and supportive member, and participation in the group had satisfied many of her needs. There are many possible explanations. The point is that she was basically broadcasting what she sensed was a healthy path for her; I need only have heeded and supported it.

Not all messages from clients are so clearly broadcast. Over the years, I have learned to listen better, and to listen with more than my ears. Clients often communicate much more than they can put into words. Moreover, the literal meaning of their words may be less important than the messages that lie between and beyond their words. I have learned, for example, that many questions are really impassioned statements: Why did this happen? How could they have done that to me? What did I do wrong? Questions such as these are often expressions of anger, anguish, and confusion. Although a client may be asking for help in making sense of what has happened, she may also be posing questions as a way of communicating her sense of feeling overwhelmed. In these moments, her questions are not requests for answers so much as they are exclamations or lamentations. Often, such questions are reflections of transitional episodes of intense bodily (emotional) experiencing and oscillations in exploratory activity. My professional goal in assessment is to attune respectfully to a client's oscillations, personal rhythms, and styles of experiencing.

CONSTRUCTIVE THEMES IN ASSESSMENT

The primary purpose of constructive assessment is to help a therapist better understand what it is like to be the client. I want to know how he experiences himself and his world. In the interest of safety and social responsibility, of course, I not only want to evaluate immediate risks in terms of his health and behavior, but I am also listening and looking for things that the client may feel that he cannot do. I often find it useful to conceptualize the ongoing process of assessment in terms of the five themes of constructivism.

Theme 1: Activity

In the realm of activity, I am interested in learning about a client's daily patterns. What is a typical day like for her? What does she do first? What is her inner life like as she goes through her day? What are common thoughts or images? Attention is important in healthy functioning.[8] Where is her attention drawn most frequently? Are there things she is doing that she wishes she were not? What is she not doing that she wishes she were? Some of these questions are addressed by direct questions and in homework exercises. Others begin to become more apparent in the course of our interaction. The way a client is and acts with me is likely to reflect her patterns of experiencing in other relationships in her life. I pay attention to her ways of communicating, the tones in her voice, and the topics that seem to be the focus of her attention.

Theme 2: Order

In all of this, of course, I am also listening for the meaning systems by which she is living. I am trying to enter her world, at least for moments, and to imagine what life is like for her. What are the dimensions in which she finds meaning? As she describes her current concerns, I listen for the apparent structure in her life (e.g., daily routines, roles, responsibilities). My focus reflects my interest in whether there have been felt shifts in her life order. Is she seeking, for example, to find more or different meaning in what she is doing? Does she feel constrained by her life patterns or, alternatively, is she seeking more structure or direction in her life? Because emotions are such powerful organizers of experiencing, I am particularly attuned to her emotional presence and her ways of communicating it. Although her words are extremely important, I am often very interested in the cues offered by her facial expressions, her gaze, and modulations of her voice.

Theme 3: Self

In the realm of personal identity or selfhood, my assessment focus is on the client's presentation of himself. In early sessions I may ask questions about how he feels about himself or his capacities. My primary interest is to get a sense of his coherence or stability, as well as his capacities to experience from a perspective different from his own. I also want to understand his general patterns of self-relationship: Does he engage in self-attack as well as self-defense? Is he comfortable with questions about his current body sensations or inner life? Is he skilled in self-comforting? The preliminary answers to questions such as these are likely to become apparent as a trusting relationship develops between us.

Theme 4: Relationship

In this theme of social–symbolic processes, my focus is on human bonds. Depending on a client's immediate focus, this may take the form of childhood memories, a history of an important relationship, or concerns about a current relationship. I look and listen for themes of trust and open communication (or their contrasts). I try to be sensitive to my client's images, metaphors, and symbols of expression. I want to learn to listen and speak in her language. Are there analogies or metaphors that she prefers? If so, these should be incorporated into my communications with her. Importantly, I want to learn about the sources of her life support. Who are the people she entrusts with her feelings? What are the sources of her inspiration? Where does she find or renew her strength?

Theme 5: Development

The final theme of constructivism is developmental, and it embraces and retraces the preceding four themes. As I begin to know a client, I am particularly attuned to the signals he may be giving about where he is in his cycles of experiencing and what he needs first from me. Many clients arrive with needs for comforting and reassurance. They may want me to be a compassionate listener. They may want or appreciate clear gestures or statements of support or encouragement. These same individuals may also want challenges or at least structured suggestions for things they might do outside the therapeutic session. I emphasize homework—experiments in living—as crucial to personal development. I pay attention to the cycling of their attention, both within and across sessions, and I informally monitor the frequency, intensity, and range expressed in such cycles. I try to respond across the spectrum with a clear assurance of my commitment and caring, as well as a sensitivity to the specific instants of our exchange.

PROBLEMS, PATTERNS, AND PROCESSES

What I am interested in doing with a client—beyond offering him a secure base and generous encouragement—is to help him to elaborate a sense of himself and his life that will serve his future development and well-being. To accomplish this, I must do my very best to "meet" him, as Martin Buber would say—to engage him in a consensually authentic process of human presence. I must try to know him, but not as a scientist examining a biological specimen or a doctor ministering to the requests of the ill. I must meet him on his own grounds, on his own terms, in his own current life. To serve him optimally, I must know how he experiences himself—how he relates to himself, what he sees as his strengths and weaknesses, how he believes he is seen by others, what he sees as his options, how he views his past and what seems both possible and impossible for his future. I need to know in whom he can confide and how he has been helped and hurt. I need to know his sensitivities, how he copes when he is challenged, and the sense he has of what all of this means. I want to know how he manages to keep going, what offers him strength, and what allows him to enjoy himself.

I find it helpful to imagine that there are at least three interwoven levels of focus that can occupy our attention in psychotherapy: (1) problems, (2) patterns, and (3) processes. The level of the problem is perhaps most familiar, because it is the level that brings most clients into therapy. It is also the level at which many clients like to focus.

A problem is a felt discrepancy between the way things are and the way they are expected (or "supposed") to be. In the technical language of the modern sciences studying complex dynamic systems, problems are "perturbations"—violations of a system's balance or direction. Problems are expressions of a living system's attempts to protect itself and to pursue directions that feel immediately satisfying. What this means, among other things, is that problems are often attempts at solutions. If ineffectual, they may be poor or costly solutions and may create more new problems than they solve. The temporary nature of these solutions is often at the essence of their problematic nature. One of the classical realizations of early research on behavioral self-control was the "reversing consequences gradient" (see Figure 5.1 in Chapter 5). On the one hand, behaviors that may bring immediately positive effects are often associated with consequences that are ultimately negative (as in use of addictive drugs, alcohol abuse, and overeating). On the other hand, behaviors that require immediate or sustained effort and moderate discomfort may ultimately result in more positive results (as in bookkeeping, exercise, and housework). An important practical implication of this point is that many individuals "with problems" may be well served by developing skills that (1) bridge the difference between immediate and delayed consequences, and, (2) alter the meaning of the activity in accordance with this larger frame of time and well-being.

Problems do not exist in isolation. They are usually expressions of patterns. The word "pattern" comes from the Latin *pater*, meaning "father" and implying a model. Patterns are repetitive, like waves or ripples on the surface of water. Pattern is the level of recurring and related problems. A client working at pattern levels may still be trying to solve specific problems, of course, but she is also examining the bigger picture. This may be reflected in her search for causes and explanations: "Why do I always find myself falling back into bad habits?", "Why am I the only one in my family who struggles with self-esteem?", "Why is it so hard for me to trust people?" These questions reflect quests for understanding, as well as change. Such questions are sometimes (though not always) asked by clients who tend to be more "psychologically minded" in the sense of being motivated to analyze themselves. For many, making sense of their patterns of distress or dysfunction is an important step in being less frightened by their phenomenology, forgiving themselves for their problematic styles of coping, and beginning to explore actively more constructive ways of adapting. Depending on their interest and our time frame, I sometimes employ techniques that encourage life review and narrative reconstructions of the history of a pattern (Chapter 6).

Problems and problematic patterns are always expressions of processes. Processes are literally the engines of our experiencing. The word "process" comes from the Latin *pro cedere*, meaning "to go forward." As already discussed, we are always in process—always moving forward in the sense of time, anticipation, and ongoing change. We are rarely—and even then only minimally—aware of the processes involved in the generation of our experience. Developing skills of awareness in this dimension is neither easy nor necessarily helpful. Indeed, working at the level of process is among the most difficult challenges for therapists as well as clients. It can also include some of the most powerful and important work that can be done.[9]

Describing process levels of therapeutic work is itself an extremely difficult task, if only because so much of that work goes on at levels of experiencing that are above, below, or between words and languaging. Process work is always work in the immediate, living moment, and it is difficult to wrap such work in neat verbal packages. Some of the techniques or exercises I employ with clients who choose to do process work include varieties of meditative practices and stream of consciousness work (Chapter 8). In these techniques, clients are taught to "look inward" in a nonjudgmental way and to observe the multiple levels and movements of the activities that make up their consciousness—the arising and fading away of thoughts, feelings, sensations, images, and so on. Such introspection can sometimes be an overwhelming experience, but it can also open new realms of possibilities for the individual.[10]

With some clients, I point out that what they are doing in a given moment is an example of how they organize and interpret their own experience. "*That* is your process!" is a statement many clients have heard me say. Because we are each always "in process," of course, I am theoretically never wrong in making that statement. One client with whom I had used that remark several times was unclear about what I meant by it. In the course of our work together, he expressed an interest in the stream of consciousness technique (Chapter 8). We scheduled a session when we would have plenty of time and, after some brief relaxation and self-caring instructions, I invited him to simply observe the activity inside himself and to periodically describe his experience out loud. He was silent for almost a minute, fidgeting nervously in his chair and struggling to keep his eyes closed.

"I'm not sure what to say," he began in a tight voice. "I guess I am supposed to say whatever comes to mind . . . but . . . Jesus! I feel so nervous! I don't know if I understood you. . . . I'm . . . I'm not sure if I'm doing this right . . . " I was about to reassure him and to have him focus on his breathing when he popped his eyes open, looked at me in surprise, and asked, "Is *that* what you mean by 'process'?"

I asked, "What?"

And he said, "Here I am all upset that I didn't get the instructions right, that I'll get it wrong, that I'll screw it up! That's how I've dealt with every assignment in my life. Is that what you mean by 'process'?"

"Yes," I answered and smiled. "That's part of your process."

I gently patted his forearm. "Do you want to see some more?" I asked.

"Yeah!" he said, as he closed his eyes again. "This is weird," he continued, "and I'm nervous, but I want to see more." And he did.

It is important to remember that my thinking about psychotherapy in terms of problem, pattern, and process levels is itself a reflection of my attempts to organize my own activities as a therapist. As I have already said, I do not believe these three levels exist independently of one another or that clients' needs can be neatly divided among them. I have found these levels to be helpful conceptual scaffolding in structuring my services for many clients. When clients' primary interest is in a particular problem, for example, they are likely to want help with concrete solutions. This is where basic problem-solving skills may be most appropriate, and clients can be taught to experiment with different solutions (Chapter 5). Some problems cannot be solved, however, at least not as they have been framed by the client. The loss of a loved one or the tragic consequences of a past action cannot be reversed. In such cases, I believe that we best serve our clients by listening with compassion, by encouraging acceptance of things that cannot be changed (and self-forgiveness, if they feel that they were responsible), and by gradually helping them to shift their energies and attention toward moving on with their lives as best they can.

Process-level work shares parallels with "depth," experiential, and transpersonal approaches to psychotherapy.[11] It is not a simple and superficial tinkering, but rather a complex excursion into core ordering processes. As I later reiterate in discussing the stream of consciousness technique, deep process work is both risky and promising. Process work can be risky, because it can be so deep. Intimations of basic ordering processes can reflect and induce changes. Process work can be powerful, because it taps into the very engines of experiencing. For some clients, intellectualizing and living in their heads, so to speak, is their best bet at adaptation (given their skills development, history, current stress, etc.). Just as one should never push for strong emotions, one should never push for process-level work. Neither therapist nor client can accurately anticipate what may emerge in the process. Nor are there guarantees that exploring and experimenting with such fundamental processes of self-organization will necessarily result in positive developmental changes. Process is always present at any level of therapeutic work, of course, and clients will often signal their readiness to explore it more deeply. If the therapist initiates process-level work (Chapters 7–8), it should be done with gentleness and only after assurances of a client's capacities to maintain or regain a sense of center (Chapter 4).

Process-level work is promising because it addresses the heart of a person's life-organizing activities. Working at that level, even for a few seconds, may therefore create opportunities for more profound change. A friend described it as the "flash and flesh" dimension. One can experience flashes of a different perspective, a novel possibility. I once had a client who had lived much of her life frightened and vigilant. She was always ready for tragedy to strike. Then, during a process moment, she experienced a transforming glimpse of her own wary style. She said it was as if she had been tiptoeing into a dark and frightening attic, where she was surrounded by shadowy monsters. Suddenly, it was as if someone turned the attic light on for just a fraction of a second and then turned it off again. She was still in the dark, so to speak, but in that flash, she had caught a glimpse of a path and unmasked some imaginary monsters. The "flesh" part of process work is its intimate involvement of the body and emotions, about which I will have more to say as we continue.

CORE ORDERING PROCESSES

The five themes of constructivism help me organize my focus in assessment. By thinking in terms of problem, pattern, and process levels, I develop a sense of where clients want to invest their current energy. Another cluster that helps has to do with how clients seem to be organizing their own experiencing. Chapter 2 presents a synopsis of a constructive view of human experience and development (Table 2.1). Such a view emphasizes our active involvement in organizing our experiencing. Our nervous systems are structured so that we perceive stabilities in the world around us—stabilities that are critically important to our survival. Early Gestalt psychologists called it *perceptual constancy.* When we pass another person on a sidewalk, we experience them as a continuous (constant) entity in movement. Our experience of them is a construction of coherence created out of the changing sensations that arrive at our retinas, eardrums, noses, and so on. We need such coherence—such continuity and order—to navigate and organize our own lives efficiently.

Our everyday life and moment-to-moment experiencing is made possible by organizing processes that are largely beyond our awareness. We are not conscious of how we breathe, how we walk, or how the fragmented snapshots from our sensory receptors are woven into seamless sequences that we experience as people, objects, and the passage of time. To say that these processes are unconscious is perhaps misleading, especially given the common connotations of the term "unconscious." Pioneering constructivist Friedrich Hayek said that it would be more appropriate to call such ordering processes "superconscious," because they govern the conscious processes without appearing in them.[12] For us to "have" a thought, image, or sensation, for example, there must be processes that have literally "carved" ("edged") that particular experience out of a background (e.g., of other thoughts, images, or sensations). The very act of creating particulars—of constructing figures that can be experienced as separate from their background contexts—is an abstract, higher ordering process that we cannot deny, yet cannot observe. Michael Polanyi called it the *tacit dimension*, and it is a prerequisite for all that we consider to be conscious.[13] As I mentioned in Chapter 2, some of Hayek's insights about the tacit dimension have important practical implications. The "bad news"—if one chooses to view it that way—is that we are not conscious of a lot of the most influential organizing processes inside us. The "good news" is that such consciousness would probably get in our way more often than it would help (e.g., in routine activities such as walking, a consciousness of all levels of our neuromuscular coordination would certainly slow us down and probably interfere with our movement). Also reassuring is Hayek's insight that we are always more developed than we realize. When we realize that we have developed a certain level of skill, for example, we must also acknowledge the operation of a second, even higher level of development that makes possible our first level of realization. With continuing practice and good fortune, we may ultimately become consciously aware of the second level, but this, too, would presume the emergence of a third, still higher level to accommodate this new awareness. When you are having a bad day or feeling disappointed in your skills development, this insight can be a welcome assurance.

Perhaps because of our fascination with the power of words and language, however, we often like to talk and think about even those things we know we cannot capture in words. I confess to enjoying such conjectures. An example that has direct bearing on constructive psychotherapy is the tacit dimension of *core ordering processes* (COPs). These are the deeply abstract processes that are central to our psychological experiencing. I have found it useful to think of these core processes as involving four overlapping themes:

1. *Reality* (the construction of perceptual constancies and such dimensions as stable–unstable, real–fake, possible–impossible, and meaningful–meaningless)
2. *Value* (the construction of emotional judgments and such dimensions as pleasant–painful, good–bad, positive–negative, right–wrong, and approach–avoid)
3. *Self* (the construction of a sense of personal sameness or continuity and such dimensions as body–world, me–not-me, I–Thou, and us–them)
4. *Power* (the construction of a sense of agency and such dimensions as able–unable, hopeful–hopeless, engaged–disengaged, and in–out of control)

Note that each COP invokes contrasts as a means of creating order. This is indeed at the heart of the statement about there being two kinds of people in the world. Kinds imply contrasts and categories. Contrasts and categories create dimensions. The constructed contrast between good and bad, for example, does not require that everything be either one or the other. Developmentally, it is common to first experience a difference and then later to recognize subtle gradations. Hayek's classic work *The Sensory Order* showed this insight to be based on how our nervous systems operate; George Kelly also believed that our constructions are fundamentally dichotomous.[14]

COPs are central to human change processes. When a person changes in significant and enduring ways, what changes most are her ways of organizing her personal experiencing. What changes most, in other words, are her core processes of experiencing herself and her world. But COPs are not easy to change. Just as one does not develop a self-concept or value system in a period of a few weeks, one does not change such core processes quickly.[15] COPs are conservative and self-perpetuating. From a biological standpoint, this makes perfect sense. The story of our biological evolution involves a major theme of stability and structure. Our adaptation to our worlds has required that we develop structures that allow us to anticipate and respond in systematic ways. If we look at the structure of our body, for example, we find that its most important organs are centralized and vigilantly protected from injury or assault. The brain is encased in a thick skull of bone. Within the brain are distributed redundancies and multiple backup systems. The arteries, which carry oxygen- and nutrient-rich blood away from the heart, lie deep below the surface. A superficial wound is more likely to injure veins, which are less critical than arteries. The heart is located deep within our core, surrounded by other organs and protected front and back by bones. The rib cage also protects the lungs, and we can live with only one lung functioning. Those organs most crucial to our life support are also most protected. With a few qualifications, I believe the same is true of our psychological processes.

It is easier to change relatively unimportant or superficial parts of ourselves and our lives than it is to change our COPs. We change clothes, hairstyles, jobs, and houses more easily than we change life partners, our values, or our self-image. This is understandable, but it may not be what we want to hear when our pain stems in part from our relationships with others and ourselves. Consider again problem, pattern, and process levels of focus. A problem, in the purest sense, is an isolated challenge. When similar problems keep recurring, they suggest that a pattern has developed. The engines of experiencing are processes, however, and I find it useful to think in terms of these four core processes of perceiving, valuing, identifying with, and controlling. Process-level work involves intentional observations and experiments nearer the heart of our being. Because our most influential organizing processes are also our most tacit, we should not expect to "see" them in the same way that we can see an image of our insides [e.g., in an X-ray, sonogram, computed tomographic (CAT) scan, functional magnetic resonance imaging (fMRI)]. To the extent that we come to "know" our COPs, it is through witnessing our own actions and emotions in the process of examining them. One might call this *epistemotion*: the felt act of knowing as it unfolds.

Dream work and stream of consciousness reporting (Chapter 8) may provide important glimpses of epistemotion for both client and therapist. They almost invariably emphasize the limitations of words in capturing the richness and flow of private experience. Moving into the present moment and closer to the source of what happens next is a potentially powerful developmental move. It also tends to highlight the existence of cycles or waves in the process of all experiencing. These cycles are expressions of our dynamic quests for balance in our being (Chapter 2). They are at the heart of Herbart's and Piaget's constructive theories of human learning and development. We open (or expand) and we close (contract). We approach and then we retreat. We feel closer and then farther apart. We make progress and then we plateau or regress. Because we are made up of systems nested within systems, we are very complex expressions of interacting cycles.

An appreciation for the cycles of experiencing is an important aspect of constructive assessment. Such an appreciation can help therapists to modulate their provision of comfort and challenge according to individual clients' changing needs. For clients, an awareness of cycling may help them to understand the nonlinear and tacit aspects of their development. It is also important for clients to appreciate the wisdom of waves in their change processes. Some clients become frightened by how much or how rapidly they are changing. Other clients may despair at how little or how slowly they are changing. In long-term intensive psychotherapy, it is not uncommon for the same person to feel both of these patterns at different points in time.

ATTUNEMENT

Early aspects of "making contact" and "coming together" are very important in psychotherapy. Whether we or our clients realize it, we each communicate subtle signals in the early moments of our encounters, and particularly in our first meeting. Enthusiasm, hope, tension, and fatigue may all be communicated in our gestures and facial expressions, voice, walk, and how we sit down. In my practice, the first ("intake") interview is always a mutual exploration of compatibility. I want each client to feel free to explore his sense of me and my capacity to help him. I also want that same freedom. In this first interview, I do not work from a clipboard or a standardized intake form, and I seldom take notes during the session itself. I do, of course, listen for and inquire about issues that may require immediate attention. However, I feel that it is most important for me to be as present as possible to the client and to focus my attention (visually and otherwise) on how he is presenting himself. I do not believe that it is necessary to "track" everything that a client says, and my experience has been that clients often repeatedly return to their central themes of concern throughout the course of a session or therapy. I take my time, and I encourage clients to do the same. Our first meeting may last 90 minutes or 2 hours. I ask familiar questions such as "What brings you here?" and "How can I help?" As I listen to their responses, I try to attune to them with my whole body. Their words are important, to be sure, but so are the intonations of voice, eye contact with me, what they do with their hands, and so on. In my early years as a therapist, I could easily get lost in possible interpretations of these experiences as they occurred. Gradually, I began to learn to relax my need to interpret, and I am now more comfortable in letting the session unfold spontaneously.

If I doubt whether I can serve this person well, I tactfully tell her so. I believe the skill of referral is one that deserves more attention in our profession—not only the skill of recognizing when a client would be better served by someone else, but also the skill of how to communicate that decision. I am careful to emphasize the fact that my recommendation for referral is aimed at her receiving the best possible help. I honor and affirm her seeking help, and I remind her that she has both a right and a responsibility to find the best possible help for herself. My intention here is to encourage her self-caring motives. If she presses for reasons as to why I do not feel I can serve her well, I am careful to honor what she may be feeling and how she may be giving meaning to my decision. My decision to refer her to a colleague could feel like rejection to her, for example, or she might jump to the conclusion that I consider her "hopeless." I try to be sensitive to her possible feelings, even (perhaps especially) angry reactions, yet I return to an emphasis on the importance of an optimal attunement in helping relationships. I honor her search but tell her that I feel less qualified than some of my colleagues, whose names and phone numbers I offer her. Thus, if there is a failing in our not being well suited to work together, that failing is mine, not hers. I make it clear that I am trying to serve her in my referral, and I assure her that if she does not feel satisfied with her work with a colleague, she can call me again for alternate referrals.

When an intake interview leads to a mutual sense of possibility, I invite collaboration. A sense of possibility means I feel competent to serve a client; I feel myself drawn toward her in a caring manner, and she feels hopeful and interested in working with me. I emphasize the importance of her experience of me and how comfortable she feels talking to me. The venture into psychotherapy is an important one. I invite questions and I encourage clients to take their time in deciding whether they would like me to be their therapist. Many individuals appreciate having some time and privacy to reflect on that decision, and I often suggest that they take at least a day before calling me for another appointment. If they choose to enter therapy with me, I ask them to return with a completed consent form (Appendix B) and the first part of a self-report on their present experience, personal concerns, and highlights of their developmental history (Appendix C). Some clients long for a label for their suffering, and others arrive with a diagnosis already in mind. Without agreeing with its accuracy or finality, I think it is wise to honor the label toward which they have gravitated. What is important is that they have recognized some of their own patterns in something they have read, heard, or been told. Their attempts to organize their experience should be respected.

Recall that a fundamental assumption of constructivism is that human beings are active participants in organizing and making sense (meaning) of their own lives. They do most of this at tacit (nonconscious) levels by repeating patterns of activities such that they become so familiar as to seem automatic and fundamentally "real." These patterns include thoughts, feelings, daily routines, styles of perceiving and interacting with others, and so on. These are the patterns that make up the world as they experience it, and, indeed, their personal identity. A primary function of assessment is to develop approximate sketches of these patterns, so that their effects can be appraised and their interrelationships can be guaged. With such approximations, a therapist can help clients to realize how such patterns may be limiting their functioning or well-being and, more importantly, how they might begin to explore initially small and then progressively bolder experiments in alternative ways of being.

There is an important sense in which assessment *is* intervention in constructive practice. It marks the beginning of an evaluation process in which the client—with the therapist's help—is closely examining and evaluating how he feels, who he experiences himself to be, the nature of his current challenge(s), and the options and resources available to him. When I begin working with a client, I am usually prepared to hear his initial preoccupation with a specific problem and his desire to focus on its immediate solution. At the same time, I am aware that any given problem is likely to be part of a pattern that is generated by self-organizing processes. Therefore, when time and the client's patience permits, I prefer to launch our collaboration on all three fronts; that is, I try to be sensitive to the immediate demands of his presenting problems and the challenges that these problems may be creating for his everyday adaptation. At the same time, however, I like to begin collecting information on his lifelong patterns of self-organization and his in-the-moment styles of processing novelty.

I experience attunement as an appreciation of connectedness; in this sense, it includes and embraces my bodily sensations and my intuition. Our knowing is much more subtle and profound than our logical, linguistic, and mathematical consciousness can imagine. The scientific evidence for tacit or unconscious processes in knowing is now overwhelming, and much of this evidence implicates embodiment (bodily sensitivity) as fundamental.[16] Oscillations in the popular preference for thinking versus feeling are likely to continue for some time, but the dynamics of these swings should not distract us from some very basic resources in our processes of knowing. This theme is a central one to constructivism, and there is undeniable difficulty in expressing it via common language. If the proper goal of assessment is to know someone in a way that may serve them (i.e., in immediate coping or in eventual development), then it is important to appreciate that the processes of knowing another person and knowing one's self are intimately related.

This is where there is clear wisdom in the literatures offered across the spectra of consciousness studies, ego and self psychology, object relations, intersubjectivity, and transpersonal studies.[17] Many practitioners struggle to suppress or ignore their own experiencing while they are in the role of a therapist. Although I agree that one must be vigilant about projecting one's own assumptions and issues onto a client, I think it is both impossible and unwise to ignore one's inner processes in interpersonal exchanges. I must use good judgment in how I respond to my own reactions, of course, but I find that my internal reactions to my clients valuably inform my experience of them and the counsel I can offer. My knowledge of myself is therefore not an impediment to my professional services but rather is a valuable contribution to them. And when the therapy process unfolds optimally, both the client and I emerge with refinements in our self-knowledge.

It is relevant here to revisit our human penchant for kinds. Note, for example, the frequency with which research on assessment is classified as either quantitative or qualitative, subjective or objective, empirical or not, and so on. The issue of objectivity was central to the formalization of science as a method of inquiry, but it has come to be used as a formidable constraint on science's recent development.[18] All words containing *ject* refer to a process of throwing (e.g., eject, inject, project, reject). The prefix *ob* means to thoroughly throw down or away, so that one can stand apart or against that which is thrown. Being objective means being separate and at a distance. *Sub* means "under," and being subjective implies that one has "underthrown." Clinical objectivity is supposed to reflect a detachment. There is, however, a difference between detachment and nonattachment. I strive to embrace the polarity of objectivity versus subjectivity in my clinical work. The result, when I achieve it, is "diajectivity" (working "through the thrownness"), more popularly known as intersubjectivity. I believe this to be an integral style of inquiry.

I routinely ask my clients for certain kinds of information at various points in our collaboration. These reports are given as homework assignments and are meant to stimulate reflection and dialogue. Samples of forms that I now use for informed consent, presenting concerns, and personal experience patterns can be found in the Appendices. I join clients in periodic reviews of our progress and process. Some clients are helped by counting the frequency of impulses or actions, and self-monitoring is the single most effective component of self-regulation. Some clients find it useful to rate their feelings on scales (e.g., 1–10 or 0–100, with anchors to which they can relate). I try to be sensitive to their ways of making meaning in the navigation of their lives. Like George Kelly, however, I am more interested in the dimensions that they find meaningful than in the absolute numbers that they assign. For valuable discussions of constructive assessment, I strongly recommend Kelly's classics and Greg Neimeyer's excellent casebook.[19] I present here and in the following chapters some of the patterns that have developed in my practice over the years. I emphasize several methods that I have found most useful. The spirit of constructive assessment is fundamentally creative, however, and—like constructive therapy itself—the primary purpose is to explore and experiment in service of the client's development.

NOTES

1. Crosby (1997); Davis and Hersh (1986); Lakoff and Johnson (1999); Lakoff and Núñez (2000).
2. Lyddon and Alford (1993); G. J. Neimeyer (1983); Neimeyer and Raskin (2000); Snyder and Ingram (2000); Wright (1991).
3. Ballou and Brown (2002); Bergner (1997); Bowker and Starr (1999); de Angelis (2001); Fischer (1980, 2002); Follette (1996); Horwitz (2002); Livesley, Schroeder, Jackson, and Jang (1994); Thakker, Ward, and Strongman (1999).

4. See Gillham (2001) for an interesting analysis of Galton's mission.
5. Gallagher and Shear (1999); Hargens (2001); Kirsch (1999); Markus and Nurius (1986); Varela and Shear (1999).
6. Bohart and Tallman (1999); Hoyt (1998).
7. My reservations in her case were probably influenced by my sense of the local chapter, which seemed to be particularly strong on emphasizing "character flaws" and the impossibility of social drinking for "true" alcoholics. For a discussion of the consequences of such categorical assumptions, see Marlatt (1998), Peele (1985, 1999), Smith (2000), and Weil (1972, 1983).
8. Greher and Mahoney (2001); Mahoney (1991).
9. Bohart and Greenberg (1997); Bugental (1965, 1978, 1981, 1987); Greenberg, Watson, and Lietaer (1998); Kwee and Holdstock (1996); Mahrer (1983).
10. Goleman (1988); Levine (1979); Murphy and Donovan (1997).
11. Hunt (1995); Walsh and Vaughan (1980, 1993); Wilber (1999).
12. Hayek (1952, 1964); Mahoney (1991); Weimer (1977).
13. Polanyi (1958, 1966).
14. Hayek (1952); Kelly (1955).
15. Rapid "quantum" shifts in experiencing can and do occur, however (Miller and C'de Baca (1994, 2001). I discuss these in my later synopsis of how and when people undergo dramatic changes (Chapter 11).
16. Abram (1996); Ackerman (1990); Arciero and Guidano (2000); Bakal (1999); Bechara, Damasio, Tranel, and Damasio (1997); Benthal and Polhemus (1975); Berman (1981, 1989); Csordas (1994); Fischer (1980); Gallop (1988); Gendlin (1996); Johnson (1987); Lakoff (1987); Lakoff and Johnson (1980, 1999); Mahoney (1991); Nisbett and Wilson (1977); Polanyi (1958, 1966); Reber (1993); Shevrin, Bond, Brakel, Hertel, and Williams (1996).
17. Bernstein (1983); Gendlin (1996); Harding (1961); Hargens (2001); Hunt (1995); Kernberg (1975, 1976, 1995); Kohut (1971, 1977); Lamiell (1987); Levine (1979); Marquis (2002); Merleau-Ponty (1942, 1962); Ram Dass (1970, 1971); van Maanen (1990); Vaughan (1979, 1986); Walsh and Vaughan (1980, 1993); Wilber (1999).
18. Bernstein (1983); Mahoney (in press-a, in press-b). See also Keller (1983, 1985) and Shepherd (1993).
19. Kelly (1955); Maher (1969); Neimeyer (1993).

CHAPTER 4

Basic Centering Techniques

There are two kinds of clients in the world: those looking for a safe place to fall apart and those looking for help in putting their lives back together. Like all dichotomies, this one is a simplification that has at least a hint of truth to it. Many people enter therapy because they have lost their balance. Others may seek professional help because they feel stuck and unable to move out of destructive or dysfunctional patterns. It is not uncommon for people to report mixtures of these two caricatures. As discussed in Chapter 2, I believe development always involves cycles or spirals of movement between old and new. One of the dimensions to which I attune in my ongoing assessment of clients is their recurring needs for comfort and challenge. People vary considerably in their developed capacities to regain their psychological balance when life circumstances have thrown them off center. With some clients, our primary work involves their quest for a sense of center. For them, I serve as a guide, and my sense of balance is important to their search. Even with clients who have well-developed skills in coping, however, basic and novel centering exercises may be very useful. For this reason, I often begin my services with exercises that are intended to develop and refine centering skills.

This chapter presents some of my favorite techniques for teaching centering. Before I proceed, however, I offer a brief comment on techniques themselves. I have discussed the "tyranny of technique" elsewhere. Abraham Maslow used to call it the law of the hammer. If you give a child a hammer, he will find many things that need pounding. The same is true of psychotherapy techniques. We develop proficiency in certain techniques and then apply them rather generously to a variety of situations. For the sake of maintaining a practical focus in this chapter, I condense the main points of my views about techniques. First, *constructive psychotherapy is not defined by techniques*, but by an overall conceptualization of human experience, knowing, and development. A constructive practitioner can therefore draw on the full spectrum of therapeutic and teaching techniques. More importantly, he or she need not be constrained by that spectrum. As I elaborate later, an essential element of constructive practice is exploring, experimenting, and otherwise "risking" novel experiences that challenge old patterns of activities. This often requires creativity and a spirit of adventure on the part of the constructive practitioner.[1] That creativity and spirit cannot be formalized in a particular procedure.

A second contextual theme is that *constructive practice recognizes that the power to change lies in processes* rather than specific procedures. Yes, these processes require the active engagement of the client. But the processes themselves can be engaged by any number of particular exercises. The process of relaxing, for example, can be learned by means of many different techniques (e.g., autogenic training, imagery, progressive muscle relaxation, meditation, hatha yoga, and so on). The purpose of these techniques is to activate whole-person processes that serve momentary adaptation, as well as ongoing development. With practice, an individual becomes less dependent on a particular technique and more skilled in activating the operative processes in new and challenging circumstances. Skills development is therefore a central aspect of constructive practice, and the skills involved tend to be broad spectrum living skills rather than circumscribed proficiencies.

A third related point is that *techniques can be viewed as specialized forms of communication*. Techniques are like languages. The more languages one knows, the more people with whom one can communicate. We should not mistake the language for the message, however. One can communicate the same message in many different languages. But one can know many languages and still not have anything important to say. My point is that techniques are tools to help us teach living skills. In Table 2.2, I included them among the third "R" of Jerome Frank's "three R's" of helping (relationship, rationale, and ritual). Techniques are rituals in that they are prescribed forms of activity that are set apart from casual or usual conversation. The term "ritual" has taken on connotations of mindless repetition or pathology, which is unfortunate given the importance of rituals in everyday life.[2] Rituals can be healthy routines of activity that symbolize and facilitate important dimensions of experience. They are distinguished from other activity patterns by their significance, which may have special meaning.

Because they are set apart as something different, techniques or exercises may need special introductions or emphases in a session. One can do this in a variety of ways, of course, and clients respond in their own unique fashion. I usually preface my introduction of a technique with a comment to the effect that "Perhaps this would be a good time . . . " or "I would like to suggest that we explore an exercise . . . " The rationale for the technique may be briefly elaborated, but I try not to prolong my discussion of its purpose unless the client seems to need reassurance. I find it important to move into the experience of the exercise (e.g., a role play, an imagination experiment, a meditative focus) as quickly as possible, if only to encourage the client to risk an excursion into a safe unknown. With some clients, it eventually becomes possible to move spontaneously in and out of experiential exercises without a preparatory rationale.

Finally, it is important to remember that *individuals differ in their responses to the same technique*. This fact often illustrates the power of meaning construction in personal realities. Progressive muscle relaxation can actually induce anxiety in some clients, perhaps because they experience it as a loss of control. Likewise, with various visual images, I have had clients for whom the image of a sunny beach has brought up memories of painful sunburn or personal trauma. The bottom line is the client's reaction. This is why trust and honest communication are so critical to the counseling process. I want clients to be able to tell me when something I have suggested is not working for them. Together we can experiment with alternatives until we get closer to what feels appropriate and effective for them. This often requires both patience and creativity on both our parts. To illustrate client reactions in a concrete manner, I have included some of their remarks throughout this chapter.

BREATHING EXERCISES

The essence of centering is a process associated with safety, peace, and well-being. I know of no more reliable method for engaging that process than breathing meditation. Breathing is fundamental to life support. It is connected with heart rate, muscle tension, alertness, energy levels, and emotional experiencing. All vocal expression is based in breathing (crying, laughing, yelling, speaking, singing). It is not surprising that many approaches to consciousness and spirituality have encouraged the regular practice of breathing exercises.[3] These exercises may focus directly on breathing or they may influence breathing through a related activity (e.g., chanting, prayer, or singing). The breath is considered the "golden portal" of consciousness because of its mixture of voluntary and involuntary components. One can exert conscious control over one's breathing, yet respiration does not require consciousness for its continuation. Altering one's breathing can quickly and consistently alter one's consciousness. Rapid, shallow breathing (hyperventilation) will reliably produce many of the sensations associated with anxiety or panic (e.g., racing heart, dizziness, numbness or tingling in the extremities). Slow, deep breathing (as I soon elaborate) can have the opposite effect.

For ease of use with clients, I have condensed these exercises into a handout (Appendix D). The best teachers of relaxed breathing are sleeping babies. They naturally breathe with a rounding of their abdomen, "soft belly" style, and their breathing is slow and deep. It may be occasionally punctuated by a balancing yawn or sigh. This relaxed, natural process can be contrasted with the shallow, rapid, "hard belly" chest breathing of many uptight adults. Posture is important to breathing because of its effects on the movement of the diaphragm, the ribs, and the openness of the abdominal area. This is why many meditation traditions encourage an erect spine when the person is sitting. The process of bringing air into the lungs (inhalation) is actually achieved by creating a partial and temporary vacuum.

There are many more muscles involved in exhalation than in inhalation, and this makes it a better target for conscious control. When working with individuals who experience episodes of panic, the technique of "*pause breathing*" may be particularly helpful. Pause breathing is easier to demonstrate than to describe, but it essentially focuses on inserting a brief (and gradually longer) pause between the end of each exhalation and the beginning of the next "in breath." A person in the midst of panic is very likely to be hyperventilating (and, as noted earlier, the subjective experience of panic can be induced by intentionally breathing rapidly and shallowly). This results in an excess of oxygen (relative to carbon dioxide) in the blood, and the body–brain complex reacts strongly to such changes in blood gases. In a state of panic, persons may mistakenly breathe more rapidly, "trying to catch their breath," and this only complicates their dilemma. The old trick of breathing into a paper bag can help (because, after a few breaths, the air in the bag has a lower oxygen ratio than the outside air). One can also breathe into cupped hands for a similar effect. However, pause breathing is generally more effective.

Here is how to pause breathe: Focus on letting your lungs empty. When it feels like all of the air is out of them, count slowly "one thousand, two thousand, three thousand, four thousand." Do not take in another breath until you reach the second or third count. Try to exhale slowly. It may help to purse your lips while you exhale (as if you were blowing air over a cup of hot coffee or soup). Lip pursing helps to equalize the pressure inside the chest. Continue this exercise as long as necessary, with special emphasis on slow, regular exhalations, each followed by a pause of 2–5 seconds. The calming effect will usually be felt in less than a minute, but it may take another few minutes to relax into trusting in your breathing and well-being. Pause breathing is recommended not just for people who suffer bouts of panic. It is useful for just about anyone as a basic bodily relaxation exercise. Because we often respond to stress by accelerating and compacting our breathing cycles, many of us drift closer to hyperventilation than we may realize.

> When I first started practicing this, I became very aware of my heartbeat. After a couple of pause breaths, though, I did start to calm down. Now I try to do it several times a day and anytime I recognize myself as feeling stressed. I was amazed at how much my breathing mirrored my work pace. The faster I worked, the faster I breathed. It's nice to know I can do something simple that slows me down.

A similar exercise that I like to teach clients is called "*release breathing*." In release breathing, one takes a comfortably deep breath and then—at the very top of the inhalation—one simply releases the air with an open mouth and throat. This may produce the soft sound of an "Aahhhhhh," as if one were settling into a tub of water that is at just the right temperature. A release breath may also feel like a sigh of relief. When I demonstrate it to clients, I make an audible sigh and allow my shoulders to drop as the air exits my body. In a release breath, it is important to avoid forcing the air out of one's lungs or prolonging the process of exhalation. The point is to take in what one needs and then, like a natural valve being opened, simply to release it. Along with pause breathing, I recommend release breaths at regular intervals throughout the day.

> When you first showed me how to do this in the office, I thought I would be too embarrassed to yawn or sigh out loud in front of my coworkers. I started practicing it when I was alone in the car on the way to and from work. It seems like making the sound makes a difference! I've started to do it more often when I'm doing chores at home. I just wish I would remember to do it more often.

A third breathing exercise is something I call "*alternate control and surrender breathing*," and it is actually a combination of several basic breathing skills. It can be practiced in several positions, including sitting or standing, but I prefer the form in which one is lying on one's back. Alternate breathing takes a few minutes, and it practices the contrast between controlling and letting go of control. Like all other techniques, I recommend individualized tailoring of the specifics to suit each client and his or her current skills development. The essence of alternate breathing is the alternation between an active and passive attitude toward one's breathing. During the active phase, I recommend pause breathing. A person may perform three to five pause breaths, for example, then a release breath, and follow this with a minute or two of simply watching (but not controlling) his or her breathing. The number of breaths and the lengths of the pauses can vary, of course. In my experience, "simply watching" is often reported to be the more difficult part of this exercise. This can be a valuable source of personal lessons about balance between effort and surrender. If clients become enmeshed in worries about their limited capacities to "let go," I invite them to join me in a release breath as we prepare to talk about their experience.

> This alternation thing sure feels like it is taking me somewhere I need to go. Maybe it's my issues around trust. I don't know. But I started using it at night when I can't sleep. At first, I got hung up on pausing too long or seeing how long I could go before I needed another breath. That didn't help! So I set a limit of a four count after exhaling and only doing four of those breaths. Then I got hung up on how long I should just watch my breathing in the other part of the cycle. I decided to set a limit of nine. Am I obsessive or what? Of course, there were all sorts of thoughts wanting my attention, too. But after a while, it seemed to get easier. You didn't tell me this might help my insomnia!

These breathing exercises are not a remedy for everything, but they are impressively consistent in their helpfulness. As I emphasize in other chapters, I believe part of their benefits derive from focusing attention and simply slowing down.

BODY BALANCE EXERCISES

Another technique I like to use in teaching centering skills is one that literally involves balance. As a physical exercise, it has the advantage of moving beyond the limits of language and coming back to a basic bodily sense of equilibrium. I usually describe and demonstrate this exercise in my office and then suggest that clients experiment with it on their own at home. Instructions for clients are summarized in Appendix E. Standard precautions regarding safety and responsibility are appropriate (e.g., clients should not perform this exercise if it does not feel safe or reasonable to them; they should assume responsibility for their own body and action; they should consult a qualified specialist if they have vestibular problems or experience vertigo; they should practice it in a place where an unexpected loss of balance can be safely corrected). All of these precautions may suggest that I am about to ask them to walk a tightrope over the Grand Canyon. In fact, what I ask them to do is simply to stand up!

The "*standing center*" exercise is as follows: Stand in a comfortable position with your trunk and head erect and your hands by your sides. Focus your gaze ahead of you on some object or area at eye level. Take a deep release breath and relax. Very slowly and gently begin to lean slightly forward (somewhat like a ski jumper in the middle of a jump, only with much less of an angle). Take about 10 seconds to reach your farthest forward angle. If you lean so far forward that you need to take a step to avoid falling, you have gone too far. As you lean slowly forward, you will feel more pressure on the balls of your feet (just behind the big toe). Spend a couple of seconds near your most forward point of balance. Now, reverse the direction of your lean and slowly shift your weight backward. You will pass through your original position and begin to feel more pressure on your heels. If you have to step backward to avoid falling, you have again gone too far. Spend a second at your farthest backward point and then reverse direction and repeat this cycle at least three times.

Take about 10 seconds in each direction, and slowly rock forward and backward. After doing this several times with your eyes open, experiment with closing your eyes either partially or completely. You may notice two things with your vision reduced: (1) that it is easier to feel the sensations in your soles (and other parts of your body), and (2) that it is a little more difficult to balance. Finally, with your eyes open or closed (whichever you prefer), begin to pay special attention to the sensations in the soles of your feet. They are likely to include a combination of the balls, heels, and the outside edges. Perhaps the sensations will remind you of the indentation your foot makes in soft, loose sand. When you are standing still, your center is always moving, even if ever so slightly. Your weight is distributed between the front and back of your foot and then from side to side in the area of your arch. If we could hang a tiny plumb line from the middle of your arch, it would trace a gently swaying pattern on the floor as your body continuously compensates for slight movements. Call this middle region your center or base. It is your gravitational home. Invite yourself to stand comfortably relaxed and let your body rock gently through it. Slowly let yourself settle into a comfortable sense of stillness. Feel it deeply as a familiar and secure base.

> I admit that when you demonstrated this in your office I thought it was weird. I mean, I've been in therapy before and all we did was talk. Well, I guess I talked and they listened. And I've never been comfortable with my body, so this was not a welcome assignment. In fact, I didn't intend to do it. It sort of just happened. I was trying to change a light bulb in a ceiling fan, and it reminded me of it. I was alone, so I figured "what the heck." What surprised me most was how familiar and strange it was at the same time! And I see what you mean about other messages in it. My center is always there, even when I forget that. And when I'm at my edges, I tend to get frantic and flail about.

Besides its being simple and physical, I like the standing center exercise because of the many metaphors that it can convey about the complexities of life. This exercise makes it clear, for example, that there are limits to how far one can go without falling. Likewise, it provides a basic bodily example of the fact that one recognizes a sense of center most dramatically when it is lost. We often take our sense of center for granted until something comes along and throws us off balance. I also like the fact that one can easily witness the fact that balance is a dynamic process. Even in the middle—at one's balance point—there are rhythmic waves or pulses that the body is constantly using to maintain an equilibrium. We need the edges to find the center. The technical term for it is "postural sway" and one can feel it in a kneeling position or even while sitting, if the torso and head are free to move. There are soothing effects to rocking slowly back and forth (e.g., in a swing, hammock, glider, rocking chair), and I encourage people to find forms of rocking that feel comforting to them.

What may be most important about this standing center exercise is its simple and concrete demonstration that one recognizes the experience of centeredness and that one already has the capacity to find it. When I later discuss the exercise with clients, I encourage them to consider the possibility that this may also be true of their emotional and psychological balance—that they may already know what it feels like and how to get there. It may be most apparent when it is lost, but its being lost does not mean that it no longer exists. Likewise, I suggest that clients consider the possibility that, with practice, they will develop skills that enlarge the size of their center. This will make it easier to stay balanced and to regain their balance when they lose it.

A second exercise that I recommend to some clients is the "*one-leg stand.*" This is more demanding than the standing center exercise, and one can find versions of it in popular methods of stretching, yoga, and a variety of martial arts. People with ankle or knee problems should approach this exercise cautiously. (It is frequently used in physical therapy for rehabilitation after injury to these joints, but such therapy should be supervised by a qualified health professional). As with any other body balance movement, it is wise to practice it near a wall in case one needs support quickly. Begin by standing in a comfortably relaxed position with your back straight and your head level. Release breathe. Focus your gaze forward at eye level. Your goal is eventually to stand safely balanced on one leg. Approach this goal very slowly, gently, and with a keen awareness of what you feel as you do this. Imagine yourself to be wearing a baseball cap with a string hanging from the center front of the visor. When you are standing on both feet, the string would hang directly between your eyes, in front of your nose, and touch the ground between your feet, probably just in front of your big toes.

With your back remaining straight, begin to shift your weight slowly from one foot to the other, in an alternating and very slight, sideways rocking motion. Continue the gentle, sideways rocking for perhaps 30 seconds and focus on the sensations in your legs and feet. Then, choose which foot you will lift. As you begin to shift your weight to the other foot, your physical sense of center will also shift. The bottom of that imaginary string will slowly begin to shift toward the foot on which you will be standing. Notice the very subtle adjustments you make in your pelvis and hips. Feel a gentle change in the pressure on your weight-bearing leg (particularly in the knee, the ankle, and the sole of that foot). Be aware of the changing feelings in the foot you are about to lift. Notice that you are slowly pushing it off the floor and that the last part to leave the ground is the ball of the foot and the big toe. You may need to touch down several times with that toe before you feel steady and balanced on the other leg. Again, notice that your center of balance is dynamic in the sole of your stationary foot. Breathe slowly and notice what else is happening in your upper body during this exercise. As you feel ready, experiment with the differences you feel if you slowly move your elevated leg slightly behind or in front of you. See how long you can balance on one foot before needing to touch the other one on the ground. Experiment with the different feelings produced when you alternate the foot on which you balance.

> This reminded me of my dance lessons when I was a little girl. Without even thinking about it, my arms went up and out to the side, and I could feel myself smiling. It's been so long since I've done that. Too long! It made me want to dance again. Of course, not in front of anyone! But what's the harm in a little dancing in the dark by myself? Is that OK? Was that what you wanted me to discover?

Many clients have presumed that I knew what they would discover when they did this or other exercises. (I wish I were as clever as some have thought.)

The one-leg stand is rich in metaphors, as well as lessons in physical skills. Shifting your center is not as easy as it sounds. It requires adjustments throughout your whole being. Many of the adjustments you make are so subtle and automatic that you must pay close attention to notice them. At first, your new center feels strange or awkward, and there is a strong tendency to return to your more familiar stance. It is "touch and go" for some time, and the smoothness is punctuated with wobbles of instability. The smaller the base (your area of contact with the ground), the more difficult it is to balance. Breathing slowly and relaxing into the process is often helpful. Self-criticism and hurrying interfere. Concentration helps. With patience and practice, the new balance becomes easier to achieve and maintain.

I have used the one-leg stand as an assessment and a skill development exercise with numerous athletes in a variety of sports. It requires and reflects considerable concentration. For athletes who desire more of a challenge, the exercise can be made more difficult by closing the eyes. Some Olympic athletes can balance on either leg with their eyes closed for half a minute. We then increase the challenge by asking them to carefully tilt their head back, so that their head (with closed eyes) is facing the ceiling. This reduces the valuable equilibrium feedback from their inner ear, and they must focus more exclusively on sensations in their body. Some athletes and dancers are capable of briefly balancing on just the ball of one foot or, in ballet, on the reinforced tip of one big toe! These more advanced movements are not appropriate for most clients, of course, but they illustrate the possibility of creatively edging toward ever greater degrees of challenge.

For individuals with more limited abilities in physical balance, I recommend explorations of what is available to them. Slow-motion walking, for example, involves some of the same transitions used in the standing center and one-leg stand exercises. Many practitioners of Zen alternate sitting meditation with slow, mindful walking. Individuals confined to a wheelchair or bed can also develop creative exercises in balancing small light objects (e.g., a Ping-Pong ball on fingertips). The specific form of the movement is less important than the process and the practice.

RELAXING INTO CENTER

"Letting go" is, of course, the essence of relaxation, which involves a slow surrendering (letting go of unnecessary resistance, surrendering to basic rhythms of life support). Relaxation is fundamentally a process of acceptance that cannot be achieved by "trying harder." Effort is the opposite of relaxation, as is the process of being judgmental (which is, literally, a "judge's mentality"). Relaxation involves a trusting in the wisdom of one's body and the natural processes of rest and recuperation. Long before the city of New Orleans adopted the nickname, relaxing has been a natural "big easy." It is easy once it is relearned and practiced, of course, but it is also easy to get caught up in habits and a hectic pace that get in the way of relaxation. I emphasize with my clients that they are not just now learning to relax; they are relearning. Again, a sleeping child is a good teacher. Their breathing will be slow and deep, their face muscles smooth and relaxed (sometimes to the point of drool dropping from their open mouths). Their hands will be softly cupped (rather than clenched or tensely splayed). We all know how to relax. The challenge is to apply that knowledge regularly in the face of high-pressure challenges in our lives and worlds.

As a young behavior therapist, I was trained in progressive muscle relaxation. This method highlights the role of contrast by alternately tensing and relaxing muscles. One asks the client to tightly clench his fist, for example, and to focus on the sensation of tension as he maintains the clench for several seconds. Then, on the cue word "relax," he is asked simply to stop clenching and allow his hand slowly to resume a normal, relaxed state. By focusing on the differences in the sensations of tension and relaxation, an individual can learn both how to recognize muscle tension and its release. This can be very helpful.

As I matured as a therapist, I incorporated more diverse aspects of imagery and breathing into my relaxation exercises. I also learned to avoid negative instructions (e.g., "*don't* worry," "Try *not* to tense," etc.). Negatives seem to contribute to (rather than relieve) tension. My instructions became much slower, and I believe this is important to note. Rushed instructions delivered in a tense or hurried manner are not likely to achieve the desired result. The method is taught most effectively by modeling and induction. In other words, teaching relaxation and centering is best accomplished by actually relaxing and centering in the presence of the client. Verbalizing a memorized script is much less effective than is entering and trusting a process that embodies the central message.

> I really appreciated your being so human about teaching me to relax. When you said you were about to ask me to close my eyes, I started to get uptight. Then you said that you would be closing your eyes, too, and joining me in the exercise. That felt a lot better. Your voice is so soothing.

I often use soft music as a background for my instructions. When clients feel helped by this exercise, it is not unusual for them to ask for an audiotape to help them practice at home. After making dozens of individualized tapes, I finally went into a recording studio and created a version that I could share more widely. Although I can reproduce the script of my "Invitation to Relax," the written word does not convey the importance of pauses and inflections (Appendix F).

From my earlier remarks, it should be clear that I do not recommend reading this script to a client or memorizing it and repeating it verbatim. Such strategies would be less likely to reflect a counselor's personal style or to invite the underlying process that is the aim of the exercise.

In relation to this process, note that I like to use present participle ("ing") forms of verbs and verbs that suggest invitation, acceptance, allowance, and trust. More recently, I have found it useful to include metaphors that convey safety, familiarity, and ease of being. For example, I may suggest that a client think of relaxing as a process of "coming home inside themselves" or "coming home to their heart." Images may include being held lovingly or memories of being gently rocked by a trusted caregiver. I invoke associations with a favorite armchair or couch, and I invite clients to "sink into" or "curl up inside" their own center. Some clients report that they find it helpful to use religious metaphors (e.g., being held in the hands of God, resting in the lap of Buddha). Others have said that they needed to change certain words (e.g., if they associate their childhood "home" with trauma, or if they are worried about a "heart" ailment). I encourage their improvisations. Again, these illustrate the power of the process over the procedure, as well as the precious sense of internal navigation into which each individual can tap.

In the process of relaxing, many individuals experience plateaus and minor muscle tremors, especially in the small muscles around the eyes and mouth. Such twitchings are natural, as are the plateaus (periods when there is no apparent deepening of relaxation). Such episodes are to be honored and incorporated into the overall process. The individual should be encouraged to accept occasional episodes of tightening as natural and healthy expressions of their own self-protective tendencies. As these tendencies are more progressively trusted, the process itself is facilitated and deepened. To the extent that the counselor is willing to explore such trust in the living moment of being with a client, the client is more likely to pursue that same exploration. As one of my teachers once remarked, much of what we teach in psychotherapy is neither explicit nor technical so much as it is an "induction" of an experiential process.

Relaxation and centering are fundamental skills in emotional regulation. They warrant regular practice. Recall my repeated discussion of the essential tension between old and new ways of experiencing. The old ways are familiar, and they feel safe and stabilizing. The new ways are unusual and may feel risky and destabilizing. Both are necessary for healthy development. When new experiences destabilize one's system, it is valuable to have skills in restabilizing and returning to a sense of safety and security. The more often one practices and refines such exercises, the more confident one feels in risking excursions toward the edges of unfamiliar experiencing. Although relaxation and centering skills are often thought of in terms of preparing clients for coping with stresses outside the consulting room, they can also be used as a form of "entry meditation" at the beginning of therapeutic sessions. I find it useful with many clients, and particularly with those who have trouble getting focused on therapeutic work. The first time I remember using it in this manner was with a client I had been seeing for more than 4 months. More than half of every session had been consumed by "small talk" and "continuing complaints"—the traffic, the weather, world news, her in-laws' insensitivities, and the changing demands of her work. When we did get down what she was feeling, it was usually with little time left in the session. Several times, she seemed to move toward a "transformative edge," an experiential cliff that signaled a different level of focus and processing. But time became the usual excuse for not getting too close to that edge, and—to be honest—there was a part of me that was glad we kept running out of time before she got there.

Then, one session, I decided to suggest that we open the session with an "entry meditation" that would help both of us settle into where we were and what we were about, and to let go of other distracting details. She agreed, and I invited her to close her eyes. Like so many other clients I had observed, her eyelids flickered with the effort to stay closed, and her face showed that this was not an easy experience for her. I said something like "I will close my eyes as well [which I did], and we can each relax into the privacy of our own interiors. Breathing deeply and honoring the multiple activities that are going on inside us." As I allowed myself to relax, I invited her to do likewise: "to let go of my needs to understand . . . to relax my needs to control what is going on inside me . . . even to relax my need to relax. Simply coming home inside myself, relaxing into a sense of safety and center, relaxing into being myself just the way I am in this moment."

The purpose of a centering meditation is to seek or return to a sense of center and safety, and to experience from that sense. When used with a client, it is both an act of entering into our special kind of relationship and a means of encouraging each of us to find a current sense of center from which to engage one another. In some clients, the exercise itself may take 10–15 minutes or more (e.g., my audiotape version is 23 minutes), and I try to gauge its future length by clients' past comments on its helpfulness. For clients who tend toward the end of the spectrum emphasizing needs for comfort, this may well be the most important part of the session. This, I believe, should be deeply respected. The entry and centering exercise can be substantially condensed to only a few minutes for clients who learn centering and presence more quickly—or who feel that there is more value in devoting session time to other activities.

FINDING STABILITY IN RELATIONSHIPS, PLACES, AND PATTERNS

The main purpose of centering exercises is to help recover a sense of meaningful order. This is equivalent metaphorically to "getting a grip," having something or someone to hold on to, or coming back to a safe base. Some of the common synonyms for stabilizing or balancing are worth noting: steadying, anchoring, mooring, grounding, settling, rooting, fastening, assuring, leveling, collecting, adjusting, aligning, securing, and harmonizing. Different clients will be drawn to different words and metaphors. The underlying processes are related, however.

The previous exercises have emphasized breathing, bodily balance, and a symbolic "coming home" meditation. Even with all its limitations and imperfections, the concept of "home" usually has safe and supportive connotations. I remember paraphrasing a line from Robert Frost when I once said to my mother, "Home is where, when you go there, they love to take you in." Frost had said "have to." And what are the most stabilizing aspects of an ideal home? I believe there are at least three: relationships (particularly people and pets), familiar and significant places (a porch, a chair, a room, a tree, etc.), and familiar patterns (daily routines, regular cycles of sounds, etc.). These can be important sources of stability throughout life and far away from home.

Relationships are a significant source of emotional and psychological stability throughout the lifespan. This was the primary emphasis of my overview of constructive practice in Chapter 2. Many people are fortunate enough to have felt loved by someone (perhaps many people) early in their life. But even individuals who did not experience consistent childhood love manage to discover and develop relationships that become important sources of support for them.[4] And pets, bless their hearts, are often precious participants in healing relationships. My point here is that it is important to learn what resources a client has in terms of supportive relationships. Some may say that they don't have "a friend in the world," and many clients report that they have entered counseling because they just can't talk to the people in their lives. As professional helpers, we are often asked to be a keeper of their secrets. But it is important that they learn to find stability and support in other relationships as well. This can be done in many ways, some of which are illustrated in other chapters. Community groups, churches, libraries, and clubs all provide opportunities to be around other people, which can be calming and stabilizing in itself. The Internet is also a rich source of potential connections. All of these require exploratory ventures on the part of the client, of course (Chapters 5–9), and explorations are easier when one already feels securely based.

Another source of relationship that deserves emphasis is the written word. I talk (write) about the power of writing one's own words in Chapter 6. What I wish to emphasize here is the use of reading as an exercise in centering. Once again, the content may be as diverse as the people we counsel. Mysteries and science fiction are sources of relaxation for many. Self-help books can help.[5] Personal accounts of coping are plentiful and often strike a resonant cord with readers who are struggling with similar challenges. Spiritual and inspirational books are consistently among the most popular.[6] Poetry can touch a reader in powerful ways. And a tangible book can become symbolic of something to hold on to in an act of self-care.

Places can also be sources of psychological stability. Familiar buildings or landmarks are examples. I sometimes explain this in terms of the common habit of welcoming the sight of the familiar when one has been away from it for some time. For persons in the throes of felt chaos in their life, it can be helpful for them to notice the familiar and consciously enjoy its stability. The specifics of the place are again less important than the meaning it can represent. It might be a large tree, a public building, or the view out a particular window. It might also be a durable object. I have given some clients small, smooth rocks that are meant to represent endurance and to symbolize my faith in their own durability. Some people find it helpful to designate a particular place as their own (e.g., a park bench, a table at a restaurant). They may also identify their home or their room as their base. With regard to the latter, however, I sometimes need to remind them that the function of a base is as a place to come from and go to. If one seldom leaves it, its function is compromised.

Finally, patterns or routines can be valuable sources of a sense of order. When I am working with clients who feel that they have lost their balance in a psychological sense, I often ask them to describe their daily and weekly routines in great detail. Sometimes I also ask them to sketch informally their living quarters. Their responses to my requests give me a better idea of the degree of structure or order in their lives. There are, of course, a range of individual differences. Many individuals are unaware of having developed mundane routines (e.g., which side of the bed they sleep on, the sequence of their first acts upon awakening, which chair they sit in at a table or in a living room).

Although I am asking them for details, my primary interest is in their overall pattern of changing and unchanging activities. An awareness of that pattern may be very important in later phases of our work together, when explorations of novelty are our focus. If individuals seem to be unaware of what they do regularly, I may ask them to pay attention to their activities and write them down. For some clients, I may also recommend at least a temporary increase in the regularity with which they do things (e.g., awakening and going to bed, meals, and movement routines). I may also suggest that they introduce new rituals into their daily routine. If they are leading a supercharged lifestyle, the ritual may be to pause breathe or release breathe once an hour. If clients are feeling overwhelmed by sudden changes, I may recommend that they clean or organize something familiar (their closet, garage, silverware drawer, etc.). The sense of agency and order that comes from this is often calming. I also encourage clients to discover and use music as a means of centering. Music can evoke strong emotional reactions, and I inquire about musical preferences and their felt meanings. Listening to the same piece of music can be equivalent to a lullaby or soothing sounds, and it can become part of a daily ritual of self-care.

The most important part of developing a new habit is consistency. This was noted by William James more than a century ago, and it now has substantial scientific evidence behind it. In the early stages of developing a new pattern, it is valuable to practice it regularly. If an occasion is missed, or if a mistake is made, it is important to return to the desired pattern as quickly as possible. I am suggesting not perfectionism but commitment to consistency. Such consistency is often aided by cues that serve as reminders. Persons who are trying to slow down and reduce their stress, for example, may benefit from gentle reminders. These can take almost any form: a special attachment on their key chain, a note in their wallet, a small bell hanging from their rearview mirror, and so on. I often encourage clients to purchase something for themselves (including jewelry) that will serve as a reminder to practice a new pattern. Small items kept in a pocket can also work (e.g., a "worry stone," prayer beads, a special coin).

Daily events can also be given new meanings as reminders. A stop sign or traffic signal can, with practice, become a reminder to pause, to take a deep breath, or to note what one has been thinking. A radio or television commercial can be designated as a cue to stretch. Other frequent sights and sounds can be similarly redefined. The problem with such reminders is that they often work for a limited amount of time. Most of us have had the experience of placing a reminder on the refrigerator, on a desk, or near a doorknob. It works well when it is new. But when the novelty fades, so does the salience of its message. This is where an ongoing creativity is required.

But beyond the cleverness required by coming up with ever-novel reminders, it is often useful to establish a daily routine or ritual that is associated with something that does not change. Examples include practicing meditation or prayer the first thing in the morning, using sunset or bedtime as a signal for a comforting contemplation, noting the changing phases of the moon and its regularity in repeating those phases, and so on.

NOTES

1. Gergen (2000); Hoyt (1998); Leitner and Faidley (1999); Lyddon (1993); Ronen (1997, 2003); Rosenbaum (1990, 1998).
2. Emmett (1998).
3. Haruki, Homma, Umezawa, and Masaoka (2001).
4. Lewis (1997); Mahoney (1991); Snyder (1999).
5. Norcross et al. (2003).
6. Buber (1958); Camus (1955); Carlin (1997); Chödrön (1997); Huxley (1944); Kapleau (1980); Kazantzakis (1960); Kornfield (1993, 2000); Lash (1990); Leder (1997); Leonard and Murphy (1995); Lesser (1999); Levine (1979); Merton (1968); Miller (1999); Muller (1992); Nepo (2000); Norris (1998); O'Donahue (1997, 1998); Pargament (1997); Ram Dass (1970, 1971); Russell (1992); Steindl-Rast (1983, 1984); Walsh (1999); Watts (1966).

CHAPTER 5

PROBLEM SOLVING

Basic Behavioral and Cognitive Techniques

All change is relative to something that is not changing, and this is why I have emphasized the refinement of stabilizing skills prior to experiments in change. But change is what the majority of clients are seeking, and psychotherapists are presumed to be specialists in fostering change. This chapter begins with a discussion of basic problem-solving skills. I believe personal problems are felt discrepancies. They are, in other words, contrasts: the way things are is felt to be in conflict with the way they should be. There are two kinds of solutions to problems: Change the way things are or change what you need them to be. My discussion of basic problem solving focuses here on changing the way things are. This was the essence of early behavioral approaches. The early cognitive therapies emphasized changing one's perceptions of things or expectations about how they should be. This is dealt with under the heading of cognitive restructuring. Cognitive and behavioral strategies are now commonly combined and are often helpful in personal change projects. Indeed, from a constructive perspective, it is hard to imagine any form of human development that does not include cognitive, behavioral, and emotional components. But not all change is as simple and straightforward as a planned intervention with a single strategy. Much change emerges from trial-and-error activity. This is what a constructive view would predict. Because we are dynamic, open systems that are continually reorganizing, new patterns develop out of exploratory ventures. This will be the emphasis in the technical exercises I discuss in Chapter 6.

PROBLEM SOLVING

Because many clients enter psychotherapy with a specific problem in mind, it is not surprising that they often want help with problem solving. The problem with problem solving is that it is such a broad categorization. Most self-help or self-improvement books are directed at specific personal problems rather than at the overall process of solving problems. There are some exceptions, however, and these tend to share a common core that expresses the heart of scientific experimentation. Albert Einstein used to say that science is nothing more than a refinement of everyday thinking, and the refinements are generally what make problem solving systematic rather than haphazard. In George Kelly's personal construct psychology, the similarities between science and everyday life were also emphasized. For Kelly and other constructivists, people are embodied theories that constantly generate and test hypotheses. Much of the inflexibility associated with personal problems may stem from a failure to realize this. A professional counselor can serve as an expert consultant on the process of being a personal scientist.

Problem-solving skills involve capacities to make careful observations, to generate ideas, and to conduct experiments. In my own early efforts to organize the essence of problem-solving skills, I used the acronym SCIENCE such that each letter of the word represented a different phase and skill in the problem-solving process[1]:

S Specify the problem
C Collect information
I Identify possible causes
E Examine possible solutions
N Narrow solutions and experiment
C Compare your progress
E Extend, revise, or replace your solution

Specifying the problem is a way of delimiting what one is tackling. For individuals who are drawn to concrete issues and particulars, identifying the problem is a large part of the solution.

Without getting sidetracked by abstractions, it is important to recognize that misidentifying the problem can also create or intensify difficulties. A common example of this occurs in relationship counseling. It takes the form of a total externalizing of the source of difficulty: "The problem is my spouse." A relationship is a dynamic and developing pattern. It is more than the sum of two isolated elements, one of which is bad. (The inverse of total externalization is total internalization, in which the client feels solely responsible for the difficulty.) Each individual makes unique contributions to the shared burdens and blessings. The problem, I believe, is always a felt sense of discord or discrepancy. It is never completely "out there" (in another person, a job, or a situation).[2]

Assuming that a problem has been accurately identified, the next phase is the collection of information on it. Here, again, there are two kinds of clients in the world: those who like to count things and those who don't. The latter are "no accounts." Quantification is a valuable method of organizing experience. The power of numbers was recognized long before the Scientific Revolution, and since then, the relationship between science and mathematics has been extremely strong. The challenge, of course, is to find equal units that are meaningful and relevant. In early studies of self-regulation, people were asked to count anything that seemed important to the problem they were addressing: calories, thoughts, cigarettes, impulses, and all manner of behavioral acts. The act of simply observing and recording one's own experience is itself influential. Much like the Heisenberg principle in physics, the process of measurement influences the phenomenon being measured. Some problems are more easily divided into countable units than others, but this difficulty can be surmounted by using a rating scale. Thus, if a client's identified problem is qualitative (such as mood, well-being, or quality of sleep), he or she can rate it on a convenient scale at regular intervals. In my experience, clients prefer 1–10 or 0–100 scales that are anchored with dichotomies (much like what is presented in the Personal Experience Report, Appendix C).

Whether a target behavior is being counted or a quality is being rated, this process provides an important reference point for evaluating subsequent change. On their own and in collaboration with me, clients can begin to identify the possible causes of their problem and potential solutions. In considering the latter, it is important that they be encouraged to brainstorm creatively. This often means coming up with some solutions that are impossible, impractical, or unfeasible. The opening to creative novelty is key here, and it requires a temporary suspension of critical foreclosure. Once a number of options have been generated, the list can be narrowed to candidates for experimental testing. In formal scientific research, the testing phase has meant isolating the experimental factor (called the "independent variable"), so that its effects can be confidently estimated. The need to isolate causes is less pressing in personal domains; therefore, I encourage clients to experiment with as many as two or three combined strategies at once. It is important that they consistently apply these changes, however.

In evaluating the effects of a personal experiment, the careful record keeping becomes important. Without such records, evaluation becomes very imprecise. Consider one of the most commonly asked questions in psychotherapy: "How was your week?" Although most clients believe they are reporting an overall rating, their responses are likely to be most strongly influenced by their present mood and their most recent emotional experiences. This is why rating scales and daily notes (including personal journaling) can be such important components in evaluations of both process and progress. After giving a solution a reasonable period of time, clients can compare the frequency or quality of their problem before and after the experimental intervention. If the new pattern is helping, they continue to use it. If it offers partial relief, they can revise it or add another of their optional strategies. If it is not helpful, it is time to go back to the drawing board and consider other possible solutions.

Recall my suggestion that there are two kinds of solutions to a specific problem: Change the way things are, or change the way you expect (or interpret) them to be. Behavioral methods have generally focused on changing the environment, and cognitive methods have focused on changing our interpretations of events.

THE ESSENCE OF BEHAVIORAL METHODS

My early training was in behavior modification and cognitive therapy. Cognitive-behavioral methods are now among the most extensively researched forms of psychotherapy, and it is clear that they are helpful to many individuals with a variety of personal problems. Most therapists are likely to be familiar with these methods, and there is an abundance of good resources on their practice and effects.[3] What merits emphasis here are their basic practical strategies. Because cognitive and behavioral therapies are now well integrated, my separation of them is simply for ease of presentation.

The first principle of constructivism notes the importance of activity in human experiencing, and activity lies at the heart of behaviorism. B. F. Skinner liked to emphasize the importance of a "motivated organism." Motivation is inferred from movement, and teaching is fundamentally a process of developing, maintaining, and changing movement patterns. I believe the most important practical messages of the behavioral tradition are the following:

1. Activity is important.
2. Behavior takes place in an environment.
3. Consequences matter.
4. Small steps are important.
5. Practice begets consistency.

These are crudely abbreviated, of course, but they contain precious crystals. The importance of activity has already been addressed as a central tenet of constructivism. The statement that behavior takes place in an environment helps remind me of the power of "stimulus control" and the intentional engineering of life circumstances. In an evolutionary sense, we have not only adapted ourselves to our environments, but have also adapted our environments to suit our needs and preferences. I often ask clients about their living circumstances, and I am particularly interested in how they are influencing the environment that influences them. No one has total control over the medium in which they exist, but many of us exercise only a small portion of the options we do have. We can make and break habits more easily, for example, by anticipating choice points at which we are likely to face competing alternatives. A little foresight in "stacking the deck" can make a large difference in how that competition plays out.

There is everyday, practical importance in recognizing that our activity patterns are sensitive to our stimulus conditions. I sometimes illustrate this with clients by asking them to look at the salient cues in their daily paths of movement. If an individual is trying to diet or to eat healthier foods, for example, I ask her what kinds of food are most visible in her refrigerator or supply shelves. When tempting foods are salient and easily accessible, they are more likely to be consumed. This illustration can be extended to the process of grocery shopping. Both quantity and quality of food purchases are influenced by the shopper's current hunger (particularly blood sugar levels). The internal cues are powerful. One can change those cues by eating a high protein snack 15–30 minutes before grocery shopping. There are, of course, many other ways of arranging one's environments to encourage desired patterns.

I do not lecture clients on the differences and similarities between classical conditioning (sometimes called respondent or Pavlovian) and operant conditioning (also known as instrumental or Skinnerian). What I try to emphasize is that we are biologically wired to make associations and that we are often unaware of that process. An everyday illustration is that we often find ourselves remembering an experience associated with a particular physical location. In the commute to and from work, for example, the sight of a particular building or billboard may remind us of a thought we had at that same location on some previous viewing. We may not have been aware that we had linked the two (our internal experience and a specific location). We often use our tacit awareness of such connections to prompt our memory. A common mnemonic strategy is to use physical location as a memory aid. Suppose one thought of something he needed to do, and this thought occurred while he was in the kitchen. Minutes later, he may have forgotten the task he had set for himself. He might find himself in another room, with a felt sense that he had an idea moments earlier but has now forgotten it. One of the most reliable ways of "re-minding" ourselves of what it was is to go back to the physical location in which the idea first occurred. (Note that "re-membering" literally means to reconnect a missing member.) The relatively unconscious power of association has important bearing on many of our everyday activity patterns. We develop strong emotional associations to pieces of music, for example. I suggest ways of tapping this resource in a later discussion of life review techniques. For the moment, however, it is worth noting that we are stimulating ourselves whenever we choose to listen to a particular kind of music. Indeed, we are stimulating ourselves all the time, and this is also one of the central messages of the cognitive therapies.

The next essential message from behaviorism is that consequences matter. This also has important practical implications. Our actions produce consequences, and these consequences influence the direction of our future activities. Pleasure and pain are not all there is to life, but we are life forms with a fine-tuned sensitivity to this dimension. Reward is associated with pleasure, and pleasure beckons movement or continuing engagement. Reward communicates encouragement and is informative in a positive sense (it tells us what to do). Punishment is often associated with pain, and pain signals what *not* to do. It is informative in a negative sense. Reward and punishment are not mirror images of the same process, however. In teaching, parenting, and relating to others in general, the overall ratio should greatly favor the positive (reward, pleasure) over the negative (punishment, pain). This very simple strategy is often overlooked or unexercised, however. As is apparent in contexts ranging from traffic jams to divorce court, negativity is too often met with escalations of negativity.

I am reminded here of a humorous example of misunderstanding behavioral principles and their application. A mother consulted a would-be behavior therapist for advice on what to do about her two young sons' frequent swearing behavior.

> The behavior therapist began his therapeutic program with a brief synopsis of two learning principles. "First," he said, "it is important that you use immediate and severe punishment each and every time the swearing behavior occurs. Second, you can maximize the impact of your punishment by making sure that both children are present whenever one of them is punished. This is called 'vicarious learning'; the second child will learn from example." Enthusiastic over this refreshingly straightforward recommendation, the mother returned home to implement her newly acquired knowledge. At breakfast the next morning, she sat down, ready and raring to modify behavior. The older son opened the day with the request that she "pass the fucking Cheerios." With lightning fury, the mother lunged across the table, hit her son, and sent both the boy and two chairs sprawling to the floor. The younger son helped her replace the furniture and the two of them sat back down. Pleased with her skillful execution of modern learning theory, she turned to her second breakfast partner and said, "Well, what will *you* have?" With ample indication that he had learned something from the preceding slaughter, he sagely remarked, "You can bet your sweet ass it isn't Cheerios!"[4]

As cognitive therapists emphasize, the perception of contingencies is often more powerful than the contingencies themselves.

Actions have consequences. This is another basic message of behaviorism (as well as Buddhism, where this connection is called "karma"). Some of those consequences are predictable, and some become apparent only historically. The delay between actions and consequences is, in fact, an important source of many struggles for self-control. Bad habits are often behaviors that have immediately pleasant effects but ultimately painful consequences (e.g., addictions, compulsions, impulsive reactions). On the flip side are behaviors that may involve short-term pain (or effort) and long-term benefits (e.g., exercise, study, investment). Figure 5.1 depicts these two patterns in what is termed the "reversing consequences gradient." Part of what is involved in behavioral self-regulation is a balancing of the dimension of time, so that ultimate consequences are made more salient in the present. Once again, an emphasis on ultimate rewards is more effective than the threat of eventual punishment.

The importance of small steps in skills development is also something that behavioral methods emphasize. This is illustrated in the procedure of "successive approximation," also known as shaping. Having recently acquired a darling puppy named Babe, I have been reminded of how small those steps may need to be. I have been teaching her to ask to go outside. This has meant paying close attention to patterns in her behavior. After drinking water or eating, for example, she is likely to be "inspired" to eliminate. At first, I regularly took her outdoors immediately after feeding. Each time I took her out, I paired our actions with an enthusiastic pronunciation of the word "outside." Gradually, I increased the amount of time I delayed this trip after she had eaten. I wanted to start shifting the initiative to her. I began by catching her in the act of anticipating my moves. She

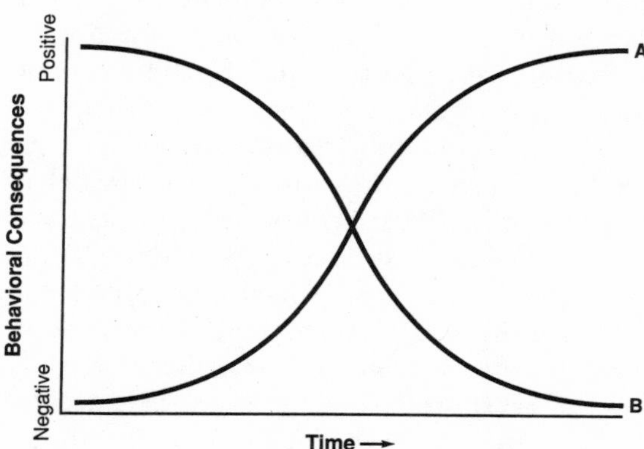

FIGURE 5.1. Positive and negative consequences often reverse over the course of time. Copyright 1989 by Michael J. Mahoney.

would look at me and look toward the door. I would quickly pair her look with an enthusiastic question and praise: "Outside? Good dog!" Gradually, I gave her more and more responsibility for initiating the request. I also hung a Christmas bell on a string near the door, so that it jingled whenever she walked past it or the door was opened. Then, I devoted some of our play time to teaching her to ring the bell. Now, a few weeks later, she nudges the bell with her nose to get my attention and then we venture outside.

As Humberto Maturana emphasizes, the signaling that goes on between Babe and me is a kind of languaging. We have learned some of each other's patterns, and we act accordingly. (The sound of an open refrigerator door has recently begun to pique her interest; clever dog). When the communication is between humans, our symbolic processes allow even subtler and more efficient transmissions. Albert Bandura's work on vicarious learning has shown that we develop many patterns of action by first observing them being performed by others. For better and for worse, our children tend to do what we do more often than they do what we say. In his investigations of self-efficacy, Bandura has also shown that small steps and performance aids are extremely valuable components of personal change projects.[5] The emphasis in these projects is on starting where you are and making small, regular excursions toward the current edges of your capacities. For someone rehabilitating from a stroke or an accident, these excursions may be miniscule, yet each step is an important bridge in building a pattern.

The final message emphasized in the behavioral tradition has been about the importance of consistency. Patterns become patterns because of regularity. I mentioned in Chapter 4 William James's advice about consistency in the early stages of habit development. One can think of this in terms of momentum or developing a groove in ongoing activity. Consistency also contributes to the experiencing of patterns and a sense of structure. Structure is the root of constructivism. Even though early behaviorists were not fond of talking about anticipation, this is a large part of what consistency permits. In the early phases of teaching a new behavior in animals, consistent reinforcement is critical. At first, the consistency must be focused on the initial elements of the desired response. Gradually, the standards of acceptability are increased. Once the behavior is learned, a different level of consistency is optimal. Instead of every response earning a reward, it may take several responses. Interestingly, this was discovered by accident when B. F. Skinner ran low on rat pellets one weekend. He decided to stretch out his supplies by rewarding every other response rather than every response. To his surprise, the rats began responding at higher rates. Thus began the now-extensive investigation of schedules of reinforcement. Intermittent reinforcement leads to higher rates of activity. This phenomenon is what makes gambling such a profitable business. An occasional small win will encourage continuation of the gambling behavior. When I see a noisy room full of people playing slot machines, I cannot help but remember the pigeon and rat laboratories where I first studied reinforcement contingencies.

COGNITIVE RESTRUCTURING

Skinner pioneered studies of superstitious behavior in pigeons, but we humans are notorious for our capacities to perceive connections where none exist. We are also, by the way, good at overlooking connections that later become obvious. This is the area in which research on cognition has made valuable contributions in understanding how we participate in our own experiencing. I believe the most important messages in the cognitive therapies are that

1. We live much of our lives in and from our heads.
2. Thinking influences feeling and acting.
3. Self-talk is an important domain for awareness and change.

The message about life in and from the head is one that bears emphasis. I believe a constructive approach to life and psychotherapy encourages balance among the domains of mind, body, and spirit. As I elaborate later, this quest for balance often encounters formidable challenges in changing minds and mental patterns.

Cognitive methods for influencing emotions are hardly new. In a scholarly analysis of ancient Greek and early Christian approaches, Richard Sorabji has shown that many of the methods used by modern therapists have their roots in exercises recommended by the likes of Pythagoras, Socrates, Plato, Epictetus, Epicurus, Zeno and the Stoics, and Augustine.[6] These exercises encourage the formation and strengthening of patterns of thinking and imagery. The patterns being formed are intended to compete with or replace patterns that are associated with distress, emotional imbalance, and inappropriate action. As a student and teacher of the history of ideas, I find it interesting that 20th-century cognitive therapists have followed similar lines. In his development of rational–emotive therapy, for example, Albert Ellis noticed that many of his clients contributed to their own suffering through their "stinking thinking" patterns.[7] These patterns often reflected some core beliefs that were unrealistic or irrational (e.g., that one *must* be loved by everyone, that one *must* have perfect control over things, that a failed performance *must* mean failure as a person, etc.). The frequency of the imperative "must" in these beliefs led Ellis to call them "must-erbation," which he discourages.[8]

Aaron T. Beck developed his early ideas about cognitive therapy while studying dream processes in depressed individuals.[9] In interviews with these people, he also noted that they tended toward a "negative triad": negative self, negative world, and negative future. As later studies have extensively shown, perceptual and cognitive distortions are common in many different patterns of psychological disorder (e.g., anxiety, eating disorders, obsessive–compulsive activity). Distressed individuals tend to be selective in what they notice and remember, and they also tend toward generalizations that fuel distress. The essence of cognitive methods for relieving such distress involves a recognition that the thought is not the same as the thing. Echoing the famous phrase of the Stoic Epictetus, we are not disturbed by things, but by our view of things. The therapeutic formula is stated simply by Beck: "The therapist helps the patient to identify his warped thinking and to learn more realistic ways to formulate his experiences."[10] How does the therapist do this?

> First, [the patient] has to become aware of what he is thinking. Second, he needs to recognize what thoughts are awry. Then he has to substitute accurate for inaccurate judgments. Finally, he needs feedback to inform him whether his changes are correct. The same kind of sequence is necessary for making behavioral changes.[11]

There is a step prior to awareness of thinking, however, and this is the awareness of a felt sense of discomfort or distress. This is where I believe the experiential therapies add valuable components. To summarize the practical stages in teaching cognitive restructuring to clients, I often list them as follows[12]:

1. Pay attention to what you are feeling, especially when it seems to be changing (toward either better or worse).
2. In that moment, focus on your most recent thoughts and images. (What have you been thinking about or imagining?)
3. Evaluate the merits and direction of your train of thought or imagery (e.g., Does it make sense? Where is it leading? What does it mean? What are you are anticipating? Would you wish that kind of thinking on someone you love?).
4. If you don't like what you are feeling (or the direction your mood is moving): Can you imagine counterarguments to your thinking? Can you think of alternative interpretations of your situation? What action might you take to shift your attention and redirect your stream of feeling? What are your options?

Sorabji suggests that the cognitive therapies, like their Stoic predecessors, are most useful for the reinterpretation of situational reactions.[13] This means that they are probably valuable for changing the meaning assigned to specific events (e.g., the loss of a job or relationship, the portent of somatic sensations).

I believe training in introspection is also a helpful adjunct to cognitive methods. In order to change self-talk and automatic imagery, it is helpful first to be tuned in to their occurrence. Many contemplative methods have been developed across cultures and spiritual wisdom traditions. A brief summary of mindfulness meditation is offered in Chapter 7 and Appendix G. There is recent evidence that such meditation may add to the benefits of cognitive therapies, particularly in terms of long-term effectiveness and avoidance of relapse.[14]

Cognitive methods generally presume that individuals are aware of their self-talk and that this is the most accessible dimension for an attempted change. Not all clients respond well to a cognitive focus, however. I was once asked to consult with a man named Ira who was severely depressed over the loss of his job as an auto mechanic. Ira came from a very traditional background in which the husband was the "breadwinner," as he termed it, and the wife stayed at home and raised their children. When Ira suddenly found himself without a job, he experienced a reactive depression. He felt ashamed and suicidal. Not wanting his working-class neighbors to know his plight, Ira would not leave the house during the work day. His wife offered to seek employment for herself, but that only added to Ira's sense of worthlessness. After establishing some rapport and a "life engagement" (nonsuicide) contract, I focused on Ira's interpretation of his situation. He was a very skilled mechanic, and his job loss had been due to company "downsizing" rather than something he had done wrong. I used a straightforward cognitive approach, inviting Ira to review his thinking and to challenge his self-diminishing interpretations of being laid off.

Ira did not respond well to this focus on his thinking. He seemed to have trouble detaching himself from the contents and emotional correlates of his thoughts. When I used Socratic method to lead his thinking in a less negative direction, he experienced difficulty seeing any other possible interpretations. He then interpreted his difficulties as signs that he had a bad mind or was stupid. After several sessions of trying to adjust my level of concreteness, we were still making no progress. I decided to move back to more behavioral basics. I gave him the assignment of leaving the house at least twice a day during regular work hours. It did not matter what he did on these excursions so long as he got out. He usually ran errands or just drove around for a few minutes. On one of these excursions, however, he saw a notice on a bulletin board for a basic course in auto repair at a local community college. In his state of depression, Ira feared that he had forgotten all he knew about automobiles. When he asked my opinion about whether he should take the course, I encouraged him to enroll. I sensed that it was at least a venture in the direction of life engagement. A serendipitous event turned the tide on Ira's low self-confidence.

The course instructor had demonstrated how to take apart and rebuild a carburetor. However, the instructor couldn't get the engine to run after his demonstration. Ira made a timid suggestion and the instructor invited him to try it. Ira quickly had the engine running again. The instructor's failed demonstration turned out to be an opportunity for Ira to gain confidence in himself. He took several other courses over the next few months and ended up finding work in an auto parts store. Neither of us could have anticipated or predicted that this would be the result of the simple assignment that he get out of the house twice a day.

Ira's initial failure to respond to cognitive therapy may have been due to many factors. I believe that it illustrates the importance of remaining flexible and sensitively attuned to what is (and is not) working for a client. It also reminded me of how easily we therapists can get into patterns of using the same techniques almost mechanically. Vittorio Guidano liked to tell a joke about a man who went to see a rather mechanical cognitive therapist. The man's problem was that he believed that he was a mouse. Using what was meant to be a Socratic method, the therapist asked the man how many legs a mouse has.

"Four," the man said.

"And how many legs do you have?"

"Two," the man said.

"And a mouse—where does it have hair?" asked the therapist.

"All over its body," said the man.

"Do you have hair all over your body?"

"No," said the man.

"Do mice have a tail?"

"Yes."

"Do you have a tail?"

"No."

"You see!" the therapist exclaimed. "It is absurd to think you are a mouse! Just look at the evidence!"

The man, taken aback by the strength of the therapist's statement, said, "But, doctor, what if I still *feel* like a mouse?"

"Well, it is very simple. When you find yourself feeling like a mouse, just stop yourself and correct your thinking. Let's practice it right here in the office. Say to yourself 'a mouse has four legs and I have two. . . . A mouse has hair all over its body and I don't. A mouse has a tail and I do not. I am a *man, not a mouse*! *I am a man, not a mouse*!' "

They rehearsed this sequence several times and the man began to feel more confident. He shook the therapist's hand and thanked him for his help. The therapist sat down at his desk, and the man walked to the door to leave. Just before closing the door behind him, however, the client opened it and timidly said, "Doctor, thank you. Thank you. Can I possibly just ask one more small question before I go?"

The self-satisfied therapist said, "Sure, what is it?"

And the man said quietly, "Well, doctor . . . um . . . the cats . . . do the cats know that I am not a mouse?"

WHEN PROBLEM SOLVING DOESN'T WORK

Let me now offer a few final words about problem solving. Sometimes *that* problem wasn't *the* problem. I recall working with a woman who had struggled with agoraphobia and panic. After patiently developing her skills in recovering her sense of center, she set off to test herself against a formidable challenge. She survived the challenge, and I thought she had handled her distress extremely well. However, she was very upset by the paradox that presented itself. I remember her saying to me, "That wasn't *it*." When I asked for clarification about the "it," she said that her panic was about not surviving. Because she had in fact survived, she concluded that she must not have really faced her demon.

Another common occurrence is that sometimes the problem improves for a period of time and then returns to its previous level. Alternatively, sometimes solving one problem creates others. These are not uncommon patterns. I have also worked with a number of clients for whom problems played a central role in their life organization. I do not believe that they were insincere in their problem-solving efforts or that their distress was ingenuous. I recall one man who arrived at a session in a state of seeming confusion. He usually arrived with a particular dilemma to discuss, and he often expressed a sense of urgency about each week's dilemma. This particular week, however, the dilemma he had planned to discuss with me had suddenly resolved itself just a few hours before our session. We were both struck by his sense of feeling lost, and I remember his saying, "I don't know what to do without a problem. What does that mean about my life?" We spent several productive sessions exploring that question.

The foregoing example also illustrates the relevance of "solution-focused" expressions of constructive psychotherapy.[15] These are approaches that emphasize the client's resourcefulness and the potential benefits of looking at the positive side of adaptation. Rather than focus on what is wrong with clients or their lives, such an approach emphasizes and explores how they have managed to cope, what they have done when there were exceptions to their problematic pattern, and how they might reframe their constructions of possibilities. Alfred Adler's so-called "miracle question" is sometimes employed: "What would your life be like if a miracle occurred during your sleep and you woke up without your problem?" For the client I described above, this was not only inconceivable but intensely discomforting to imagine. His life had become organized around his problems, and his energies were crisis-driven. The solution for him required problems and crises for its coherence. In his case (and that of many others), the problem was not so much an obstacle to his well-being as the need for a problem from which to orient and organize his actions.

Finally, it is worth remembering that problems exist at different levels than do solutions. Problems motivate us to seek solutions, but the solutions emerge from processes that are much more abstract than the problems themselves. This point is made in several Asian wisdom traditions, and I recall Friedrich Hayek noting it in his reflections on spontaneous developments in open systems. Albert Einstein emphasized this when he said, "We will never be able to solve our problems at the same order of complexity we used to create our problems."[16] Problems are experiences (and patterns of experiencing) that do not fit with our assumptions or expectations. They are life's "misfits."

As noted in my earlier overview of constructive psychotherapy, I sometimes organize my own approach to therapy in terms of three overlapping levels of focus: problems, patterns, and processes. Problems are the most common things that clients want to address. But problems rarely exist in simple isolation. More often, problems reflect habitual patterns of experiencing. These patterns are the results of ongoing processes that literally generate the order and meaning in our lives. Problems are often the things that knock us off balance or prevent us from feeling centered. This is why I emphasize centering skills throughout the course of therapy. Basic behavioral and cognitive strategies can also provide a sense of structure and agency for people struggling to recover their balance. For individuals whose distress or dysfunction has become a pattern, however, situational remedies may not be sufficient. It may be important for us to look at the patterns in their living (past and present). If they find themselves "stuck" in ruts of unsatisfactory being, explorations of alternatives may be their best options. Let us therefore turn our attention to some of my favorite methods for encouraging pattern recognition and exploring novel experiences.

NOTES

1. Mahoney (1979).
2. On this point, I differ with some therapists who recommend the general strategy of externalizing the problem (see Hoyt, 1998). This strategy may be useful for some clients at some developmental stages, but I question whether it always serves a useful function in the client's assumption of existential responsibilities.
3. Alford and Beck (1997); Aron and Aron (1987); Bandura (1969, 1986); Bandmaster (1991); A. T. Beck (1976); J. S. Beck (1995); Beck, Rush, Shaw, and Emery (1979); Caro (1997); Kazantzis, Deane, and Ronan (2000); Mahoney (1974, 1995a); Philippot and Rime (1998); Salkovskis (1996).
4. Mahoney, 1974, p. 164.
5. Bandura, 1969, 1977, 1986, 1997.

6. Sorabji (2000).
7. Ellis acknowledges his indebtedness to the Stoic and Epicurean traditions in philosophy, as well as to Karen Horney's ideas about the "tyranny of the shoulds." I recommend reading his account of how his approach developed.
8. Ellis does not discourage masturbation, however. In his book *Sex without Guilt*, he candidly recommended sexual indulgence as healthy. I once jokingly asked him if he had considered writing a book on guilt without sex. This led to reflections on cultural patterns of guilt. I maintain a bemused conversation with some Jewish friends about whether Jews or Catholics can claim the gold medal on guilt proneness. To date, we seem to agree that there is a stereotype that depicts Catholics as feeling bad when they feel good and Jews as feeling good when they feel bad.
9. A. T. Beck (1976).
10. A. T. Beck (1976, p. 20).
11. A. T. Beck (1976, p. 217).
12. For more elaborate practical methods, I recommend the manuals developed by Christine Padesky and her colleagues (Greenberger & Padesky, 1995; Padesky & Greenberger, 1995).
13. Sorabji (2000).
14. See particularly Segal, Williams, and Teasdale (2002).
15. De Shazer (1994); Hoyt (1998).
16. Quoted in Kegan and Lahey (2001, p. 5).

CHAPTER 6

PATTERN WORK

The problem with which a client presents is likely to be only part of the picture. There is often more than one problem, and these multiple areas of dissatisfaction may be complexly related. This is neither unusual nor unfortunate. The presenting problem may have been the proverbial straw that made the client's life burden too much. Seeking professional help is a healthy and self-caring response to feeling overwhelmed. And the fact that the primary problem is not the only one is simply a reflection of the fact that our lives as open systems are delicately balanced and intricately interwoven. As I elaborate in a later discussion of the personal experience of change, none of us can realistically hope to arrive at a level of development that is free of problems. Challenges are part of the fabric of life as an open system. The next problem is always in the mail. Fortunately, this is also true of the next solution and the next blessing. Difficulties become opportunities for development. Development creates new levels of difficulties, to be sure, but development also begets enlarged capacities for embracing the overall process.

A woman named Karen was instrumental in teaching me that a presenting problem is not necessarily *the* problem. She phoned me to inquire whether I would help her lose weight. Eating disorders had been something I had focused on early in my career, but I had grown dissatisfied with the oversimplifications of existing treatments. Calories may be a final common dimension of energy exchange, but I had learned that there was more to weight control than the physiology of metabolism. In my clients, I had encountered considerable complexity in personal and relationship factors that made it difficult for them to balance food intake and activity. When Karen contacted me, I explained that I was no longer specializing in weight problems. She said she understood and asked if I would see her for a single session, so that I could make an informed referral to a colleague. I agreed.

Karen arrived at my office at the appointed time. She was very personable and conveyed strength and confidence in her manner. We began by discussing her overall health and her history of failed attempts to diet. She had been moderately overweight all her life, but she reported a recent weight increase that had caused her concern. "All I want to do is lose 30 pounds and keep it off," she said. I asked, "And how would your life be different after you lose those 30 pounds?" To my surprise as well as hers, she began to cry. "I'm sorry," she said, wiping away tears. I waited, wondering what was going on inside her. "I'm just afraid that my life won't be any different even if I do lose the weight!" She explained that it was her husband who wanted her to lose the 30 pounds. He thought that she would feel more "romantic" if she were thinner. Besides being overweight, Karen said that she had been depressed all of her life. She had developed a public persona of being formidably strong and assertive, and she had never talked to anyone about depression. We scheduled another appointment. Karen's weight problem led us to explore her feelings about herself, and these were reflections of longstanding patterns. Our exploration of those patterns eventually led us into some very powerful process-level work, which I discuss later.

This chapter is focused on methods for examining patterns in personal experiencing. The essence of a pattern is a relational structure. Recall that the origin of the word pattern is *pater*, literally "the father" of that which has been created. We most often notice patterns by means of their repetitions, however. Individuals have the sense that they have been "here" before (dealing with a species of problem). Indeed, one of the sure signs that a client feels trapped in a particular pattern is the frequent use of the word "always" (e.g., "I always fall in love with the wrong people"). Another marker of interest in the pattern level of personal development is a puzzlement over causes (e.g., "Why did it have to be this way? How did I get so messed up? When did I start hating myself?"). Such questions are signals of quests for meaning. Indeed, the search for meaning and reconstructions of meanings are fundamental to pattern work.

In the trio of levels that I have proposed (problem, pattern, process), it is important to remember that all three exist simultaneously. A client may move through cycles of interest in a particular problem or pattern of problems. These cycles, as well as particular problems and patterns, are constantly being generated by self-organizing processes. One can think of pattern work in terms of the dance between experiencing and explaining (Chapter 2). Discovering patterns in one's life can be an important step toward self-awareness, and it can be instrumental in developing a greater sense of agency in determining future directions.[1] It would be a mistake to assume that pattern work is nothing but intellectual puzzle solving, however. The search itself is often motivated by strong emotions, and discoveries may bring waves of mixed feelings. Constructive therapy honors the waves and trusts the process of the developmental dance. This is seldom an easy task. One cannot know in advance what clients will find in their self-examination, and witnessing their intense emotions cannot help but touch a helper's heart.

PERSONAL JOURNALING AND BIBLIOTHERAPY

Individuals vary tremendously in their awareness of their inner life and the tonality of their self-relationships. I often find it helpful to ask my clients to make notes to themselves about things that feel important to them—not only their problems or their moments of distress but also thoughts, hopes, and questions that we might explore together. The structure and formality of their notes are not important, but many find it helpful to focus them into a private diary or personal journal. What is important is that they develop or refine their skills in paying attention to what is going on inside and around them. There is also something important about the process of attempting to communicate their experiences in words. The positive effects of writing and verbalizing about painful experiences is now well documented.[2] The power of language in human life has only begun to be appreciated. As Freud put it, "Words were originally magic and to this day words have retained much of their ancient magical power."[3] Words bring other worlds to us, and words express our own voice in these exchanges. We call out to the others worlds and the words that bring them to us, and sometimes—it seems—we may be heard. Walter Anderson reminds us that the Latin origins of the word "self" or "person" invokes the ancient *persona*, which is a combination of *per* ("for") and *sonare* ("sounding").[4] Besides being the "masks" that hide our true identities from our assumed roles, our "personae" thereby become the instruments of our voice—the means through which we make sound.

Although personal journaling may eventually lead toward the weaving of a life story, it usually begins as a daily ritual of self-reflection. Some clients are very reluctant to write. They may not know how to write, or they may be embarrassed about their spelling or their grammar. I try to work with each at their own level and pace.[5] What I want from them are expressions—doodlings, drawings, single words in the language of their own life experience. For clients who seek some degrees of structure for their personal journaling, there are some wonderful resources available, many of them products of the women's movement and feminist studies.[6] Two of my favorite resources are Christina Baldwin's *Life's Companion* and Tristine Rainer's *The New Diary.*[7] Rainer recommends specific techniques that include making lists (ranging from the familiar lists of things "to do" to written lists of fears, annoyances, and blessings). She also suggests writing character portraits and creating imaginary dialogues (e.g., among parts of the self or between oneself and a past or present loved one). Baldwin's book is a more explicitly spiritual guide to self-awareness and self-relationship, and she encourages the reader/writer to define "spirituality" in terms of a personal sense of what is sacred:

> The spiritual quest is that part of life which is the path within the path [p. 3]. . . . Consciousness is our life's companion, the company we keep inside ourselves. When we take up pilgrimage, consciousness emerges as an ongoing intimate dialogue within the self [p. 7]. . . . Writing bridges the inner and outer worlds and connects the paths of action and reflection. Writing is sorting. Writing down the stream of consciousness gives us a way to respect the mind, to choose among and harness thoughts, to interact with and change the contents of who we think we are. And that is what the spiritual journey is: a major change over time, in who we think we are, followed by a corresponding change in what we believe ourselves capable of doing [p. 9].

Baldwin has two rules for journal writing: (1) Date your entries as you go, and (2) don't make any other rules. I like her style and her emphases on guidance from the body, from dreams, from disorder, and from wonder. Besides the sacred art of paying attention, she encourages four major practices (love, forgiveness, trust, and acceptance).

For many clients, the process of reflecting and writing about their personal life is a more challenging task than they can initially accommodate. It is here that bibliotherapy—therapeutic reading—may help to bridge a gap. I have collected files of readings to share with clients—poetry, short stories, philosophical reflections, excerpts from writings in the spiritual or wisdom traditions. I sometimes recommend books—fiction, nonfiction, self-help.[8] I also ask what my clients have been reading and what they are drawn to in magazines, newspapers, on the Internet, and so on. They often feel that others have written passages that reflect aspects of their own experience, or they report seeking writings that touch on their personal concerns.

When clients do venture into writing about their own lives, it is often a very private excursion. I have seen many clients initially reluctant to write who then later exhibited giftedness in their expressions. Indeed I have had many clients—and I chuckle as I reflect on them—who became so prolific in their writings that I could not keep up with reading everything that they had written. In such cases, I have had to ask them to select the passages that they wanted me to read. In my clinical experience, it has not been unusual for clients to tell me that they have written things in their journal that they would not be comfortable letting me read. I respect their need for such privacy and emphasize that their writing and reflection are the most important parts of this exercise. At times, clients will bring one of these "secret" entries into a session and ask me if I would like to read it. It has been my experience that the content of the secret is often less important than their feelings and anticipations about my reaction to learning it. Again and again, our work comes back to experiential process, and our challenge is to engage authentically in that process to the best of our abilities. I occasionally ask clients to read selections from their journal to me while we are in session. This is often a powerful experience for them, perhaps because it is unexpected, and reading one's own words aloud—in the presence of a trusted other—adds significance to their meaning. Reading aloud may also bridge a metaphorical gap of privacy: They wrote their words in the privacy of their own space and I am now asking them to reexperience what they have written by literally giving voice to it.

Writing does not need to take the form of a personal journal in order to be therapeutic, however. I believe that almost any form of writing can be helpful. Poetry, letters, short stories, riddles, single lines of philosophical reflection, descriptions of everyday events—I invite my clients to experiment with writing and to share with me what they wish. One of my favorite structured assignments is that of the "unsent letters," which I discovered in Kopp[9] and is described in Rainer's book. It can be presented verbally to the client or given to them in written form, such as the following:

> The purpose of this exercise is to explore your own private psychological experience as you write three (3) versions of an "unsent letter"—that is, *letters that you will write but never actually send.* Begin by choosing someone in your life (still living or deceased) with whom you have shared an important relationship—it could be a parent, sibling, lover, grandparent, teacher, and so on. *Most important in choosing this "someone" is that there were things in your relationship with them that were left unsaid, unfinished, or unsatisfactorily resolved.*
>
> *Phase 1*: In a private, safe place, *handwrite* (do not type) *a letter to that person expressing your authentic and uncensored feelings* about them, about your relationship with them, and about incidents that were important to you. Be aware of your feelings as you write. Also be aware of any tendencies you may have to "take care of them" or otherwise "pull your punches." Remember that they will never read the letter, so do not hesitate to be as candid as you possibly can.
>
> *Phase 2*: Now shift your perspective and imagine that you are momentarily the person to whom you have written your unsent letter. Imagine that he or she has actually received it. *Write a letter from him or her to you that feels like the most likely response he or she would have rendered.* Would he or she have expressed anger, apology, guilt, indignation, resentment, sadness, surprise, tenderness? Let the letter flow as if he or she were actually writing it.

Phase 3: Once again, assume the role of the person to whom you wrote your unsent letter. Imagine again he or she has actually received your very candid letter. This time, in a safe and quiet place, *write a letter from him or her to you, but let it be written from his or her highest human qualities*—gentleness, compassion, openness, candor, wisdom, and so on. Let it be the letter you wish you could receive from him or her and, again, let it flow as if it were his or her hand and head and heart that were writing it.

These letters are often a very challenging assignment for clients. We frequently spend time discussing their reactions, their reluctance to write certain things, and the feelings that were evoked in the process. Some clients are more challenged by one of the letters than by the others, and they may be perplexed by this. Sometimes they need my help in writing one or more of the letters—most often the first and the third.

The difficulty of this assignment was apparent in my work with a 64-year-old bookkeeper named Luther. He had been in therapy several times over the course of his life. His most common diagnosis was depression, but he had also struggled with social anxiety, loneliness, and chronic health problems that included obesity, hypertension, colitis, and insomnia. Luther was very reserved emotionally. He had begun to show more expressiveness in his diary, however, and the unsent letter exercise accelerated his process of opening to some intense feelings. His first letter was written to his father:

Dear Father,

I know you have been dead many years, but still I want to say things to you. Even though I know you cannot do anything now, I fear that you will beat me for what I say. Perhaps you are in Hell. Maybe you can see me writing this and you will punish me. My hands are shaking and it is not because I am 64 years old. It is because I am still scared and angry!

That is how I always felt with you. You beat me so often, so bad. Do you remember? Do you remember the time you stood me up on the table in the kitchen and you stepped back far away and told me to jump into your arms? I was so little, and I was scared that it was so high and you were so far away. I didn't think I could jump that far. I cried, "Father, I can't do it!" And you yelled at me. You called me a baby. You said I must try. I was trembling all over. You said, "Come on, jump! I'll catch you." I began to cry louder, and you yelled, "Jump, God damn it!" And so I jumped. But instead of catching me like you promised, you stepped back and laughed as I hit the floor with my face. You said, "That will teach you a lesson in life, you little bastard! DON"T EVER TRUST ANYONE!" My nose was bro-

> ken, and my mouth was all bloody and I couldn't breathe. You just laughed and said, "You are a stupid boy. They will eat you alive out there."
>
> I hate remembering things like this, Father. How could you be so cruel? You were like a crazy animal. I remember how you used to hit Mother with your big hard fist. It was even worse when you were drunk. I could hear you hitting her in bed at night. I tried to close my ears. But you yelled so loud, and when you threw her against the walls, it shook our whole house. Sometimes I was so scared I wet my bed. . . . You would beat me if you found my bed wet. So I learned to sleep on the bare floor.
>
> I hate you for what you did to me. I hate you for making me hate. I have been scared and angry all of my life. I do not trust people, and I am a lonely old man. I blame you. Damn you to Hell! I hope I never do anything so bad that I have to see you again.
>
> Your Son,
> Luther

He wrote in his diary that he was angry with me for "making him" write that letter. Luther did not share that journal entry with me until weeks later. His second letter was easy to write, he said, because he knew exactly what his father would have said:

> Fuck you, you little piece of shit! You are not my son. Your whore of a mother must have been fucked by a jellyfish to have borne such a spineless child as you.
>
> I will get you, you little whining bastard. I will haunt you. I will make you trip over things and hurt yourself. I will make you sick. I will make people hate you. And when you die, you will come to Hell and I will beat you and spit on you for eternity! I am waiting for you.

Luther said that the third letter was impossible to write. His father had no human qualities, he said, and he did not want to imagine something so absurd. I suggested that we work on it together in a long session. This was when his anger toward me became apparent. I responded with respect and appreciation for his willingness to express that anger, which I viewed as a healthy response to his pain. There were long silences in that session. Luther said that he saw a pattern in how easily he could be angered by minor inconveniences in his life (e.g., a bus being late, a noisy neighbor, cold coffee). Anger had become part of his daily way of being; he said he was tired of it.

I suggested that we try that third letter. He was irritated by my suggestion and then quickly realized that this was part of the pattern he had just acknowledged. His quick response indicated that he was already moving into process-level work (Chapter 7). Luther accepted my offer of a pen and paper, after which he sat motionless. I could see that he was at a loss for how to start so I suggested the line: "My dear son, Luther."

He flinched at this and said, "He would *never* write that!"

"No," I said, "but you would if it were your son. Write it from your highest capacities."

His eyes watered and his hand trembled as he printed those first words. The letter emerged slowly in carefully printed letters:

> My Dear Son, Luther,
>
> Thank you for writing to me after all these years and after all that I did to you.
>
> I am so sorry, Son.
>
> You did not deserve to be treated so badly. I cannot explain why I acted like that with you and your dear Mother.
>
> If I could change it, I would. I would take it all back. I would be a good father and your friend.
>
> Please forgive me for what I have done to you and your life. But if you cannot find it in your heart to forgive me, I will understand.
>
> What is important now is that you do what you can to be happy. Like writing that letter to me and finding people who can help you see that you are a good person. You deserve many good times, and I am sure that you will go to Heaven, where you belong.
>
> I hope that you can forgive me, Son, or at least forget me. I am so sorry for your pain. I wish you happiness.
>
> Love,
> Papa

As he printed the word "Papa" Luther wept. "Papa" was what he had wanted to call his father, but it had not been allowed.

We sat together for several minutes without speaking. The exercise was over but the ordeal was not. Luther later said that he was weeping for many reasons. He wept for the pain he had endured, he said, and also for the loss he felt for the life he never had. "There was so much I wanted to forget," he said, "and yet I find myself now wishing that I could remember." Sometimes the remembering is an invaluable part of moving beyond old patterns of being.

LIFE-REVIEW EXERCISES

The primary purpose of reviewing one's life is not to discover a single traumatic event that explains an entire lifestyle. Nor is its purpose to assign blame or to live in the past. Life review is undertaken to give meaning to present circumstances and to create new possibilities for future experiencing. I say this at the outset because there seem to be two kinds of psychotherapists in the world: those who attribute everything to the past and those who attribute nothing to it. This is an exaggeration, of course, but it captures a common stereotype about therapy. Because of Freud's preoccupation with early childhood experiences, it is often assumed that all psychotherapists are involved in archeological digs. Indeed, the early behavioral and cognitive therapies distinguished themselves from psychoanalysis by emphasizing their lack of emphasis on the past. Because of the developmental essence of constructivism, I believe a constructive approach to therapy embraces a balance between historical lessons and present action. One can counsel constructively without conducting a life review, of course, and I do not recommend reflective exercises with all clients. When clients find themselves stuck in a pattern of experiencing, however, it may be useful to trace the pattern backward in time. This process can be particularly helpful for individuals who are mercilessly blaming themselves for their current patterns.

There are many ways of reviewing a life. Some are very brief and sketchy; others are detailed, long-term projects. A format for a sketchy life review is offered in Part 2 of the Personal Experience Report (Appendix C). Many of the questions there are aimed at evoking capsule summaries of a client's early experiences. I ask about the clarity of childhood memories and the overall happiness that clients associate with having been a child. Which emotions were considered "good" and which were discouraged or devalued? Using a simple check mark as an indicator, clients are asked about dimensions such as trust, stability, friendships, parental presence, and love. They are also asked to name the people by whom they first felt loved, and by whom they were hurt. These lists may overlap, of course, and this is something to which I attend. Two brief essay questions invite clients to share their happiest and most painful childhood experiences. Some clients initially leave many of these questions blank and I respect their choice to do so. Others begin to elaborate a life story.

An intermediate level of life review might be called the *life story method*, because it asks individuals to describe their life in a short story. The length of that story is less important than the process of writing it and the basic patterns that the story conveys. I recommend that my clients write the story in such a way that the main character (themselves) is described with third-person pronouns (he, she, they). I encourage them to author this story as if the part of them that is writing were an intimate but invisible witness to the life they are describing. In other words, I ask them to presume that they know themselves (the main character) better than anyone else ever could, because they were there throughout everything that happened. I also recommend that they write honestly, without concern for privacy or anyone's reactions. My emphasis is on the process of the writing, not the product. Therefore, if a client tells me that he is concerned about my possible reactions to his story, I encourage him to postpone his decision about whether he will actually allow me to read it. What is most important is that he fully engage himself in the act of describing his life as it now seems to him.

Writing one's life story can feel a bit daunting. One way to start is to set aside 10 minutes and ask the client to write down possible chapter titles.[10] These titles then serve as the focal themes of the chapters. This exercise may sound very simple, but it is rarely an easy undertaking. Some clients are reluctant to write at all, let alone to write about the secrets of their heart. As one woman put it, "I don't want to remember the pain. I went through it once. Why make myself go through it again?" The goal is not simply to relive the pain so much as to harvest new meaning from it and to put it in a new perspective. Early experiences may have ossified into memories with exclusive or unnecessary meanings. The process of changing meanings is itself an emotional one. I have had some clients ask if they could tape-record their life story, and I think this is a worthwhile consideration. Again, it is the process of reflecting, remembering, and "languaging" about their experiences that is essential.

Like meaning making in general, "languaging" is a relational activity. Another life review exercise that highlights this process is something I call the *musical memories method*. Like many of the exercises I describe in this book, this one was inspired by an experience with a client. Mark, a surgeon, was renowned in the medical community for his skills in remaining controlled in the face of the most gruesome traumas in the emergency room. I had been asked to help him and his wife improve their communication. Our consultation had just begun, however, when the unexpected occurred. Mark came home from the hospital one day to find an empty house. With the help of several friends and two moving companies, his wife had totally stripped the house. More tragically, she had disappeared with their 3-year-old son, Martin. A week later, Mark learned through an attorney that his wife had moved to an unspecified location in another state, where she planned to file for divorce. Living alone in an empty shell of a house, his heart was breaking. He missed his wife terribly, and the loss of his son brought unspeakable grief. I encouraged Mark to talk about what he was feeling, but his well-developed emotional control got in the way.

In our second session after the trauma, Mark was at a loss for words. After several minutes of silence in which he was struggling to express himself and make contact with his anguish, he suddenly said, "Wait a minute." He went to his car and brought back an audiotape. It was a live recording of a rock band whose music he had enjoyed for years. But the piece that Mark had intuitively been drawn to play for me was not a rock song. It was something spontaneous that had been recorded while the band was taking a break. One of the backup musicians had just gone through a painful divorce. It had resulted in his being separated from his own young son. Perhaps to express his own grief, the musician had written a song from the perspective of his little boy. Mark put the tape in my office stereo and pressed the play button. What I heard and felt is etched in my memory. The simple, slow, and plaintive beginnings of a dirge were followed by a father's faltering voice as he anguished through the falsetto of a frightened little boy. The tonality was torture; the words were something like this: "Please . . . some . . . body . . . hold . . . my . . . hand; I'm scared . . . and I feel real shaky. . . . ; Please somebody, understand. . . . I just now lost my Daddy. . . . Daddy said "good-bye" today. . . . I miss him so already. . . . I love Mommy very much . . . but mommies can't be daddies . . . "[11] Tears were running down my face, and Mark began to cry. The lyrics had touched the tenderness of his suffering, and the music was able to express what Mark could not yet say.

After that experience, I began to ask other clients for samples of music that had touched them. Most relevant to life review, I also began asking clients to construct audiotapes or compact discs of the music that had been most important in their lives. This has turned out to be a powerful experience for them as well as me. To give the exercise some focus and boundaries, I suggest that the tape or CD be no longer than 60–90 minutes. I do not ask for explanations of the meaning of specific songs or pieces. Some clients worry about which pieces to choose, how to arrange them, the quality of their recording, and what I will think of their musical tastes. These worries are, of course, reflections of patterns in how they organize their experiencing (of our relationship, novel challenges, etc.). Our work together is deepened by honest discussions of such worries. I am sometimes moved by new pieces of music, and I frequently discover dimensions of my clients' lives that would have been unknown to me without this exercise. Moreover, the process of compiling musical memories is usually an emotional journey. Clients frequently report becoming absorbed in the project—reflecting on earlier periods in their life and searching for copies of songs. Music has strong emotional associations. In the process of remembering and replaying music, memories are activated.

When I was first experimenting with life review exercises in psychotherapy, I encouraged my clients to collect these memories for the creation of a *life collage*. One way of doing this is to recommend that they devote several weeks to collecting cues and mementos. I encourage a balance of spontaneity and planned recollection. A client who is 40 years old, for example, may begin with 41 envelopes—one for each year since her conception. As she recalls things about a particular age or year, she writes a brief note about it and places it in the appropriate envelope. Photographs and other relics of the past may also be filed. In the early stages of this process, I may caution a client to avoid analyzing any particular memory. The completion of the life collage project is a tangible presentation. We set aside a double session for this life review. Some clients may "lay out" their life before me by arranging their envelopes on the floor and then slowly—often emotionally—walking me through their story. Some clients create drawings, sculptures, poems, music, enacted scenes, and combinations of all these. The life collages are never the same. They are always very personal. The story of the life that clients tell in that session is very much told by how it is shared.

Another pattern-work exercise that I like to use is the *origins pilgrimage*. A pilgrimage is usually thought of as a journey to a sacred place, but it is also a quest for meaning and self-awareness. In his opening remarks for Phil Cousineau's book on the sacred art of pilgrimage, Huston Smith writes:

> To set out on a pilgrimage is to throw down a challenge to everyday life. At home or abroad, things of the world pull us toward them with such gravitational force that, if we are not alert our entire lives, we can be sucked into their outwardness. The art is to master today's unavoidable situation with as much equanimity as we can muster, in preparation for facing its sequel tomorrow.
>
> In the course of this training we come to see quite plainly how essential it is . . . being centered in ourselves, not somewhere in the outer world.[12]

An origins pilgrimage is a journey to the places of one's birth, childhood, and earlier life. Such a journey can evoke intense emotions, and I recommend that it be undertaken solo, if possible. Having done such pilgrimages over the course of my life, I also recommend taking a camera, a personal diary, and perhaps old photos and a tape recorder. The purpose of this trip is not to capture the past but rather to record in rich detail one's immediate associations and memories. In my first such pilgrimage, I was struck by strong contrasts (e.g., the farmhouse kitchen was very different than I had remembered it, the smells of the school gymnasium were remarkably familiar, and my bodily reactions were powerful).

An origins pilgrimage may include conversations with family or friends, and this may require visits to cemeteries. My clients and I have found, however, that there is wisdom in Huston Smith's advice. Even though the origins pilgrimage is organized in terms of externals (places and people from one's past), its function is to stimulate an internal journey. The goal is to forge new meaning. Things will have changed, of course. As one pilgrim put in her journal,

> The old schoolhouse was gone and my first reaction was anger. How could they do that to my memory? The space was now consumed by an ugly parking garage. I sat on a concrete bench and just stared. Then my anger became sadness that nothing was the same. The red brick building was gone. The playground was gone. My childhood friends were gone. But then I heard some children laughing down the street and it reminded me of the sounds that used to fill the playground at recess. I remembered my favorite

> teacher and bologna sandwiches on Wonder Bread. And I smiled. I don't eat meat—I haven't for years. I have changed too, but I'm not gone.

You cannot go home again (Thomas Wolfe) or step into the same river of time (Heraclitus). But you can return to the places that represent earlier moments in a life journey.

Eventually, of course, the culmination of the life collage project or an origins pilgrimage is clients' attempts to display their lives in some finite expression. I continue to be amazed at the range of diversity in these displays—literal collages of photography and newspaper clippings, sculptures, poetry, quilting, and so on. Many clients will be at a loss for how to pull their life story together. This is where our skills as a constructive therapist may be stretched and strengthened. Some clients want to have their life story told to them (rather than *by* them). They honestly believe that psychotherapists can actually cast them as classical types in a fixed number of human life stories. There are two kinds of people in the world.

NARRATIVE RECONSTRUCTION

Our fascination with kinds, types, and stories is itself a reflection of our strong desire to organize our experience. Early in my career, I was frustrated with clients who wanted me to figure out their lives and make difficult decisions for them. Many of those clients were frustrated with my reluctance to assign them a diagnostic label or to agree with their fatalistic views of their plight. Slowly, it seems, we began to grow toward a middle path. My clients, as a cast of changing characters, have become more agentic and exploratory. And I have become more patient and understanding of their desires for simple stories and clear choices.

One of the most powerful developments of recent years in the field of psychotherapy has been the realization that human beings are embodied stories and creative storytellers. The "narrative turn," as it has been called, has been a central theme of constructivism. We are not simply the bearers or vehicles of our lives; we are also the authors. We write each moment at multiple levels, for the most part unaware that we are generating the very story in which we are living. Among other things, this means that psychotherapy is fundamentally an endeavor in which therapists are attempting to help clients reclaim their *author*-ity and write different and more fulfilling dimensions into their lives.

I do not here defend or detail the narrative turn in constructive psychology and psychotherapy.[13] As Gonçalves has put it, psychology has moved from viewing the person as an *object*, through a phase of making the person a *subject*, and on to the postmodern view of life as a *project*. We are subject and object at the same time that we are an ongoing project. The stories that we tell ourselves about ourselves become the fabric of our existence and the literal meaning(s) of our lives.[14] Recall that a basic assertion of constructivism is that we organize our experience. We make meaning. What changes when we change, psychologically speaking, are meanings.

It is helpful to understand something about the basic structure of narratives in order to best work with them in therapy. Drawing on classical works on narrative, Bruner and Kalmar suggest that a narrative is an interaction of the following components: a character or characters with some degrees of freedom, an act or course of action under way, a goal toward which the main character is committed, resources, setting(s), and a problem or series of problems that must be overcome. This problem is often pivotal in the decision to seek professional counsel. As these authors note, "The *engine* of narrative is Trouble."[15] The function of the narrative is to give meaning to the whole. I agree with the views of Arciero and Guidano and Baumeister that loss of coherence lies at the heart of psychological disorder.[16] Among other things, psychotherapy is a quest for coherence in the presence of trouble.

Consider some of the common ways clients render their life stories. Their characterizations of themselves are often negative, and they frequently do not view themselves as having much agency or freedom. Many lack a clear goal or a strong commitment to a goal. They often view their resources and personal capacities as limited. Their presumptions may vary considerably, but common among them are some of the irrational or unrealistic ideas made famous by Albert Ellis[17] (e.g., that life should always be fair and painless, that one must be universally loved and perfectly successful, that one can do little to change the way things are, or that there should be a simple and easy solution to every problem). Moreover, many clients believe that their troubles started with a single event that threw them off course and, because they cannot "undo" that event, that they are helpless and adrift.

Narrative reconstructions of meaning seem to follow a nonlinear course. Recent research on changes in narration during psychotherapy seem to converge on an overall dialectical process.[18] The retelling of stories may be important, especially when each retelling allows for variations in the felt sense or significance of the specifics. Thus, it is important for therapists to be patient with clients' needs to repeat their accounts of life episodes. Such repetitions are central to the process of "assimilating" what has happened, "accommodating" these experiences into larger and usually more complex systems of meaning (relatedness), and utilizing this new equilibrium as a base camp for launching novel projects into the adventures of a life in process.

In reflecting on the development of narratives in my own clients, I am struck by the frequency with which early renderings tend to portray the characters and problems in a polarized manner. In these preliminary renditions, it is as if there were only "good" and "bad" characters, favorable and unfavorable circumstances, and acts that were clearly wise or foolish. With some clients, these polarized renditions persist. Sometimes the clients assume the role of the guilty party, and their movement forward is one of accepting the fact that they "fucked up" in their past. This construction of meaning can be adaptive if they accept responsibility for their mistake, forgive themselves (which is usually an ongoing rather than a finally achieved process), and move on with their lives. That same construction can be very dysfunctional, however, when it is rendered as a definition of their identity and their future (e.g., "I *am* fucked up and so is my future").

An alternate construction involves blaming other characters in one's life story and casting oneself as a victim of their abuses. This apparently externalizing construction is often part of a similar internalizing process (i.e., one in which the original blame is placed on an other but the ultimate consequences are incorporated into a negative view of the self and the future). If a client sees his fate as inevitable and unalterable, he is less likely to explore new options.[19] Exploration is again a key theme. Clients who move beyond the preliminary polarizations begin to explore other possibilities. They begin to wonder and to question. They become less intent on classifying and explaining than on opening and asking. In my experience, such explorations are much more likely to generate transformations in ways of viewing the self, the past, significant others, and future possibilities.

In my experience, more successful or helpful retellings of life stories tend to share the following features:

1. Oscillations in the level of focus (e.g., sometimes emphasizing a detailed description of events, sometimes focusing on the emotional experience of those events, and often suggesting shifts toward different possible explanations for either the events or their emotional consequences).
2. Oscillations in the activity of blaming (self, others, or circumstances), with an eventual softening of the need to blame and an increase in acceptance and forgiveness (of self and others).
3. A "thickening" of the complexity of the characters (particularly the self) and the plot.
4. A shift in emphasis from past to present events and future possibilities.
5. A movement toward a more positive and agentic portrayal of the self.

With regard to this last point, the work of Markus and Nurius (1986) on "possible selves" is noteworthy.[20] Particularly important was their finding that many individuals do not see the self as protean or flexible. Some thought that the chances of there being a nuclear war were greater than would be changing their sense of self. Thus, the "impossibility of selves" may be more to the point (i.e., that many individuals experience themselves as very limited in their mutabilility). Many people have foreclosed on their flexibility as a continuing identity, and their options for future development are accordingly limited. One of the primary functions of constructive practice, in my opinion, is to gently but persistently challenge such foreclosure.

With all due respect for past identities and the ways they have served the functioning of the person, there must always be constructive alternatives. There must be options, and an openness to embracing them. In its most precious role in systemic self-organization, the self must remain an ongoing and always unfinished story—a central mystery:

> We suspect there is something both culturally adaptive and psychologically comfortable about "keeping one's options open" where one's self-narrative is concerned. Fixing the story of one's life, with a limiting conception of Self as major protagonist, may have the effect of shutting down our possibilities and opportunities prematurely. A fixed-in-advance omnibus life story creates . . . a tragic "figure" with no options. In any save a highly ritualized social world, the more firmly fixed one's self-concept, the more difficult it is to manage change, to deal with local contingencies. It is "staying loose" that makes negotiation possible. Not so surprising, then, that turning points are so characteristic of the autobiographies we finally write or tell: They are the points in a life where, faced with difficulties, one may be forced to fashion a new omnibus Self to cope with the jeopardy in which we have been put.[21]

The narrative reconstruction of meaning is a lifelong project of becoming. It is not something accomplished within psychotherapy, although it can be valuably structured and accelerated in that context. The stories we tell ourselves (and others) are temporary constructions of a life in progress. Exercises in life review are themselves quests for coherence. The self is cast as the main character and, hence, with characteristics. There will be contrasts in the unfolding of a story line. When a client is describing his life story—whether via a collage or music, after an origins pilgrimage, or any other life-review method—I try to listen for these characteristics and contrasts. What are the dimensions used to describe the self and other people in this life? How evident are themes such as good and evil? Strength and weakness? Health and illness? Malice? Virtue? Guilt? Fate? What are described as having been turning points in life? I sometimes invite a separate *turning points* exercise to clarify this. This exercise can be as simple as the question itself (i.e., "What have been the turning points in your life?"). It can also be elaborated as a graph with time (in years) on the horizontal axis and well-being on the vertical axis. I am particularly interested in depictions that take the form of "Everything was fine until *X*" or "My life was horrible before *Y*." I am also interested in attributions of motive or causality, as well as global portrayals that are unidimensional (e.g., "Grandmother was a saint" or "There was never any love in our house").

I do not view my professional role as that of critic or corrections officer, however. Nor am I just listening to a story. I am bearing witness to a unique human life. The act of sharing it with me, even partially, is an act of tremendous trust. I treat it as such and often express my appreciation explicitly. In encouraging my clients to review their lives and share their stories with me, I am also expressing my faith that we humans can make sense of our troubles and—importantly—that we can do so in ways that create new possibilities for our patterns of being. The process of revising a life story is not one of denying facts, diminishing the reality of past suffering, or—to put it graphically—"blowing sunshine up the ass." It is, however, an exploration of alternative interpretations and evaluations. This means that narrative reconstruction necessarily suspends prior conclusions. Remember George Kelly's principle of constructive alternatives.[22] The good news is that there are always alternative ways of viewing bad things or their effects. The bad news is that the converse is also true of good things. And the balanced news is that there is ample room for choice and agency in how one navigates the news.

COMING HOME TO PROCESS

Recall that techniques are languages that can help us communicate with clients. Some of my favorite techniques are summarized in Table 6.1. I have clustered them loosely, and I again caution about reading a linear sequence into them. We should remember that categories are convenient tools that serve only a limited set of tasks. Beware of the law of the hammer. Don't pound things that need to be tickled. Techniques are rituals of enactment. They serve to structure or initiate activity. Activity is key.

At the heart of all living is process. The same is true of psychotherapy. Each client's current focus of attention is a reflection of his or her processes of self-organization. The same is true of us as therapists. We are all always "in process," and everything we think, feel, and do is an expression of this fact. There are many levels of processes, of course, and many different ways of conceptualizing them. Partly out of respect for tradition, I next discuss process work on the inner (*intra*-personal) level. This will inevitably bring us into the interpersonal realm of human relationship, which is the ultimate crucible for most personal development.

TABLE 6.1. Selected Techniques in Constructive Psychotherapy

Bibliotherapy

How-to guides
Personal accounts of similar experiences
Inspirational
Pleasure reading

Relaxation

Centering attention
Rituals and routines
Familiar relationships
Familiar places (e.g., Wal-Mart retreat)
Sacred places

Breathing exercises

Pause breathing
Release breaths
Alternate (control vs. surrender) breathing

Problem solving

Self-monitoring
Possible solutions brainstorming
Personal experiments
Stimulus control
Self-reinforcement
Shaping small improvements

Cognitive restructuring

Therapeutic writing

Personal journaling
Unsent letter
Life review
  Life story method
  Musical memories method
  Life collage
  Origins pilgrimage

Narrative reconstruction

(continued)

TABLE 6.1. ***(continued)***

Body-focused techniques
Balance exercises
Standing center
One-leg stand
Range of movement
Stretching
Yoga
Resistance exercises
Isometric (dynamic tension)
Weight (strength) training
Rhythm
Finding a beat (tapping exercises)
Walking meditation
Following a flow (e.g., Tai Chi)
Music appreciation
Music performance (instrumental)
Dance (creative and choreographed)
Touch
Handcrafts (e.g., painting, sculpture, woodwork)
Self-massage
Massage therapy
Petting pets
Voice
Laughing/crying meditation
Vowel movement exercise
Yelling exercises
Singing
Voice play
Process work
Role plays
Dramatic enactment
Fixed role therapy
Fantasy
Dream work
Meditation
Mirror time
Stream of consciousness
Spiritual skills exercises

NOTES

1. Volk (1995).
2. Bowman (1994); Brand (1980); Pennebaker (1990, 1995, 1997); Rimé (1995); Van Zuuren, Schoutrop, Lange, Louis, and Slegers (1999).
3. Quoted in de Shazer (1994, p. 3).
4. W. T. Anderson (1997).
5. Goldberg (1986); Lee (1994).
6. Belenky, Clinchy, Goldberger, and Tarule (1986); Brand (1980); Efran, Lukens, and Lukens (1990); Goldberg (1986); Goldberger, Tarule, Clinchy, and Belenky (1996); Hermans and Hermans-Jansen (1995); Lee (1994); McAdams (1993); Pennebaker (1990, 1995, 1997); Tobias (1997); Ueland (1987).
7. Baldwin (1990); Rainer (1978).
8. For a review of therapists' ratings of self-help books, see Norcross et al. (2003).
9. Kopp (1972).
10. I am indebted to Bob Neimeyer for teaching me this exercise.
11. Mangione (1978), *Children of Sanchez.*
12. H. Smith (1998, pp. xi–xiv).
13. Bakhtin (1975, 1986); Bruner (1979, 1986, 1990); de Rivera and Sarbin (1998); Neimeyer (1995a); Polkinghorne (1988); Rennie (1994); Sarbin and Keen (1998); Schafer (1992); Smith and Nylund (1997); Spence (1982); White and Epston (1990).
14. Carlsen (1988, 1995); Gonçalves (1994, 1995); Gonçalves, Korman and Angus, 2000); Gonçalves and Machado (1999); Gonçalves and Gonçalves (1998); Hoshmand (1993); McAdams (1993); Messer, Sass, and Woolfolk (1988).
15. Bruner and Kamar (1998, p. 324).
16. Arciero and Guidano (2000); Baumeister (1991).
17. Ellis (1962, 1998).
18. Angus (1996); Angus and Hardtke (1994); Luborsky, Barber, and Digeur (1992).
19. Fosha (2000, 2001); Lewis (1997).
20. Markus and Nurius (1986).
21. Bruner and Kalmar (1998, pp. 323–324).
22. Kelly (1955).

CHAPTER 7

BASIC PROCESS WORK

Meditation and Embodiment

Heraclitus and Buddha seemed to agree on the fluidity of things, including human experiencing. "All that is is becoming." One can say the same of process. Everything we experience is fundamentally our process, our way of being in the flow of time. Lao Tzu, the legendary founder of Taoism, made it clear that the Tao (literally, the "way" or "path") that could be captured in words was not the one he meant. More than two millennia later, constructivist philosophers such as Ernst Cassirer and Alfred North Whitehead would use words to explain why words cannot fully grasp process. Words are wonderful tools for some tasks. They can symbolize what is not present (and hence *re*-present it). When words are shared in a community of language, they can serve to connect and coordinate experiencing. But words can also get in the way and separate rather than connect. In the distinction between experiencing and explaining (Chapter 2), for example, there is an implied separation between living in the body and in the head. One of the perennial functions of poetry is to bridge that gap and to bring us into a dynamic tension between head and heart. As we enter the poem, it enters us. Boundaries soften. Time and self float. Not only are body, mind, and spirit momentarily seamless, but the moment itself also seems temporarily paused. As Stanley Kunitz (1995) puts it,

> The moment is dear to us, precisely because it is so fugitive, and it is somewhat of a paradox that poets should spend a lifetime hunting the magic that will make the moment stay. Art is the chalice into which we pour the wine of transcendence.[1]

Process-level work in constructive therapy is closely related to the art forms of poetry and dance. It is a dynamic and emergent flow and it can be tantalizing in its elusiveness. I recall a conversation with Vittorio Guidano in which he spoke of his experience. He would feel himself getting closer and closer to the heart of process, only to find it evaporating as he reached to embrace it. His description reminds me of some poetic lines:

Each day, again and again,
    I begin to teach myself
The first step of a dance which,
    The night before,
I dreamt I had mastered.[2]

Process work in therapy is often like that. No matter how often you do it, and no matter how good you get at it, you are always beginning. There are metaphorical glimpses of an organic loom weaving very intimate patterns from threads of meaning, memory, values, and more. There is a developing sense of another level of order and other ways of experiencing. There are felt shifts, some subtle and a few dramatic. As undeniable as they are, these shifts are often undescribable.[3] It is more than mildly amusing that thousands of volumes have been written about something that cannot be captured in words. One can perhaps get closer to the phenomenology of process with a visual metaphor, and I sometimes use the figure of a Necker cube to illustrate such shifts to clients (Figure 7.1). The apparent orientation of the cube will abruptly shift, so that the corner in the center of the figure sometimes appears to be nearest you and other times appears farthest away. If you try to force the shift, your act of effort may actually postpone or prevent the change you want. You are more likely to see the cube differently if you blink, relax your focus, or look away and then take a

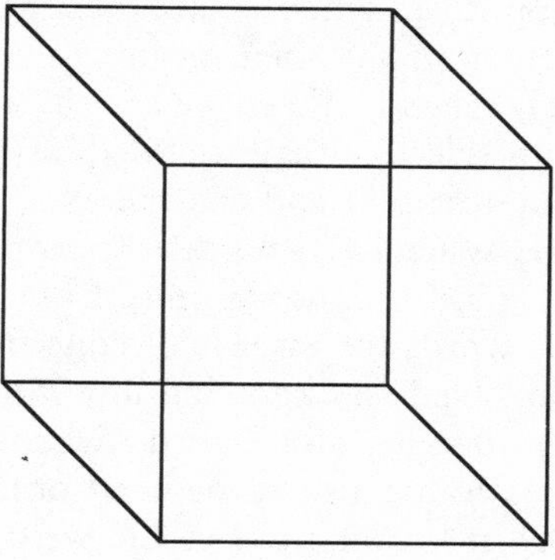

FIGURE 7.1. The Necker cube.

fresh look at it. I like the metaphorical messages in these strategies, because they also have relevance for many everyday perceptions of life situations.[4] Also noteworthy are the facts that one cannot see the cube both ways at the same time, and that once it has been seen differently, it becomes impossible not to have it flip once in a while. Thomas Kuhn used the Necker cube phenomenon to describe shifts in scientific paradigms. What shifts during a scientific revolution is rarely external, and I believe a parallel statement can be made about personal revolutions. The stars in the heavens were the same for Copernicus as they were for his predecessors. The lines on the page that make up the Necker cube do not magically move. It is our perception that shifts—our processes of organizing our sense data. The perceived relationships change; hence, we see possibilities for new meanings in old patterns.

Process work involves an attunement to shifts in experiencing and a refinement of the skills that allow those shifts to take place. Not surprisingly, those skills are intimately related to the processes of centering and edging (Chapter 4). Clients may differ considerably in their readiness for and interest in process work. Such work is very demanding for both client and therapist. In my experience, it has also been among the most powerful in transforming lives. Process-level work requires creativity and the courage to examine oneself in the heat of the present moment. This means that the psychotherapist must be willing to take risks in the process of encouraging clients to do the same. In this chapter, I briefly describe some of the practical exercises I have found useful. Most of these exercises focus on active witnessing of a client's inner world. The role of such witnessing skills in personal change is also addressed in later discussions of psychological development and psychotherapy process.

MEDITATION

Much of what we therapists do when we are most helpful to our clients involves shifts in their attention and their meaning-making processes (which are, of course, intimately related). When we are paying attention, we are investing life energies in a selective manner. Meditation practices foster the development of skills in attention and can therefore be a valuable component of personal change. When I was resident sport psychologist at the U.S. Olympic Training Center in Colorado Springs, Colorado, I was once asked to summarize in simple words the essence of concentration. I said, "There are three basic skills involved: (1) knowing how to hold on, (2) knowing how to let go, and (3) knowing which to do when with what." I believe those simple-sounding skills are also at the heart of living life well. Meditation is ultimately aimed at learning to live life well.

How does one teach meditation as a part of psychotherapy? When I sense that a client is interested in exploring his own inner activity, I may suggest one or two resources from the vast literatures on spiritual wisdom traditions and the multiple varieties of meditation.[5] I may also give him a copy of some brief instructions to try at home (Appendix G). More importantly, I invite him to join me in-session in 5 minutes of silent reflection. We assume a comfortable position—preferably sitting so that the spine is erect, and the abdomen and diaphragm are free for easy breathing. I invite him to close his eyes or at least to lower his gaze, so that visual stimulation is minimal and constant. I join him in this. I then encourage him to breathe slowly and simply to witness his "stream of consciousness" and the shifting activity of his attention. Then, I remain silent and direct my attention inward toward my own stream. Because I am the mentor in this process, part of my awareness remains attuned to the client (e.g., the sounds of his breathing and body movements). After approximately 5 minutes, I take an audible release breath and open (or lift) my eyes. I wait for him to do the same. When he does, I may ask, "What was that like?" or "What did you notice?" Clients' responses will vary, of course. Some report that they thought nothing. Others will have been struck by how much "mind chatter" was taking place. Still others say they felt awkward with the silence, and many ask what they were supposed to have noticed. All of these responses are normal. I reassure people that such reactions and questions are not unusual. Research on spontaneous reports of consciousness suggest considerable complexity, many individual differences, and shifts of focus occurring every 7–15 seconds.[6] Clients seldom report any adverse reaction to this brief exploratory exercise. A far more common response is curiosity and questions about how to learn more.

As is apparent in the extensive literature on meditation, different traditions emphasize a variety of rules and rituals for meditation. Some are strict and highly structured. Others are less formal. I recommend the latter for people just beginning to explore the practice of contemplation. In the early stages of basic skill development, encouragement should be generous. I assure beginners that meditation does not require sitting on the floor or assuming a lotus position. There are many ways to meditate. Virtually all of them emphasize breathing and posture. As noted in Chapter 4, breathing is important for at least two reasons: (1) It directly influences many other bodily processes, and (2) it is an automatic process that can, with attention and will, be voluntarily altered. Posture is important, because it influences the alert state that is necessary for optimal attention and learning.

Meditation is different from relaxation. In relaxation, the goal is to surrender to the body's basic wisdom in resting and letting go of unnecessary muscle tension. In meditation, the goal is to practice alert awareness. The easiest postures for alertness are standing, kneeling, and sitting upright (with the spine erect). Meditation while lying down is possible, but it is often more challenging in terms of remaining alert. For beginning meditators, the position of the hands is not important. The hands can be folded on the lap, rested on the arms of the chair, folded in a prayerful position, or placed on the abdomen. An erect spine is probably the single most important feature of meditative posture. When that is maintained, alertness is more likely. The rest of the body can find comfortable positions, but the back should be straight.

Mindfulness meditation (also known as *vipassana* meditation) is one of the simplest forms, and its positive effects are well documented. As noted in Appendix G, the basic goal of such meditation is to practice a gentle witnessing of one's attention. Using a breathing-related sensation as a reference point, one practices a disciplined alertness to the straying of one's focus. The analogy is that of a river. Thoughts, images, memories, and sensations may flow through one's consciousness in the same way that ripples move along the surface of a gently moving river. The meditator is asked to use her reference sensation as a bridge that allows her to rise above and witness her stream of consciousness. From time to time, of course, something interesting will "hook" her and draw her downstream. Each time this happens, she simply returns to the bridge. Counting "out breaths" (exhalations) is used as a repetitive way of maintaining a perspective in the midst of the flow.

> When you told me to just sit up straight and count my breaths, I thought it was too simple and easy. It wasn't! Even the sitting up straight was a challenge. I would slowly start to relax my back and end up in a slump with my shoulders rounded and my head down. And the counting!? I thought you said that it was hard to get to 9. So I was real proud of myself the first couple of times I made it. But then I realized that I was counting on one level and doing all sorts of daydreaming on another. It reminded me of saying prayers in church when I was a kid. I could say the memorized words so automatically that there was a lot of freedom to talk to myself and think about other things while my lips were moving to the prayers. It was the same thing with the counting. When I really started to get absorbed in what my breathing felt like, I also found a lot of mental stuff competing for my attention. It reminded me of the kindergarten kids I work with . . . lots of them waving their hands and shouting for my attention."

This is a graphic description of the complexity and inherent internal competition that is often recognized during process work. One begins to realize that there is a lot going on inside all the time, and that much of it is simultaneous. In cognitive science terminology, these are called "parallel processes." Learning to maintain a fixed focus in the presence of such complexity is a difficult challenge, but it is also a skill that is valuable for many important life tasks.

> I thought this was going to be pretty easy because I am always so scattered in my life and my mind just jumps around. What I am beginning to learn is that I am just beginning to know my own mind. Like I would

> try not to get hooked by anything, and then minutes later I would find that I had gotten snagged on my impatience for the time to be up or questions I was going to ask you (like "What am I supposed to be getting out of this anyway?"). And then I'd get upset with myself for having lost my flow. It reminded me of walking through an old-time carnival where all the carnies are trying to get your attention and pull you over to their booth to blow your money on a ring toss game or something. Or maybe the telemarketers who try to get you into a conversation just so they can sell you something you don't want. Wow! I'm not sure yet, but I think the things that keep pulling me off are the ones that are trying to warn me that I'm missing something good or forgetting something important.

This is an unusually insightful comment on the richness of the lessons that may be offered by this practice. Mindfulness meditation is very popular, and there are a number of places worldwide that offer instruction and opportunities for its practice.[7]

Silent and stationary meditation methods are valuable for developing skills in self-awareness and attention. Some clients are frustrated in their early experiments with meditation. These are often individuals who are impatient to see dramatic changes in their lives. Part of what these forms of meditation may teach is patience and persistence. Slowing down and paying attention are worthwhile goals for many of us. Clients may ask how often and how long they should meditate. I gauge my response according to my felt sense of their current needs for structure and progress. To some I may say, "That's a very individual matter. You should experiment with different lengths of time and see what works best for you." This statement is true. Other clients may need to hear, "I recommend that you meditate at least once a day, preferably in the morning. If you have appointments or a schedule to keep, set a timer so that you don't have to check your watch or a clock while you're meditating. Ten minutes is a good length. If you can afford 20, that is fine. If you are rushed, get in the habit of at least devoting 1 minute to the exercise. It will be a symbolic expression of your intentions, and even a minute will help to slow you down and get centered before a busy day." Eventually, of course, the goal is to transfer the active attention of stationary meditation to the tasks and situations of everyday life. Heavy traffic, for example, presents frequent opportunities to practice alertness and patience, as well as forgiveness and generosity.

EMBODIMENT EXERCISES

Meditation need not be motionless, and those who practice sitting meditation quickly notice that their consciousness is seldom at rest. But there are forms of meditation that focus more specifically on bodily movement, and they are potentially as promising as breathing methods for changing immediate mood, self-appraisal, and well-being. I believe many cases of psychotherapy would be improved with greater emphasis on learning body awareness and regular practice of movement. The mind and its ordering processes are expressed in the body and vice versa. Movement is a primary dimension of human experience that has been remarkably absent from psychotherapy. Embodiment education is so basic and relevant to human health and well-being that I devote a future volume exclusively to this topic. Here, I can only briefly note that the neglect of the body in psychotherapy may be a reflection of the legacy of rationalism, which was incorporated into the Christian church before and during the Middle Ages. The body was then considered an earthly prison and the source of all sin. The intellect was supposed to rule over the passions. Mind–body dualism has continued to plague psychology throughout its brief history as a discipline, and one of the more positive developments in the last quarter of the 20th century was the movement toward a more holistic view of the human being. This development has direct bearing on how we practice psychotherapy.

Psychotherapy need not be just an exchange of information between two talking heads. It never could be. If you listen closely to the conversation between those heads, the one with the problem is often referring to its body. The head says that the body isn't doing what it is supposed to, or that it is feeling things that are unpleasant. The head, with the license, listens from atop its own body, which is feeling and doing in its own way. Two bodily beings are interacting, primarily through words, but also through gestures, glances, intonations, smells, sounds, and movements. At a recent workshop on constructive psychotherapy, one of the participants asked me, "But how does one bring the body *into* psychotherapy?" It usually enters just underneath the head. The body is always in psychotherapy, of course, and much of what is discussed in the therapeutic hour is focused on how the body is functioning, feeling, or looking. My point is that there are things we can do to deepen our clients' appreciation and expression of their embodiment.

Some of the most important skills we teach in psychotherapy are skills in attention, meaning making, and self-relationship. Relating to our own bodies is a crucial dimension of relating to ourselves. Indeed, some individuals are overly conscious of their bodies. The individual who suffers hypochondriacal concerns tends to be hypervigilant regarding body sensations. He often exhibits remarkable sensitivities to very subtle somatic cues—sensitivities comparable to those of an elite athlete or a master of tantric sex. However, the hypochondriac tends to interpret many sensations as signs of disease or dysfunction. His highly refined awareness thus serves a self-organizational pattern of mistrusting his body. In this pattern, the individual often contributes to the creation of the very distress (*dis*-ease) that he fears. Hypochondriasis is an example of unusual sensitivity used in the service of a constrictive lifestyle. But somatic self-awareness can also serve as an appreciation for the gifts of embodiment, such as the pleasures of the senses and the treasures of creative movement.

I have been incorporating body work into my practice with clients for many years and believe it has been important to the benefits they have derived from our work together. By "body work," I mean that I have included an explicit focus on clients' bodies in the exercises I introduce in sessions and that I recommend for homework. How I do this depends, of course, on my sense of where clients are currently in their awareness of their body, their openness to bodily sensations, and so on. Fortunately, health consciousness and what I call the "movement movement" have created increasing numbers of health centers with classes for people of all ages, interests, and abilities.

I believe that physical (bodily) awareness and activity patterns are central to processes of well-being, and I enjoy witnessing the reengagement with life that usually accompanies appreciative embodiment. In early sessions, I pay particular attention to how a client appears (complexion, energy level, posture, etc.) and to her responses to those parts of the Personal Experience Report (Appendix B) that relate to bodily experiences and activities. When I encounter a client who is extremely disembodied—in the sense of being unaware of her bodily sensations and uninvolved in activities that honor or serve bodily health, one of my first homework assignments for her likely includes some physical movement. If she is quite sedentary, I suggest something like two small (5- to 10-minute) walks per day (preferably outside) or some simple range of movement (stretching) exercises to be performed morning and evening. Sometimes I demonstrate basic stretching movements in my office and then recommend books, videotapes, or classes on stretching, beginner's yoga, or a gentle form of movement meditation such as Tai Chi or Qi Gong.[8]

There are a wide range of basic techniques for teaching body awareness and encouraging bodily activity.[9] My purpose here is to illustrate briefly how practical exercises can be incorporated into constructive therapy. An alliterative mnemonic aid for three of the main classes of embodiment methods invokes the "*three R's*" of *range*, *resistance*, and *rhythm*. To these three I add "*TV*"—not television, but the merits of *touch* and *voice*. My clinical experience has been that clients make more significant, more consistent, and more accelerated personal changes in their lives when they are involved in personally tailored projects that include range of movement (physical flexibility), resistance (strength training), rhythm (e.g., music appreciation or dance), touch (including professional massage and sexual activity), and some form of self-generated sound (singing, screaming, humming, etc.). The reasons and evidence for the helpfulness of these methods are beyond the scope of this chapter, but those interested in documentation will find an extensive literature.[10]

Range

Although there is some simplification in the saying "Use it or lose it," research on the human body and its aging processes suggest that there is more than a kernel of truth to this statement. This is particularly clear in the realm of range of movement—the flexibility of the joints and their connective tissues. Children are incredibly flexible, and their flexibility protects them from many injuries. As they grow into adults, it is not inevitable that they must become more brittle and constricted. Adults who pursue regular practices that move their joints through their full range of movement lose substantially less flexibility than their more sedentary peers. Clients can literally protect and expand their degrees of freedom by exercising them. The form of their practice seems less important than its regularity and the consistency of its challenge to the limits of their range of movement. Different methods produce similar results in maintaining a flexibility that is invaluable to the living system. Classes in these methods are offered by many public and private agencies, and they often have special classes for beginners. I encourage my clients to explore them.

Exploring the edges of one's range of movement necessarily involves experiences of center. Edges and centers are connected. The importance of balance (center of gravity) in life was noted in my earlier presentation of basic centering skills (Chapter 4). Metaphorically, at least, balance is central to what most clients are seeking. The "standing center" exercise is the easiest to teach. Recall that it also provides opportunities for metaphorical lessons about life (e.g., that we recognize our sense of center most clearly when we leave it). We live much of our lives unconsciously centered (and without much appreciation for that fact). Then, when we are thrown or pushed off center, we suddenly realize what we have left behind, and we desperately struggle to regain it. Perhaps our goal should not be to stay centered all the time, but to recognize and appreciate our center more often as we move through it. We can also hope both to enlarge the size of our center and to refine our skills in recovering the sense of balance in our lives.

Postural alignments are an important part of centering, and I believe that some of the techniques developed for exploring body part alignments can be valuable. I am not of the opinion that there is a single, universal, "correct" way to stand, sit, walk, or otherwise position oneself as a body. I do believe, however, that an awareness of body mechanics can help individuals to appreciate how their sagging head, stooped shoulders, and hip–ankle discordance may both reflect and contribute to their overall psychological posture toward life. Some of the most popular systems for teaching postural balance include Rolfing (structural integration), Hellerwork, postural integration, the Alexander technique, and the Feldenkrais method.[11] Besides practicing postural alignment in everyday movement situations, I like to use *back balls*. The equipment is simple: place two soft tennis balls into a sock. Push the balls all the way to the toe of the sock, then tie a knot in the sock to keep the balls close together. Sit down on a soft floor (carpet or exercise mat) and place these "back balls" beneath your lower back in alignment with your spine. Keep your feet and butt flat on the floor. Supporting yourself on your elbows, slowly lower your back onto the balls so that each ball is gently touching the erector muscles on either side of the spine. Take a release breath. By very gradually relaxing into the tennis balls, you put gentle pressure on some of the muscles that support the spine. I recommend going very slowly and alternating between gentle pressure and no pressure at all. This alternation strategy also permits adequate circulation to the muscles. You should spend at least 10 seconds at each "notch" (vertebral space). By moving slowly from the lower back area to your neck, you can thoroughly relax and massage many of the muscles along the spine. Needless to say, this is a technique to be used with caution and common sense. It should feel good, like a gentle back rub. From a sitting or standing position, the balls can also be used manually to massage the muscles of the back of the neck and at the base of the skull.

Resistance

Resistance is the essence of what is called "strength." There are two basic kinds of resistance exercises: those in which you apply force to something that moves (e.g., weights) and others in which the force is applied to something that remains stationary. The latter, often called "isometric" exercises, were popularized by Charles Atlas in the middle of the 20th century. You can push against a wall or door frame, for example, or use one muscle group to resist another (e.g., by holding your own wrist and either pushing or pulling against it with the other arm). The advantages of isometric exercises are that they require no special equipment, they can be practiced almost anywhere, and they yield significant results. Those results require that the tension in the muscles be considerable and that this "dynamic tension" be maintained for 6–10 seconds (with brief rests between repetitions). One of the disadvantages of such exercises is that they can raise blood pressure in hypertensive individuals. There are also limits to what isometric exercises can teach about the coordination of strength movements. Coordinated strength is preferable. For the person who does not suffer from hypertension, however, isometrics can increase muscle tone and strength with only a few brief sessions per day. Such exercises may also be used as an adjunct to weight training, and they are easy to do while traveling, or during a busy work day.

The other group of resistance exercises apply force to something that moves, and that "something" is usually a weight. Indeed, the terms "weight training" and "strength training" are often used as synonyms. There are, of course, many different methods of weight training. The increasing popularity of fitness centers and varieties of fitness equipment provide many opportunities for individualized programs of strength training. Relative to the issue of advantages and disadvantages, weight (or resistance) machines generally offer greater safety than exercise with "free" weights (e.g., dumbbells and barbells). Machines are convenient, and one can vary the resistance with the simple movement of a selector pin (without having to physically load or unload weights). The primary disadvantage of exercise machines is that they constrain movement. According to the "principle of specificity" in strength training, the body develops muscles in accordance with the specific angle of their challenges. Unless one varies the machines (or how one uses them), muscle development is likely to reflect a specialized development that is attuned to the angles allowed by a particular machine.

Free weights (weights that are not attached to a machine) allow greater freedom of movement, and this involves both risks and benefits. The risks are injuries caused by improper movement, falls, or dropping the weights on a body part. These are not insignificant risks, and I recommend professional supervision in the beginning stages of free-weight training. Lifting free weights is a concentrated experience in resistance, and it is a reminder that gravity is a consistent presence throughout our lives. Most falls in older adults are caused by weaknesses in muscles that coordinate walking and balance.

One need not be a bodybuilder or strength athlete to survive, of course, but strength is an important factor in overall health. Staying strong is wise, and both strength and muscle tone are correlated with some measures of self-esteem, confidence, mood, and well-being. There are now many studies documenting the positive effects of strength training on bone density, circulation, respiratory health, sleep quality, and immune functioning.

I defer a discussion of the myths surrounding weight training (e.g., becoming "musclebound") and the different goals of that training (e.g., bodybuilding, injury rehabilitation, etc.).[12] What is most important is regular movement against resistance. Proper form is essential, and not all certified strength trainers are well versed in the challenges and benefits of exercising with free weights rather than machines. For those seeking a structured sequence around which to organize their weight training, I recommend contacting people who know Olympic weightlifting.[13] One does not need to become a competitor to derive benefits from learning and practicing good form in movements such as the squat, leg raises, high pulls, and exercises that strengthen the lower back and shoulders. The all-around benefits of such exercises are unmistakable. The U.S. Olympic Committee states that "anytime someone runs, walks or jumps they are applying the same principles as Olympic-style weightlifting."[14] Over 90% of the sports in the Olympic games use some form of the hip extension required in Olympic weightlifting. Moreover, there are joys that can be found in repeatedly testing and celebrating one's strength.[15] Not everyone will want to do free-weight exercises in which they "throw" something heavy overhead, of course. In my experience, however, clients consistently report feeling better (emotionally, as well as physically) immediately after a workout and in the course of a long-range program of strength training.

Over many years of clinical practice and consultation, I have prescribed individualized programs of resistance exercise for clients. Many of these have involved light wrist weights and slow-motion movements. By adding slight resistance to the ends of the arms and then moving them slowly, one can accentuate the sensations of everyday movements and learn to feel the different muscle groups. I am intrigued by a clinical impression that has developed over the years. There is now good evidence that both aerobic exercise (e.g., running, swimming, cycling) and anaerobic strength training can be helpful adjuncts in the treatment of anxiety and depression. My hunch is that persons who are struggling with depression and issues of empowerment are likely to respond more positively when they regularly perform exercises that involve the largest and most powerful muscles of the body (the quadriceps and hamstrings in the upper legs—worked well by squats, walking, running, etc.—and the muscles of the upper back and upper arms—the lats, the trapezius, the deltoids, the triceps, and the biceps). In contrast, but with some overlap, of course, clients struggling with issues of anxiety, control, and balance seem to respond more positively to exercises involving range of movement, balance, and capacities to expand.

Strength training is likely to be accompanied by experiences of effort, occasional frustration, and some discomfort or pain. Beyond their physical benefits, resistance exercises can be used to explore meanings of and relationships with pain. In experimenting with their range of movement, for example, I encourage clients to "feel for" the differences between discomfort and pain. Sharp pain may signal potential injury. Movement that produces sharp pain should be avoided. But there will also be realms of discomfort that signal a gentle opening of old or tight boundaries. In resistance (strength) and endurance (aerobic) exercises, the pain at the edges of exertion and eventual exhaustion can be instructive. I am particularly interested in the sensations clients interpret as pain and the meanings that they assign to hurting. Do they express denial or self-criticism about their current physical limits? Not all pain is the same, and much of the difference lies in its meaning. Delayed-onset muscle soreness (DOMS)—the soreness that is felt 12–48 hours after an exercise session—is experienced by some as a nuisance and by others as a welcome sign of their hard work. All embodiment exercises are fundamentally engagements with one's edges, and such engagements are central dimensions of a person's lifestyle.

The bottom line is that strength is biologically important, and that clients should be encouraged to exercise regularly. They should begin where they are. The client who cannot perform an unassisted sit-up can at least learn to appreciate the muscles involved in the movement that they are attempting. A client who cannot touch his toes from a standing position can usually touch his knees, and that is an honorable starting point. The client who cannot perform a push-up—even from his knees—can at least *feel* the muscles that will need to be developed to do one. The goal is to become aware of bones, muscles, and joints. These are the "hardware" of our being, the essence of our physical structure and its marvelous capacities for movement. Even though we are much more than machines (levers, fulcrums, and such), we are wise to honor the mechanical realities of our physical existence. We are wise to serve respectfully the body that so richly serves our consciousness.

Rhythm

Life involves cyclic repetitions, some of which are harmonic and others that are not. Our pulse and our breathing are perhaps the most familiar rhythms of being, but there are many others. I encourage clients to seek out those rhythms, and to move to them as they can. Walking is probably the single most beneficial form of human movement, and it is a wonderful expression of rhythm. One can "power walk"[16] or stroll and derive valuable benefits from both. A 5-minute walk has more consistent positive effects on mood than a candy bar, a cigarette, or a cup of coffee. Mood researcher Robert Thayer has aptly remarked that knowing this does not automatically result in frequent brief walks. He and his colleagues know the benefits of walking, and they must still be creative in finding ways to motivate (literally "move") themselves off their butts. Besides its physical health benefits, walking can offer a meditative rhythm that is soothing. This rhythm is also conducive to creative imagery and thought, and is therefore particularly apt for process-level work in therapy. When it is possible, I invite my clients to go for a walk, and the rhythm of our coordinated movement becomes an expression of much that is going on inside us and between us. Therapists such as Kate Hays actually join their clients for therapeutic runs and workouts, and I believe this is a creative venture with considerable promise.[17]

Music is also a welcome source of rhythm and a universal expression of emotion. The musical memories tape is a reminder of this. I encourage clients to explore and enjoy both familiar and new music. When appropriate, I may give them a copy of music that I enjoy or believe might be interesting to them. I often have soft instrumental music playing as background during sessions. When clients request music from me, it is often a request for information about the music that was playing during our session.

> I don't know why I had to have that music, but I went to the mall on the way home and bought that CD. I kept playing it over and over that evening, and I felt calm. Maybe I felt connected with you or with that zone I get into when we're on a good run in a session. After the kids went to

bed I turned the lights off and cleared some floor space in the living room. At first I thought I was just going to stretch to the music but—I'm embarrassed to tell you this—I ended up dancing! I don't dance! But I did! Very slow movements, totally spontaneous, maybe like a ballet. It felt so good.

This is not an uncommon report, and I encourage clients to explore slow movements to music. In the privacy of their own living space, I suggest that they put on music that is rhythmic. The kind of music is less important than its invitation to move. For some, that invitation will require a "back beat," such as that made famous by early rock and roll. If you find yourself spontaneously tapping your fingers or feet to the tempo, it is a good candidate. Likewise with music that invites slow, fluid movements. Many people assume that dancing is something one does with the feet, but it can involve only a small body part (e.g., a single finger) or the whole body. Spontaneous, improvisational, or creative dance is a wonderful means of reducing stress. In a recent study completed by Margo Wade Walsh, Shelley Cushman, and myself, weekly dance sessions were associated with significant decreases in negative affect and substantial increases in self-esteem and general well-being (Figure 7.2).

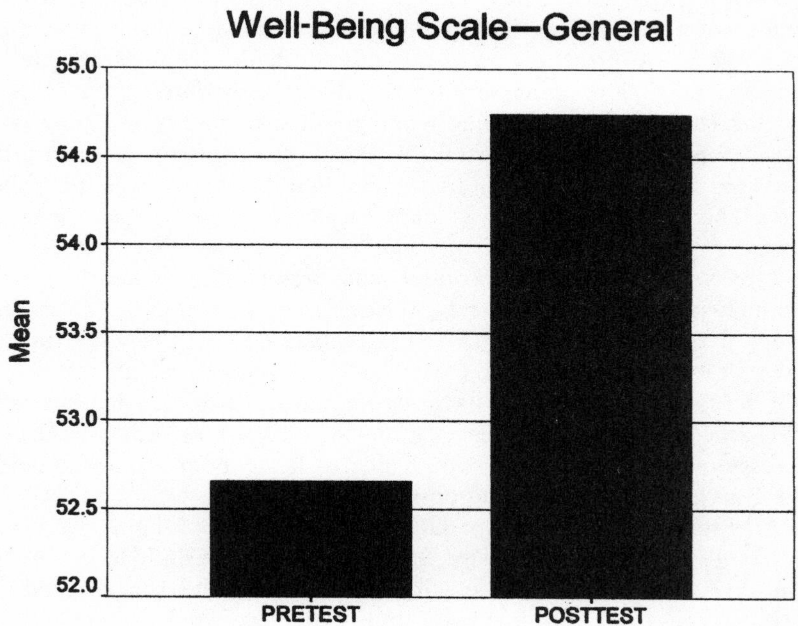

FIGURE 7.2. Measures of well-being before and after a course in expressive dance. Reprinted by permission of the authors.

To dance is to move in an energetic flow that reflects the dynamics of life. It is a healthy expression of the rhythms that are part of our human nature. As constructivist Walter Freeman and others have documented, our nervous systems seek and celebrate such rhythms.[18] Dance is a fitting metaphor for what we do in life, as well as in psychotherapy.[19] Whether we coordinate well (e.g., with others) is less important than whether we move to the drummer that we hear—a drummer who ultimately expresses our own rhythm of being. And, as Ram Dass likes to remind us, the object of the dance is not to finish; the object of the dance is to dance.

Touch

Touch is basic to human experience. There are all sorts of explanations for why this should be the case. Our skin develops from the same layer of fetal tissue as does our nervous system (our brain and spinal chord). Indeed, as Ashley Montagu has argued, the skin *is* our external nervous system.[20] Research has shown that newborns who are touched—stroked, cuddled, hugged—are generally healthier and more likely to engage with their worlds than are infants who were not touched.[21] Recovery from injuries and surgery can be accelerated by health care professionals who offer even subtle forms of physical contact (e.g., a soft touch of the forearm or shoulder, a reassuring squeeze of the hand, etc.). Massage has many benefits, and they are not just physiological. We long to be touched, and this is a natural desire. But it also presents one of the most difficult dilemmas for psychotherapists. Our clients often want more than the symbolic contact of an empathic listener. At times, they want physical reassurances. They want physical contact and bodily gestures of caring. We tell them that what they want is natural and healthy, but that it should not come from us (their therapists). This double-message was made very clear to me by one of my first clients.

Amy was a 35-year-old woman who presented with multiple problems, intense anxiety, and a desire "to learn how to cry again." In our early sessions, I tried to be respectful of her request and, at the same time, to convey a message that trying to cry—much like trying to relax or to sleep—might actually become an obstacle to the natural surrendering processes that characterize such experiences. Amy was persistent, however, and in one session she asked me if I would like to hear about the last time she cried. I invited her to elaborate on that memory.

Amy related that she was perhaps 5 years old when it happened. There was a large tree in their backyard, and she had been forbidden to climb in it. But it was an inviting old tree, with sprawling branches that reached into the sky and easy access to its lowest limbs. One day, Amy ventured into its lowest perches; she was then drawn to inch her way into higher and higher branches. A novice climber, Amy miscalculated the strength of a young limb and, when it broke, she fell to the ground. When she hit the hard earth below, Amy suffered a compound fracture of her forearm. Stunned and startled, she saw the blood gushing out where bone had broken through her skin.

Amy picked herself up and rushed into the house screaming. Her father was in the kitchen, and he reacted to her screaming and her broken arm with an angry tirade.

"God damn it! I told you not to climb that tree! Now look what you've done!" He quickly and gruffly wrapped her bleeding forearm with a dish towel and pushed her toward the garage.

"Now we will have to go to the hospital, and it will cost a lot of money. You are getting what you deserve for disobeying." He literally threw her into the front seat and began the drive to the hospital. When the blood had soaked through the towel, he yelled at her for the stains that he would have to clean off the car's upholstery. Amy could not help but cry.

"Shut up!" he shouted. "You brought this on yourself, and we'll have no cry babies in this family!"

Amy related this entire story in an almost monotonic tone, with her eyes focused on her hands and the floor. I found it painful to listen to her story. When she finished and looked at me, I had tears in my eyes.

Amy saw this and was startled. "Are you crying for me?" I felt embarrassed. I tacitly assumed that it was unprofessional to cry in front of a client.

Caught off guard and out of role, I said, "It is painful to hear what you went through . . . how your father treated you." At this moment, a tear ran down my cheek. I moved to wipe it away, but it seemed to trigger something in her. Amy buried her face in her hands and began to weep. It was as if a dam had broken, and she was flooded with years of unwept tears. She cried and cried, sobbing loudly and letting strands of mucous from her nose pour through her hands. I began to cry with her. We caught glimpses of one another as we both cried for several minutes, taking turns pulling facial tissues from the box on my desk and wiping our noses. Then, in a moment of trying to catch a breath, one of us "snorted" like a pig—"Schnagghh!" At that sound, we looked at each other's reddened faces and began to laugh. For several more minutes, we alternated between laughing and crying, passing the box of tissues between us.

Amy and I were near the end of the session, and our crying and laughing began to subside, like the whimpers of a frightened child who has been reassured. Finally, we composed ourselves, and it was time for Amy to leave. I stood up to walk her to the door. We had shared an incredibly powerful and intimate transition, and I wasn't sure what to say. At the door, and much to my surprise, Amy said, "There is no way I am leaving here today without a hug." Her vocal tone was jubilant and grateful, but I had never hugged a client before. My face apparently signaled my awkwardness, as did my body.

"My God!" Amy exclaimed. "You're *not* comfortable with that, are you?"

I felt very embarrassed. I muttered something like "Well, it would be new territory for me."

Amy was again perplexed, yet I think she enjoyed seeing this other, very human side of me. "But you are always telling me to embrace my feelings, good and bad, and to let myself express them . . . " Her voice trailed off as she looked into my eyes, which must have looked very frightened and unsure. We looked at each other for a few silent seconds, and then I heard myself say, "Yes . . . well . . . it is a lot easier to talk about some things than to do them."

Amy chuckled, and I smiled sheepishly. It was a powerful and intimate moment for each of us. Then she said, "Look. I know the boundaries. I just feel very grateful to you." I'm sure I looked down and away from her gaze. She was being much more courageous than I was able to manage. And she followed with "So, what do you think? Should we give it a try?" I said, "OK," and we hugged. It was not the best of hugs, but it felt good. After that, we hugged at the end of every session, and hugging became a more frequent aspect of my therapy. Like so many clients, Amy unexpectedly stretched me beyond my comfortable routines and familiar boundaries.

The problem for us therapists, of course, is professional boundaries. We can hug and hold and touch in reassuring ways, but we cannot responsibly allow our physical contact to move toward erotic or romantic realms. Psychotherapy is an intimate relationship in and of itself. The realm of touch—any kind of touch—is often automatically associated with sexuality in some cultures. To combine these two may be risking a synergy that can be volatile.

So what should we do? Entire volumes are now being devoted to this dilemma.[22] I do not pretend to have a perfect algorithm for whether, when, and how to touch clients or be touched by them. Much of it will remain a uniquely personal judgment call, and good judgment is a lifelong learning course. I am now much more attuned to subtle touch signals to and from my clients.[23] I am more comfortable with hugging and appropriate physical expressions, and I am more direct with those few clients who exceed my boundaries. Moreover, I encourage my clients to recognize their own needs for touching and being touched. I suggest that they pay attention to those needs in their ongoing relationships with their own bodies, with their life partners, and with their pets. For clients who have become relatively detached from their bodily experience, touch and movement are two of the most powerful avenues of reconnection. In teaching clients literally to get in touch with touch, I have found it invaluable to collaborate with the licensed massage therapists in my community.

Members of the American Massage Therapy Association (AMTA) abide by an ethics code patterned after that of the American Psychological

Association (APA), and—in my experience—they are less likely to attempt to offer psychotherapy in the process of their professional services. By coordinating with licensed massage therapists who confine their services to massage, I feel that I have been able to serve many clients better. This has often required, I might add, my becoming a temporary client of the massage therapist, if only to assess his or her style of administering services. Because I strongly recommend massage in the self-care of therapists (Chapter 11), this is hardly a sacrifice on my part. The point here is that our clients are often sorely in need of being touched in ways that stimulate their circulation, their sensory awareness, and their overall sense of being embodied. Clients who have been physically or sexually abused may particularly benefit from work with licensed massage therapists who are sensitive to clients' histories and willing to work at their individual paces of development. By coordinating with other health professionals, I believe that we can serve the needs of such clients better.

Voice

The last of the five dimensions of embodiment is voice. By "voice" I mean expression in general, but with special emphasis on vocalization. Clients come to us to give voice to their struggles, and human memory for voices is extremely powerful. Milton Erickson used to tell his clients, "My voice will go with you," and it did.[24] Our clients' voices also remain with us, along with their stories. I here forgo a review of the literature on vocalization in psychotherapy. Suffice it to say that the quantity of utterances is far less important than their emotional expressiveness. Vocal abilities probably evolved primarily to serve the expression and social communication of feelings. Although words may serve to convey some of those feelings, even the best chosen words express less than their intonation in sound. This is one of the limitations of the written word. Written transcripts of what is said in therapy reveal far less than what is expressed audibly and felt. This fact is apparent in studies that "mask" (obscure) the actual words but retain the vocal intonations of clients. Expert raters can identify the emotional tone of what was said, for example, even if it is in an unfamiliar language. How the sounds are made makes a big difference.[25]

My first experience with encouraging a client to find her voice occurred early in my career. Margo, a mild-mannered business woman, had contacted me for help with her anxiety. She was so soft-spoken that I frequently had to ask her to repeat what she had just said, because I had not heard it. In one session, she was describing her frustrations with her husband, and she ended her account with the phrase "I was so angry, I wanted to scream."

"Why didn't you?" I asked. She looked puzzled. In the process of recounting her frustration, she had become more animated and expressive. I continued, "Are you feeling some of that same frustration now?" She nodded a "yes." I said, "Why don't you scream now?" Margo was flustered. "I couldn't . . . not here." We were, after all, in an office building, and her scream might have startled some neighbors. But I made arrangements with a colleague before our next session for us to visit a speech and hearing laboratory. It had a soundproof booth that could contain just about any sound. With Margo's permission, I invited her to recall the frustrating scene with her husband and to give voice to her feeling. The first sound to emerge from her was more of a squeak than a yell. With very little coaching, however, Margo soon blasted out a whole-body scream that silenced both of us for several seconds. "Wow!" I said, and she smiled proudly. She had never yelled like that before, and it felt good.

I encourage clients to explore the dimension of their own voice. Sometimes we do this in a session. I may ask them to repeat something they have said and to focus on what they feel as they sound out the words. Because most clients do not have access to a soundproof chamber for yelling, I recommend that they use the next best option: a car with all the windows closed. My only caution on *car screaming* is safety. Intense screaming can strain the vocal chords and evoke strong emotions. On the other hand, this exercise is often stress reducing and cathartic. As one client noted, it also alters perceptions of other drivers. He had seen another solo driver apparently yelling at the top of his lungs and smiled to himself at the thought that this might be another of my clients.

For individuals who seem reluctant to express themselves, I may recommend voice lessons or a simple exercise I call *vowel movements*. The latter involves pronouncing the vowels very slowly and loudly with exaggerated movements of the mouth, tongue, and face. It is frequently used as a warm-up exercise for actors before a stage performance. Each vowel should take several seconds to pronounce, and it should be repeated several times, with an exploratory playfulness or intentional dramatization. The same sound can assume different meanings and feelings depending on how it is produced and presented. I also recommend practicing guttural productions (e.g., short and prolonged grunts) that are expressive. One exercise that can be done to emphasize this is a 2-minute *sound exchange* in session. For maximal appreciation of the emotional dimension of sound, I recommend that this exercise be done with the eyes closed or the gaze lowered. The main rule in the exercise is not to use the tongue or lips to form words. All sounds are to come from the throat only. I may begin with an inquiring "Hmmm?" The sounds that can be generated are obviously difficult to express in print, yet they are quite expressive and diverse. They include sounds similar to a menacing growl, a pleading-puppy "Please," an indignant "Hmf," and so on. Exercises such as the sound exchange are often accompanied by giggles or laughter. The goal, of course, is to more deeply appreciate the role of vocal intonation in self-expression.

Voices are also wonderful instruments of play. I encourage humming, whistling, baby talk, impersonations, and singing along with a favorite vocalist. My daughter and I play a game of *expressive gibberish*. The only rule is that we never pronounce a real word as we take turns speaking sincere nonsense. With animated facial expressions and hand gestures, we carry on conversations that have no word content but lots of emotional messaging. This can be fun to do in the presence of a friend who doesn't know the game. Another game we like to play is to substitute sounds. The "r" and "l" sounds can be softened with a "w" sound, and "f" can take the place of "th." This results in some laughter-inducing lines such as "We fwee kings of owient awe" and "Now I way me down to sweep." Laughter is itself one of the most enjoyable of vocal experiences.

The healing potential of laughter is legendary, and laughter is more than tension relief. Laughter and joy are momentary expansions that create openings. As noted earlier in the anecdote about Amy, the boundaries between laughing and crying are flexible. Indeed, specialists in *laughing meditation* are careful to note this in their instructions.[26] Interestingly, such meditation does not use jokes to induce laughter. Rather, laughter is encouraged by first performing preliminary exercises in relaxation, whole-body stretching, release breathing and yawning, and short breaths with "ha" sounds on the exhalation. In a group setting, the beginning laughter of one person often becomes a releaser for laughter in others. The process is allowed to flow naturally, without force, and laughter and crying may intermingle.

The power of collective voice is awesome. Whether as spectators (e.g., in an audience) or participants (e.g., choirs, choral groups, chant groups), there is an emotional amplification and deepening that accompanies shared vocalization. A recent example of this was my discovery of the Glide Memorial Church services in the Tenderloin district of San Francisco. I was visiting some friends who took me there for a Sunday morning service. The congregation ranged from homeless "street people" to movie stars, and the choir was accompanied by a five-piece jazz ensemble. There was standing room only, which was just as well, because we spent much of the service standing, holding hands with strangers, and singing. When we weren't singing, the choir was, and their performances (solo and collective) were simply majestic. My host, who had been a professional singer, said that she had tried to join the choir. Her application was declined despite her vocal talents, however. All Glide choir members must be former alcoholics, drug addicts, pimps, pushers, or prostitutes. This little bit of information gave me goose bumps (or, as another spiritual friend prefers, "God bumps"). It was amazing to feel the joy and gratitude in their songs and to realize the source from which they came.

I often ask my clients questions such as "How often do you laugh? Cry?", and "What makes you laugh? Cry?" I encourage them to explore their personal sources of humor and pathos. Once again, the specific source is less important than the process. All of the techniques discussed in this chapter are invitations to open toward a participation in one's processes of experiencing. I began by discussing meditation as a private excursion into the looms of inner organizing. Embodiment exercises invite other levels of awareness and attention. In the realms of touch and voice, we are drawn toward the boundaries of our physical being and the embrace of our inevitable connections with others. The techniques described in Chapter 8 continue this progression of greater challenges in the exploration of process-level work.

NOTES

1. Kunitz (1995, p. 11).
2. Sean Mahoney, unpublished poem, "Journal."
3. This is particularly true of some dramatic shifts, called "quantum changes," which characterize sudden psychological transformations (Miller & C'de Baca, 1994, 2001).
4. This illustration is not an artificial creation from a perception laboratory. It came from a real-life observation by Swiss naturalist L. A. Necker while he was studying crystals under a microscope. He described the phenomenon in a letter to a friend in 1832 (Mahoney, 1991) and noted that one can influence one's perception by strategies of selective attention.
5. Almaas (1988); Batchelor (1994); Brussat and Brussat (1996); Chödrön (1997); Garvey (1985); Goleman (1988); Grof and Grof (1989); Harding (1961); Harner (1982); Haruki, Ishii, and Suzuki (1996); Huxley (1944); Kazantzakis (1960); Kenny and Delmonte (1986); Kopp (1972); Kornfield (1993); Leder (1997); Leonard and Murphy (1995); Levine (1979); Merton (1968); Muller (1992); O'Donahue (1997, 1998); Ram Dass (1970, 1971); Russell (1992); Schwartz (1995); Taylor (1995); Vaughan (1979, 1986, 1995); Walsh (1990, 1999); Watts (1963, 1966); Wilber (1998, 1999).
6. Pope and Singer (1978).
7. For further information on vipassana (mindfulness) meditation, see the Inquiring Mind (P.O. Box 9999, Berkeley, CA 94709).
8. I recommend Bob Anderson's (1980) book on stretching as perhaps the best single resource on how to stretch safely. For other resources, see Leonard (1995) and Leonard and Murphy (1995). For philosophical discussions of the absence of the body from western scholarship, see Berman (1981, 1989), Johnson (1987), Lakoff and Johnson (1999), Leder (1990), Levin (1985), Merleau-Ponty (1942, 1962), and Stolorow, Atwood, and Orange (2002).
9. Ackerman (1990); Antonovsky (1979); Bakal (1999); Barnard and Brazelton (1990); Berman (1981, 1985); Bermúdez, Marcel, and Eilan (1995); Chodorow (1991); Friedman and Moon (1997); Gallop (1988); Gavin (1988); Griffith and Griffith (1994); Hanna (1970); Harre (1991); Hays (1999); D. H. Johnson (1994); M. Johnson (1987); Levin (1985, 1988); Marrone (1990); Merleau-Ponty (1942, 1962); Minton (1989); Montagu (1978); Nuland (1997); Ronen

(1999); Roth (1997); Van Raalte and Brewer (1996); Weidong, Sasaki, and Haruki (2000); Wendell (1996).

10. Cassilleth (1998); Gavin (1988); Knaster (1996); Leonard (1995); Leonard and Murphy (1995); Minton (1989); Murphy (1992).
11. Knaster (1996).
12. Good resources on Olympic weightlifting are Drechsler (1998) and Kono (2001).
13. In the United States, contact USA Weightlifting, One Olympic Plaza, Colorado Springs, CO 80909-5784 (*www.usaweightlifting.org*).
14. U.S. Olympic Committee (1999, p. 14).
15. During the 2001 World Masters Championships, I reflected on such joys: "Years ago someone asked me why I bother to lift weights. It is hard work, there is no money in it, and it seems stupid, they said, to throw heavy things over your head if you don't have to. I don't know why I do it except that it's fun and healthy, and I find it both grounding and inspiring at the same time. When I move with grace at the very edges of my abilities, I experience a fusion of fear and joy. In that fleeting moment when the barbell is on its way up and I am making my leap of faith to a humble position beneath it, I feel connected with everything—the platform, the center of the earth, the center of me, and the vastness of everything above. As I come up out of that bottom position with the weight over my head, I lift my eyes and arms to life itself and I feel as if I am lifting heavy loads off oppressed hearts. It feels like I'm lifting more than weights; it feels like I'm lifting spirits."
16. Power walking involves a faster pace, exaggerated arm swings, and optional wrist or hand weights to add to the challenge. Ankle weights should never be worn for extended periods of walking, because they can hyperextend the knee joint.
17. Obviously there are risks as well as benefits. There is little question that relationship issues can become pronounced and expressed in terms of competitiveness. The added physiological arousal of therapy in the midst of a workout is, in my opinion, a likely benefit. See Kate Hays's (1999) discussions of these and other dimensions of combined exercise and therapy sessions.
18. Freeman (1995).
19. Chodorow (1991); Ram Dass (1970); Wiener (1999).
20. Montagu (1978).
21. Barnard and Brazelton (1990).
22. Smith, Clance, and Imes (1998).
23. The subtlety of such signals is worth emphasizing. In recent refinements of understanding attachment patterns between parents and children, for example, levels of comfort with bodily contact are very important (Karen, 1998).
24. For a personal anecdote on how enduring his message was, see my tribute to Milton Erickson (Mahoney, 1997a).
25. For a metaphorical analysis of the role of voice in personal empowerment, see Belenky et al. (1986).
26. For resources, contact Dhyan Sutorius, Director of the Centre in Favour of Laughter, Secretariat: Jupiter 1007, NL-1115 TX Duivendrecht, the Netherlands.

CHAPTER 8

Drama, Fantasy, Dream Work, and Stream of Consciousness

We are all always in process, always actively participating in the processes of paying attention and making meaning. Although we cannot dictate them, we can influence the processes that influence us. The techniques already discussed have been aimed at centering, seeing patterns, and witnessing processes in action. Meditation and movement exercises allow valuable opportunities to observe and feel what is going on inside us. The techniques discussed in this chapter are more explicitly experimental in the sense that they ask clients to risk new experiences. New experiences are often emotionally intense. A separate book could be written on the nature of emotionality and constructive ways of working with emotions in psychotherapy. Fortunately, such a book has recently been written.[1] Even when strong emotions are not the motivations for seeking psychotherapy, the experience of change is itself emotional (Chapter 10). Therapists need to be versed not only in theories of emotionality but also in their real-life experiencing.

The techniques described in this chapter presume a deeper level of attachment, trust, and engagement in the therapeutic relationship. Problem and pattern levels of therapeutic work tend to have a built-in boundary or separation. Problems may be externalized or defined as separate annoyances. Patterns can be seen as abstract regularities. Process-level work is experience-near. One is working closer to the engines that are generating activity. In this sense, at least, there is also more potential power in process-level work. Such work also carries a greater burden of risk in that it may "perturb" a client's core ordering processes (COPs) in ways that are difficult to anticipate. Increased power implies increased potential for both good and harm. More powerful and "deep structure" techniques carry with them the risk of presenting challenges that overtax a client's current capacities. These exercises move well beyond a simple application of technology. They require courage and creativity. The making and remaking of personal and emotional meaning becomes a primary focus, and the process of being actively engaged in one's life choices becomes paramount. These process exercises can demand quite a bit from both client and therapist, and both individuals are often changed by what emerges.

I cannot offer a simple rule for when to offer which of the following techniques. In my experience, clients often give ample clues about the directions in which they are developing, and I try to respond sensitively with encouragement. If a client repeatedly uses the word "if," for example, she may be signaling an interest in exploring "what if" and "as if" exercises. At some point in our interaction, I may spontaneously suggest that we enact a role play of her hypothetical situation. Or a client may arrive at a session with fragments of a dream he had the night before. He did not plan to have the dream, and I may not have expected to do dream work in that session. So be it. Such is the complexity of our lives as dynamic developing systems. Stream of consciousness work may be a natural sequel to meditation and dream work. "Streaming," as I have come to call it, may also be a powerful means of helping clients who feel stuck. With each of these techniques, I am careful to note clients' initial reactions, and I pace our excursions into new and unknown realms. We explore a new possibility and then—again and again—come back to centering exercises. We experiment and then return to a home base. By remaining attuned to clients' needs for balance, I can minimize some of the risks involved and optimize clients' chances for developmental progression.

ROLE PLAYING "AS IF"

Role playing is a valuable means of exploring spontaneous processes of self-organization. The dramatic enactment of a past or possible challenge can stimulate the same emotional patterns as the actual occurrence. When done in a safe and experimental context, such enactments can also provide valuable opportunities for learning. This was the core idea in J. L. Moreno's psychodrama,[2] which became an elaborate theory of personal and group psychotherapy. Moreno saw the power of role enactments to change people's patterns of experiencing. We harness this power whenever we ask a client to rehearse something in our presence. A client may be playing the role of himself in an anticipated challenge. Or he may be playing the role of someone he is trying to understand. Moreno saw that personal and collective realms are interwoven in the act of acting.

> Every individual lives in a world which looks entirely private and personal to him, and in which he partakes in a number of private roles. But the millions of private worlds overlap in large portions. The larger portions which overlap are truly collective elements. Only the minor portions are private and personal. Every role is therefore a fusion of private and collective elements.[3]

George Kelly was interested in theater and influenced by Moreno's works.[4] Indeed, the technique most commonly associated with Kelly's personal construct theory is "fixed-role therapy," which is a flexibly structured experiment in self-organization and social interaction.[5]

In Kelly's fixed-role therapy, the client is first asked to write a third-person *character sketch* of himself. It is a sketch that might have been generated by an intimate friend who knows the client extremely well. The sketch is written as if the client were going to be portrayed as the principal character in a play. "The object is to see how he structures himself."[6] After the client submits this sketch, the therapist studies it and prepares what is called an *enactment sketch*. This is a character sketch of a fictional person who shares many characteristics with the client but is different in at least one important dimension. The fictional character is thus not the client's psychological opposite, but he is importantly different. The difference may be intentionally drawn from the client's self-portrait, but it is more often within a dimension that the client has not even mentioned in his self-characterization.

Part of the genius of this technique, I believe, is how it is presented to the client. He is asked to read the alternate (enactment) sketch in session, and his reaction is closely monitored. The client is asked two questions: (1) whether he feels this other character seems genuine, and (2) whether this person sounds like someone he would like to know. If his response to both questions is "yes," then the client is asked to make an important, time-limited commitment in the form of a secret personal experiment. The experiment is to act "as if" he were this other character for a few weeks. Kelly stresses that once the client agrees to the experiment, it is important that it begin immediately—in that session. He reports that it is common for therapists to feel at least as strange as do clients in their new form of interaction. Importantly, the client does not inform anyone—including his spouse—about the experiment. Clients' desires to share that secret with their friends or spouses are natural expressions of their anxiety or confusion in a novel situation. However, Kelly argues that the enactment would become simply an exercise in acting if others were aware of its temporary and pretend nature. When the client receives feedback that he seems to be acting differently or strangely, this is construed to mean that he is successful in his enactment.

A client is asked to pretend that his own identity has gone on a brief vacation and, in its place, this alternate character has materialized. He is asked to try is to enact as best he can "twenty-four hours a day, all that (the alternate person) might do, say, think, or even dream."[7] During this time, at least three therapy sessions per week are scheduled so that the client and therapist can rehearse the enactment of the alternate character and evaluate the impact it is having. The therapist is careful to protect and respect the integrity of the client's "real self," which is on an imaginary vacation. This avoids the resistance that might be evoked by a direct challenge to the client's identity. Nor is the alternate character presented as how the client *should* be. The enacted character is an experiment in being differently. In this temporary, "fixed role," the client rehearses for and enacts *five successive levels of social activity*: (1) interactions with a teacher or job supervisor, (2) interactions with peers, (3) interactions with a spouse or intimate other, (4) interactions with parents or their equivalents, and (5) interactions in situations involving religion or religious experience. This sequence is intended to be progressively more challenging, and therapy sessions every other day are designed to offer support and rehearsal for these increasing demands.

Eventually the client's "former self" must return and an integrative process begins. Honoring the importance of the processes that create "selfhood," the therapist emphasizes that it is this old self that should evaluate what has happened and choose which directions to go. Perhaps the client will see new possibilities in his life, and some of the patterns that were rehearsed and practiced in the form of the alternate character will be worthy of continued exploration. The goal of this entire venture—of experimenting with being a likeable, genuine, but slightly different person—is "to realize here and now that his innermost personality is something he creates as he goes along rather than something he discovers lurking in his insides or has imposed upon him from without."[8]

Kelly's fixed-role technique is an elaborately designed personal experiment with graduated challenges and inevitable surprises. It requires the client to make a commitment to doing more than talking about how to change himself. He is challenged to be creative, yet the entire exercise is orchestrated such that he has generous support and a feasible time frame. Old patterns of activity are respected rather than criticized, and it is the old and familiar sense of self that chooses what to incorporate from the experiment. The therapist is challenged to join the client in acting as if the client were temporarily a somewhat different person who is genuinely likable.

Although I rarely embark on something as elaborately structured as Kelly's fixed-role therapy, I employ role playing quite frequently with my clients and psychotherapy trainees. Sometimes it involves just a brief enactment of a scene from their life—an unsatisfying interaction with a friend, an upcoming job interview, an attempt to communicate something that they fear will lead to negative repercussions. We often go through several tries or "takes" (and I encourage clients to think of mistakes as "mis-takes"). Sometimes my clients come up with the ideas for our role plays. Other times, I surprise them with a challenge they had not expected. If they are thrown off balance, it provides an opportunity to practice their responses to the unexpected and their centering skills. Needless to say, they also provide me with many such opportunities.

With some clients, I also occasionally suggest that we briefly switch roles, with them assuming my chair and I theirs. I try to enact them as I perceive them, and I later ask for their evaluation of my impersonation of them. My goal is literally to enter into their frame of experiencing as best I can, and to provide them with opportunities for stepping out of their client role and into a helping role. I have found this strategy to be useful with many clients. Even though they are asking me for suggestions and assurances about their life difficulties, clients are often excellent resources in these very domains when they can access other parts of themselves.

I remember once counseling a graduate student who was in danger of being thrown out of school because he was failing an advanced course in a very technical area. Ironically, it was not a required course for his degree; he had chosen to take it as an elective and then found himself "in over his head." Realizing that the official deadline for dropping courses was still a week away, I asked him why he didn't simply withdraw from the course. Somewhat timidly, he said, "Well, my dad taught me never to be a quitter—to always finish things that I start—and I just can't bring myself to giving up on this." He sighed heavily, perhaps signifying that he saw no honorable way out of his dilemma. "Thomas," I said, "I'd like you to try a little imagination experiment, OK?" He nodded assent. "I want you to imagine that it is 25 or 30 years from now, and that you have gotten married and, in fact, you and your wife have a son. He phones you one day from grad school and says, 'Dad, I'm in trouble. I'm failing this course that I don't really have to take, and I am miserable, but I don't want to be a quitter.' What would you say to your son?" Thomas stood up abruptly, shook my hand, and said, "Thanks—I think I can make it to the Registrar's office before they close."

Role plays can be helpful in rehearsing for a life challenge, but they can also add resolution to situations that are physically difficult. Through role play, clients may be able to express strong feelings to a parent or life partner who is no longer alive or available for dialogue. Although other rituals and techniques can be used, I have found that the enactment of a brief reunion can have powerful healing value for clients. Role plays can also challenge the boundaries of our everyday reality and play with the complexity of our processes. One particularly powerful role play took place in a session with Ron Kurtz, the talented Hakomi and body therapist.[9] His client was troubled by the conflicting demands of her life responsibilities and the messages that she had internalized from her parents. These messages included statements such as "We only wanted what was good for you" and "We always gave you everything." In a masterful coordination, Kurtz arranged for two assistants to play the voices inside this client. Their task was to repeat these messages over and over again as she was trying to describe her feelings to Kurtz. The assistants sat behind her and maintained a bombardment of *sotto voce* parental messages. Eventually feeling overwhelmed by these demands, the client suddenly shouted, "Shut up! Shut up all of you!" and simply cried her heart out. Slowly and sensitively, as she regained center, the impossibility of the situation was acknowledged. It was a powerful demonstration of how assistants can be used to play parts of ourselves (much like Moreno had intended) and help to clarify the conflicts we are trying to resolve.

There is much more to say about role playing than I can possibly fit into these few pages. I believe that role playing is an extremely valuable technique for helping the movement from the realm of "just words"—talking about life problems—to the realms of feeling and action, albeit in hypothetical situations. Courage (action in the presence of fear), creativity, and imagination are at the heart of role playing. Exploring Vaihinger's "philosophy of as if" and Vico's fascination with "fantasia," the realm of "pretend" is the realm of "pre-real." Indeed, the word "pretend" originally meant "to lean in anticipation," and children do it everyday, enjoying the sense that they are preparing themselves for the realities they will encounter when they grow up. Grown-ups can also benefit from such creative and imaginative enactments.

FANTASY AND DREAM WORK

Fantasy and daydreaming are also realms of hypothetical being. Remember that possibility and freedom are central themes in constructivism. These themes are multifaceted. Vico emphasized the role of "fantasia" in our experience of ourselves and our worlds. Kant stressed the power of patterns (categories) of thought in the process of experiencing particulars. Vaihinger wrote about the necessity and power of fictions in human living. We are always living "as if" our ways of making sense of the world really do make sense. This issue is not a simple one, although critics of constructivism have often presented it as if it were (Appendix A). For the moment, what is important for constructive practice is the fact that we live from (not just "in") dynamic creative processes. We spend a large part of our lives remembering and anticipating. These processes may take many forms, including regretting, resenting, longing, worrying, hoping, and planning. Chronic patterns of distress often reflect what I call "ruts of being"—deeply practiced habits. The depressed person may not be able to anticipate anything positive, for example, and her memories may be mostly negative. The perennially angry person finds offense in everyday annoyances and may selectively remember and expect such experiences. And so on. The point is that we often live our lives primarily in these habitual ruts, yet there are ample signs of other possibilities. These possibilities are apparent in our fantasy life and in our dreams.

Attempts to understand human consciousness often divide it into kinds. Sleeping, dreaming, and being awake are common categories. The more we learn about ourselves, however, the more we realize the limitations of these three categories. Being awake is not a single or simple process, for example. This is acknowledged when people joke about not being fully awake until midday or after several cups of coffee. Research has shown that we can, if fact, dream while we are awake, and that we can be partially awake—or at least aware—when we are dreaming. Even without meditative practice, many of us are aware that there is much going on inside us all the time, and simultaneously at different levels. We may be on autopilot while performing a familiar task such as walking or driving a car. At the same time, however, we may be reminiscing, making plans, or fantasizing. Fantasy is a normal and healthy human activity, and it is among our most private conscious experiences.

I believe that sleeping dreams, daydreams, and fantasies are creative action patterns that contribute to our life quality as well as life changes. Ethel Person has also noted this synergy, and she has commented on our widespread reluctance to discuss our fantasy life:

> Why are we willing, even eager, to share our dreams, but determined to hoard and hide our fantasies? One reason is that we feel more responsible for daydreams than for night dreams. Night dreams come unbidden, but conscious fantasy, because we conjure it up and are aware of manipulating it to suit ourselves, implicates us very directly. In some ways, fantasies seem more revealing of the self—its appetites or obscure, quirky desires—than dreams or even the most intimate narratives of the lived life.[10]

Perhaps this is why I often find myself asking clients about their dreams before I ask them about their fantasy lives. The sharing of dreams presumes a level of trust, of course, but an even deeper level of self-awareness and trust is required for fantasy work.

This book is not the place to review the extensive literature on human dreaming. My synopsis of that literature is terse: Dreams and dreaming are important. We don't fully understand the why and how of dreaming, but it is clear that dreams are more than a window on the engines of our consciousness.[11] People can be changed by their dreams, and dreams often reflect current life changes. Dream functions seem to include nonlinear and nonlogical processes that connect and transcend past, present, and possible experiences. Dream processes may be viewed as

> creating a balance between the familiar and the novel, between activity and passivity, between stimulation and relaxation . . . providing a setting, night after night, where we perceive ourselves as free of social duties, of critical self-evaluations, and are able to deal creatively with waking experience. Dreams permit us to enjoy a sort of second existence, . . . to engage in novel experience, . . . to deal with the world quite playfully.[12]

Sandor Ferenczi called dreaming "the workshop of evolution," and there is evidence that the three basic processes of biological evolution are also apparent in dreaming (i.e., variation, selection, and retention). The recent surge of interest in dynamic systems theory (chaos and complexity) has invited some particularly creative thinking about dreaming. Stanley Palombo, for example, has suggested that dreams serve a constructive condensation function that permits a creative overlay of past and present experiences.[13] In this view, dreams reflect partially conscious activity at the edges of personal chaos.

The fuzziness of the boundaries in dreaming is apparent in the frequent experience of awakening in the midst of an emotionally intense dream and carrying its affective tone and imagery into waking consciousness. States of "in-between" can be fruitful sources of insight and invention. In his 1536 volume on emotions, the Spanish humanist Juan Luis Vives noted the possible importance of these transition states (which are now technically termed "hypnogogic" and "hypnopompic" processes). The processes of falling asleep and dreaming involve relaxing boundaries and surrendering. People for whom self-control is an issue often experience insomnia. Indeed, the need for boundaries may be part of what dreaming reflects.[14] Dream recall is aided by longer periods of sleep and gradual entries and exits from sleep. Clients who want to remember more dreams should therefore be encouraged to allow more time for sleep and to allow themselves to awaken gradually (e.g., without an alarm, or with several snooze periods). In such gentle transitions, the boundaries between dream and reality may be fuzzy, and the boundaries of self may oscillate.

This is illustrated in an experience I once had emerging from a dream during a difficult period in my life. I was living alone in a cold and remote trailer park on the edge of town. One morning, I began to awaken slowly from a dream in which I had apparently been expressing my distress to some unknown listener. I had a vague awareness of the chill of the room and the sound of winter winds outside my window. At some point in my slow emergence from the dream, my listener offered reassurance that things would be all right. I'm not sure if there were words to this message, but its tone was very measured and sure. Still in the dream, I angrily challenged these pat assurances with the question: "How do YOU know?! Who are YOU?!" The response that followed was quite clear even in my hazy half-asleepness: "I am the self *behind* the self that you think is in control." I bolted upright to a sitting position. I was literally shocked awake, and I sat in my bed for a long time wondering how such a response had emerged and what it meant.

Although dreams are usually more disguised than this example might suggest, assertions of alternate or mutilayered identity are not unusual in dreams. David Foulkes's studies of dreaming and development make it clear that identity and narrative are central features of adult dreams.[15] The self is the main character or reference point in the vast majority of dreams, and that self is often multifaceted. This is a working assumption in many forms of dream analysis, and it is particularly explicit in "gestalting" a dream.[16] When a client is asked to "become" a part of her dream or to speak from a dream image, the request is essentially one of Piagetian decentration. Had I gestalted my own dream, for example, I might have had several legitimate levels of selfhood with which I could have identified (e.g., a forlorn suffering being, a wise and compassionate being, and a self that needed to believe it was singular and in control). Constructive therapy would honor this diversity and emphasize my choices as an active agent in identifying exclusively with only one. Another example of identity and agency fuzziness occurs when dreamers move into a boundary region in which they are aware of the fact that they are dreaming. *Lucid dreaming* involves active witnessing and possible participation in the dream (e.g., choices to enter, exit, or remain in a dream, to change the direction of action in a dream, to change identity within the dream, and to recall dream details upon awakening). It is practiced in several spiritual traditions and has been extensively studied by Stephen LaBerge.[17]

How does one work with clients' dreams from a constructive viewpoint? One must do so carefully, with compassion and encouragement. The Personal Experience Report (Appendix C) asks incoming clients about their sleep quality, distressing dreams, and memories of childhood nightmares. In continuing sessions, when we are setting a flexible agenda for our meeting, I often ask clients if they have had any recent dreams that they would like to discuss. At the end of the session, I may also include a recommendation that they pay attention to any interesting dreams or fantasies and note them for possible discussion. Both of these practices are meant to convey my interest in and respect for this realm of their experiencing. As in many other realms of therapy, I am more interested in process than in content. I want to encourage clients' attunement to their inner experience, and I want to convey my belief that they have access to inner resources that can serve them well in their development.

The interpretation of dreams is a tricky process and one in which I emphasize collaboration and creativity. Where dream work most often goes awry is in the search for a single meaning. This search is aided by popular portrayals of dreams as coded messages from the unconscious. The single-meaning search is then abetted by therapists who are willing to assume the role of ultimate authorities. I view my role as more Socratic, and I believe that dreams share important dimensions with intuitive wisdom.[18] If a client asks me to interpret his dream, I am likely to ask him a series of questions. What images were most salient or puzzling? How did he feel in the dream? How does he feel as he now talks about it? What memories or associations does it evoke? What aspects of his current life were worked into the dream? Can he identify any things that might have triggered the dream? What intuitive meanings does he sense? If a client seems stuck on a dream as portending disaster in his life, I may encourage him to speculate on what might be done to avert such an event.

I do not believe every dream has a specific meaning, or that one should confine interpretation to the meanings listed in dream-image dictionaries.[19] Such dictionaries presume a universal system of meanings. Dream images may mean very different things to different people or in different dream contexts. Although recurring dreams often suggest a current life theme, isolated dreams are rarely the breakthroughs that are portrayed in movies. In my experience, it is seldom a single dream that turns the tide of personal development. More often, it is a series of dreams that precede and accompany major life changes. Palombo illustrates this progression with detailed dream reports by both clients and therapists over long periods of therapy. It would be oversimplifying to say that the dreams cause the life changes or, alternatively, that dreams only reflect those changes post hoc. What seems clear, however, is that dreams are not a realm totally separate from waking life. The organizing processes in dreams are much less constrained by space–time dimensions. Strangers appear in dreams with very high frequency, and novelty, ambiguity, and unknowns are common features. Dreams often reflect much more experimentation than waking fantasies, and it is possible that they are evolutionary "exaptations" involving exploratory activity.[20]

For more detailed treatments of working with dreams, I recommend books by Clara Hill and Jeremy Taylor.[21] Hill emphasizes that there should be a balanced respect for cognitive and emotional themes in dreams. She outlines a three-stage model of exploration, insight, and action. Exploration includes retelling the dream, tagging important images, pursuing associations, and feeling the dream's affective themes. The insight phase of this model emphasizes the client's creation of meaning in understanding the dream (e.g., relating it to triggering events, memories, associations, and parts of the self). Such meaning is rarely achieved in a sudden leap. It is more often the result of several reframings that may require shifts in tacit assumptions. When a particular understanding of the dream begins to emerge and feel appropriate, this leads toward the third stage, which is action. The client is encouraged to act on his understanding. This may be an act of fantasy (e.g., changing the outcome or circumstances of the dream) or it may involve a change in his behavior.

Taylor approaches dreaming with several important assumptions, namely, that dreams are natural processes that serve health and wholeness, that dreams reflect personal uniqueness and resourcefulness, and that dreams have multiple layers, many of which reflect our nested relationships with others and our world. He recommends dreamwork for personal and collective development, and offers practical suggestions that include drawing images of the dream, meditating or praying while focused on the dream, and writing about dream images with the added phrase "part of me."

Taylor also recommends actively encouraging a dream to elaborate itself. This can be done by journaling to the dream and inviting it to continue its story in future installments. This last exercise is noteworthy in its emphasis on engagement with the process of dreaming. Rather than simply being viewed as a means to an end (clues to a mystery of meaning), dreams can be respected as emergent processes in and of themselves.

The developmental progressions of dreams and fantasies remind me of the reconstructive processes apparent in life narratives (Chapter 6). There may be important differences in such things as criteria for coherence, but there are also parallels that resonate with constructivist themes. Over time, for example, individuals' dreams and fantasies may reflect changes in their core ordering processes. I listen for oscillations and shifts in clients' sense of who they are, what they feel capable of, and what seems possible to them. Such oscillations and shifts are also common in the spontaneous reporting of one's waking stream of consciousness.

STREAM OF CONSCIOUSNESS

In his classic *Principles of Psychology*, William James described consciousness as a dynamic stream that is always moving.[22] A stream is an apt metaphor for the continual activity of our inner life. Tapping into that stream has presented a fascinating challenge to researchers studying consciousness. How does one glimpse, let alone measure, the stream of consciousness of another person? Laboratory methods for *introspection* (literally "inner viewing") were pioneering developments when psychology differentiated itself from philosophy. Franz Brentano, Wilhelm Wundt, and others tried to measure the inner experience of external stimuli (e.g., the perceived redness of an apple). Sigmund Freud analyzed his own dreams as a means of understanding his complex reactions to the death of his father. His 1900 volume on the interpretation of dreams was the outline from which psychoanalysis emerged. It is not surprising that Freud emphasized associations in dreaming. David Hartley had formalized an impressive theory of association in 1749,[23] and Charles Darwin's cousin, Francis Galton, had introduced the first measures of word association.[24] *Word association* requires someone to give their first association to stimulus words. Jung, among others, noted the possible significance of long pauses in responding. Both Freud and Jung used the method of free association to attune themselves to their clients' consciousness. In *free association*, the individual is asked to report spontaneously everything that comes into his awareness. In doing so, of course, his awareness is likely to be influenced by the process of describing what is going on inside him. This is a recurring problem for first-person approaches to the study of consciousness.[25] During 10 years of studying people's experiences of sensory deprivation, I repeatedly encountered this Heisenberg-like paradox. My methods of measurement were modifying the very thing I was trying to measure.

My interest in stream of consciousness reports developed in my first years as a practicing therapist. I found myself frustrated with the overall state of psychological assessment available to me. There were the usual standardized tests, of course, which focused mostly on pathology, and there were a few behavioral and cognitive alternatives. I was already using self-monitoring, personal journaling, and some self-report forms aimed at identifying "negative self-talk." As my clinical and supervisory experiences developed, however, I felt that none of these was really tapping into the live dimensions of experiencing that were most important to my clients. So I reflected on the role of assessment in my work. What was its most basic purpose? What was I asking? What did I want to know? I concluded that what I wanted from assessment was a clearer sense of my clients' lived experience. And when I asked myself how I might do this, my first response was a simple one: "Ask them. Ask them what they are experiencing here, right now."

This began a series of explorations with stream of consciousness reporting, which I have discussed and illustrated elsewhere.[26] Stream of consciousness reporting is a technique intended to help clients explore and attempt to communicate inner life in the living moment. Although it shares obvious parallels with the forms of meditation discussed in Chapter 7, it is also importantly different. In silent meditation (whether motionless or moving), one need not attempt to package the experience in words and share them *in the same moment* with a witnessing other. This is quite a challenge. Our attention, when turned inward, can be very selective and restless. William James compared it to the short flights of a bird moving from branch to branch or tree to tree. Paying attention inwardly and noting the shifts in our attention are difficult tasks. Adding a live listener to whom one is reporting these efforts amplifies the challenge considerably. And the amplification is more than that involved in putting words to images and ambiguous sensations. Much of the increase in challenge lies in the interpersonal trust required, and this brings up an important issue.

I am sometimes asked what the difference is between stream of consciousness reporting and the free association method used by Freud, Jung, and others. My sense is that there are at least two important differences. First, I encourage my clients to respect their own needs for privacy. In other words, I tell my clients that they need not tell me *everything* that moves through their awareness. I explain that we all have our needs for privacy, and that the purpose of this technique is not for me to "pry" into their consciousness. The purpose is to invite them to really look at what is going on inside and to share with me—as they feel comfortable—the kinds of things that come to their attention. The emphasis is on the process of looking inward, the act of really tuning in to all the activity that flows through a living being. My encouragement that clients respect their own needs for privacy violates what Freud considered the essence of the "therapeutic contract"—that his clients reveal anything and everything that entered their consciousness, no matter how private or embarrassing.

A second, important difference between psychoanalytic free association and stream of consciousness reporting is the presumption of authority in the act of interpretation. Constructivists do not view themselves as absolute authorities on the meaning of what their clients report. When my clients ask for my interpretations or reflections on their "streaming," I generally respond with questions (e.g., "What did it remind you of?", "What feelings seemed most prevalent or important?", "How are you feeling now as we discuss this?", "What is your intuition about the experience?", "What do you hope or fear it means?"). I do not presume to have the "correct interpretation." I do not believe in a universal code of meaning for life experiences. Moreover, the interpretation of the contents seems less important than the engagement in the process. As a constructive psychotherapist, I am trying to help my clients find or create meaning in their lives. Those lives and those meanings are theirs. This is why it is important for them to practice and develop self-awareness. I view myself more as a coach than as a corrections officer or an absolute authority on the meanings they are making. The only times I offer alternative interpretations (of dreams, streams, etc.) are when clients become stuck on a negative or pathological interpretation of their experience.

As an exercise in developmental acceleration, streaming can be an extremely powerful intervention. In contrast to the centering exercises described in Chapter 4, streaming can have a temporary but strong disorganizing effect. The perturbing (or disorder-facilitating) effects of streaming may make it particularly useful for clients who have become stuck in routine patterns of experiencing. But the disorganizing effects of streaming can also be startling and frightening, and this is where the therapist's competence, confidence, and attunement become crucial. Streaming involves spontaneous reporting of living experience. There is so much going on inside us that it is impossible for words to capture all of it. This often leads to telegraphic bursts of isolated words and phrases. As this occurs, the orderly structure of language and grammar is temporarily lost. Letting go of language (or the familiar structures of sentences) can be disorienting. As these familiar organizing processes recede, the client may experience strong emotional responses. Altered states of consciousness and trance-like phenomena are not uncommon. In some stages of streaming, clients may experience dizziness, muscle tremors, mild nausea, or spontaneous bursts of laughing or crying. It is important to recognize these as natural and healthy expressions of responses to a temporary loss of order. Such responses demand sensitivity and balance on the part of the therapist. Some clients may want to withdraw from the experience, and their desire should be honored. Other clients may push themselves even harder at the edges of their abilities and need to be encouraged to throttle back on their efforts. Centering exercises are always an appropriate means for balancing the overall experience and for reassuring clients that they can repeatedly return to a sense of structure and stability.

I caution against using streaming in the absence of a strong working alliance. Streaming should not be introduced in the early sessions of therapy or when there may be insufficient time to process the experience (e.g., very late in a session or when only a few sessions remain). I do not recommend streaming as an exercise with individuals who are struggling to find an integrated sense of self or reality. Most importantly, I do not believe streaming should be used with anyone who is not skilled in centering, and who has not given his or her informed consent to experiment with the procedure. Before using this procedure with clients, I recommend that therapists first practice streaming on their own or as participants in a dyad (e.g., with their own therapist, or with a trusted peer). Confidence in working with intense emotions is a prerequisite for this depth of process work.

With these cautions in mind, however, streaming can be a very useful method that serves multiple functions. As with many other methods, I may mention streaming to clients in an early session. I present it as one of the options we have for exploring their inner world and experimenting with alternate ways of being. Some clients will ask more about it or show other signs of interest in taking a deep look inside. When I feel confident in our relationship and in their centering skills, I may suggest that we schedule a longer session (e.g., 2 hours) to explore their resonance with streaming as a technique. I describe it using James's metaphor:

> Streaming is an exercise intended to help me get a better sense of what it is like to be you. First I will ask you to relax and to set positive intentions for learning more about yourself. I will ask you to close your eyes and to pay attention to what is going on inside you from moment to mo-

> ment. You may find that there are many things going on at the same time and that they keep changing. Some may be thoughts, some sensations. There may be images and memories and mixtures. If we think of your inner life as a stream, this exercise is intended to help me understand what your stream is like today in these few minutes. I would like you to dip a bucket into your inner stream every once in a while and toss me some words as examples of what you caught in the bucket. Don't worry about making sense or how it sounds. If something feels too private to share, then keep it secret. Let's start with a brief streaming trip—perhaps 5 or 10 minutes—and then we will pause and take a break. We can always do more later if you want. Just be gentle with yourself and let yourself explore this as a little experiment in looking inside. Do you have any questions before we start?

I have used streaming with many clients over the years. Some of the most dramatic changes I have seen in clients have been after the introduction of this technique.

Let me illustrate streaming with excerpts from my work with a client named Apollo. He was himself a therapist who first contacted me after a workshop on therapist self-care (Chapter 11). He had struggled with episodes of anxiety and depression for several years. Exercise and medication had helped slightly, but he felt that they were not addressing the heart of the matter. In our earlier sessions, he had demonstrated good skills in relaxing and centering himself. He expressed impatience, however, at our pace and asked if there weren't some things we could do to move him "out of his rut." I described streaming and emphasized that it was both experimental and experiential. I wanted to convey the demands of this level of process work, and I wanted Apollo to be clear about the fact that it could open a Pandora's box of possible directions. My presentation was similar to the one recommended by Jim Bugental for such ventures.[27] Apollo joked about it being time to "meet his demons on the couch," and we scheduled a special session for his first exploration of streaming.

He was understandably apprehensive when he arrived for that session. I reminded him that our highest priority was that he take care of himself, and I encouraged him to halt the exercise any time he felt the need to do so. He was impatient to "get to it," however, and moved from a chair to the couch in my office. I moved my chair nearer the couch, so that I was sitting near his waist, with a view of his entire body. I joined him in a brief centering meditation (emphasizing safety, trust, and an opening to natural processes). I then invited Apollo to begin describing what was going on inside him. Like many other clients, Apollo showed signs of initial tension (e.g., muscle twitches around his eyes, restless movements trying to get settled).

"Umm . . . uh . . . Jeez [pause] . . . I am just drawing a blank. . . . " [pause]

After several seconds of silence, I asked him if he was aware of any bodily sensations.[28]

"Tension in my neck. Always tense there. Oxen. Yoke. [smile]

"Aware that I want to see your face . . . see if you're smiling. [pause] So . . . you're not going to say anything, huh?[29] [pause] I'm on my own in here? [pause, sigh] OK, I'm on my own. [pause]

"Still trying to settle in. Settle in. [deep breath] Aware of my jaws. Cheeks heavy. [voice slows and relaxes; deep breath] Don't want to go to sleep on you and miss the fun. [smile, long pause]

"[sudden grimace] Don't want to see that! [tightening of muscles around eyes] Don't want to see *her like that!* [another grimace] Damn it! [fists clench for several seconds followed by slight shake of head and deep breath]

"Think of something else. Find a way around it. [pause] Mouth dry. Mouf die [playing with sounds, slight smile] No! [sternly] I don't want to see her with him, damn it! [rapid shallow breathing]"

I leaned forward and whispered, "Gently, Apollo."

"Fuck you! [eyes still closed; turning toward the couch with his back toward me] Fuck the whole lot of you! [pause, hyperventilating] . . . I'm sorry, I'm sorry, I'm sorry. . . . " [At this point his distress was apparent in his breathing and his voice tone.]

I leaned forward and put my hand on his forearm. "Apollo, you're pushing yourself very hard. Please . . . let's take a break." He slowly sat up and I offered him a glass of water. We sat in silence for several minutes. It was clear to me that he was moving very quickly toward material that was intensely emotional. I checked out my sense of his current capacities.

"How are you doing in here?" I asked, placing my hand on my heart.

"I'm OK." Then, with a slight smile and a tilt of his head, he said, "Just dying."

"Do you want to pull back?" I asked.

"Yeah." He swallowed the last of his water. "But I won't."

"Apollo, you're pushing very hard. You don't have to go farther . . . "

He didn't wait for me to finish my sentence. He had already swiveled his feet back up on the couch, laid down, and closed his eyes. I took a deep breath and relaxed back into my chair.

"Stand by, Houston," he said with a slight smile. "Sea of Tranquility or bust!"

Apollo took his time reentering his inner stream. He modulated his breathing, beginning with soft belly breaths. Then came some waves of more rapid and shallow breaths, followed by muscle twitches in his face. Rapidly, the twitches increased in intensity and larger muscles became involved. The only sounds he made during several minutes were guttural in nature, with occasional soft groans. It was apparent that he was moving "into" something deeper, and he was exhibiting mild, seizure-like muscle contractions.

I leaned forward and put my hand firmly on his forearm. Almost immediately, he said in a halting voice, "Hayoo yoo yoo yoo st st ston, we have a prob ob bob ob blem."

I squeezed his forearm, but before I said anything, he continued in a clear and articulate voice: "No, Houston, we have . . . a tragedy." He took a deep breath with this, and I leaned closer and whispered his name. He responded immediately, still with his eyes closed, "Yes."

"Would you like to take a break?"

There was a long pause of seeming reflection, so I added, "We *can* come back—the stream may be different, but the process will be there."

He smiled and then said, "My mouth is dry." We were silent for perhaps 30 seconds and he then began to open his eyes, a very slow process punctuated with occasional blinks. When his eyes were fully open, they were motionless for more than a minute. Then, he blinked again and quickly shifted from his supine position to one of sitting across from me. He didn't look at me at first.

"How are you doing?" I asked in a gentle tone. He rubbed his hands on his pant legs and only briefly raised his face, momentarily meeting my gaze and then dropping his gaze to the floor as he spoke.

"There is something in there," he said slowly and deliberately. "Something in *here* [touching his chest] that terrifies me." I was partly delighted to hear that he was so coherent and self-aware, but I was also concerned with the physical power of what he was approaching.

"You are pushing yourself very hard, my friend," I said.

"I know," he said. Then, more softly but still with his eyes down, he said, "I'm sure you have noticed the twitching. [I nodded.] Twitching has always embarrassed me. Getting 'the shakes' is terrifying for me, especially in front of anyone else. And . . . whatever I just had was a million times stronger than the shakes. . . . "

As he said this, I sensed his need for me not to be frightened or disturbed by the intensity of his experience. I found my breathing relaxing and slowing down, and I was able to move into a more centered position, both bodily and consciously. I waited to see if he would say more.

After perhaps a minute of silence, he lifted his gaze to mine and gave me a faint and momentary smile of contact.

"What would you like to do?" I asked softly, my tone emphasizing gentleness and his freedom of choice in where we went from that moment.

"I don't know, Michael," he said. He was now looking at me unselfconsciously, his eyes meeting mine with a rare directness and consistency. "I know I am pushing . . . and I don't know if I am pushing against something or pushing away from feeling or . . . or what." He paused for a moment and then continued, "I wish you knew where this was going. . . . "

His voice trailed off, but his eyes remained deeply engaged with mine. "I wish I did, too," I said, and we both smiled slightly. I took another deep breath and said, "I don't know where this might lead, Apollo. [pause] I do trust that you will get some hints of that if you continue, but I must admit that your pushing concerns me."

His eyes dropped back down to the floor for a moment and then came back to mine. "Maybe that is part of what I'm confronting here . . . my need to push myself and some part of me that is fighting back against the pushing . . . [pause] . . . I don't know. I just know that it's scary as hell *and* it feels really important . . . [pause] . . . and that I feel safe with you . . . [pause, eyes dropping again and then slowly, intentionally returning to meet mine] . . . safe enough to feel scared . . . and for that I am grateful."

That brought tears to both of our eyes, and I reached forward with my right hand and squeezed the top of his knee. He said, "I'd like to give it one more look today."

When he lay back down on the couch, however, he found it difficult to reenter his stream, and we decided to accept that. As part of an exit meditation, I encouraged him to register a conscious appreciation for how hard he had worked in the presence of such strong feelings. I invited him to close the exercise with an acceptance of what had happened.

Apollo and I spent the remainder of that session discussing his experience. In future sessions, we explored more streaming, and Apollo again moved through a sequence of twitches and shakes, eventually exhibiting large muscle contractions that occasionally put him into a fetal position. It was a pattern that I had witnessed in other clients during streaming, and its intensity was always a challenge.

In Apollo's case, as in the others, there was an alternation between intensely emotional phases and periods of recentering, which often included attempts to describe or explain the experience. This was the dance between experiencing and explaining—a dance that expresses the dynamics of development. Like other clients, Apollo was eager to make sense of what he had experienced while streaming. The early images that he had tried to avoid were imagined scenes of his former wife in the act of making love with someone else. He eventually made peace with the fact that he did not need to visualize that scene graphically in order to accept its reality. Apollo also developed valuable insight into his intense fear of bodily twitches and shaking. His father had been a harsh disciplinarian, and Apollo was often "called on the carpet" for his mistakes or for a forced confession. If he began to twitch or shake during one of these confrontations, his father took this as evidence of his guilt and his weakness. Quite naturally, it seemed, Apollo learned to fear his own processes of feeling fear or anger and his bodily expressions of such feelings. As our work together continued, he began to incorporate this and other insights into a larger story of who he was, where he had come from, and how he might yet be.

I have found streaming to be very helpful for clients who are "stuck" in dysfunctional patterns, or who seem to repeatedly cycle through episodes of intense distress. It is also helpful in individuals who are simply seeking a more intimate awareness of self, or who want a developmental adventure. Even though I emphasize a gentleness of style, streaming is often a more intense and adventurous experience than mindfulness meditation. One of the things that I found striking was the difference between streaming and sensory deprivation experiences. Both the content and the process of inner witnessing are different when another human being is present.

The process by which streaming helps continues to intrigue me. My sense is that it is more than a single process and that the power of streaming is not exclusively associated with the particular contents of their report. In some clients, there are remarkably intense episodes that have abreactive or cathartic features. I have been repeatedly surprised by what has emerged in the course of streaming. Boundaries between memory, fantasy, and creative improvisation become ambiguous, and this may be a source of some of the power of the exercise. A few of my clients have been so incredulous about their experiences that they have investigated them to evaluate their possibility. Searching their early medical records and interviewing relatives, several were able to document what they were reluctant to believe (e.g., being victims or perpetrators of sexual or physical abuse, witnessing brutality or death, committing crimes). Some of these were reminiscent of the cases reported by John Bowlby.[30] I am particularly intrigued by what appears to be a natural titration process that often precedes complete recall. Fragments of an incident may first intrude into the stream of consciousness as puzzling images or sensations. This is *my* construction, of course, but it is almost as if these fragments are serving as a "test run" to assess readiness or capacity to handle elaboration. With some clients, these intrusive puzzles do not repeat, or the client may choose to withdraw from the exercise. In other individuals, the puzzling particulars may repeat and be elaborated in a manner reminiscent of dream reconstruction. Then, in some, there is a sudden shift in which these particulars take on meaning in a larger and coherent framework.

The primary purpose of streaming is not to search for repressed memories of early trauma. The idea that an isolated trauma is responsible for all later dysfunction has dominated and diverted too much of psychotherapy.[31] Traumatic experiences may be recalled, but they are rarely singular, and their recall is seldom sufficient for changing patterns of experiencing. Relative to action, insight is overrated.[32] I believe that much of the power associated with the technique of streaming relates to the process of the activity itself. Many people are afraid to look intensely at or inside themselves. They fear that demons and dark secrets lurk within. Sometimes, of course, they are right. But their willingness to look is itself an act of courage and integrity. And they often discover both memories and aspects of themselves that are humorous, sweet, or endearing. Every life has its own unique history of punctuations. Mixed in with the tragedies are personal triumphs and a large dose of the mundane and the comical. Psychotherapy has too long focused on the bitter without honoring the sweet. What many clients discover in the process of streaming are paradoxical mixtures.

Part of the power of streaming stems from the adventurous act of courage it requires. It is also a process that invites an opening to the complexity and the variability of one's inner life. Those who explore this exercise are often struck by how much is going on simultaneously within them and how quickly parts of it may change. Letting go of language structures—using sentence fragments and shifting focus quickly and repeatedly—can introduce unsettling variability to the experience one is trying to describe. This may facilitate a tremendous freeing at the same time that it elicits a primordial fear of leaving an established order. Memory functions may fade as present experiencing becomes central. I therefore recommend the recording of such exercises. As in dreams, time and logic may recede as organizing processes. Once again, these developments may be experienced as freeing or frightening, and they require careful and compassionate mentoring. Some of the most dramatic changes I have seen in psychotherapy have emerged out of episodes in which we used stream of consciousness reporting. These sessions have also included some of the most demanding work of my career.

Streaming asks a lot of both client and therapist. It can stretch both individuals in ways that are difficult to describe. Because of the intimacy of the adventure, streaming can deepen the relationship of the two people involved. With many of my clients, the content of the streaming has been of minor significance relative to the process of witnessing it and sharing it with me. The experience brings up issues of trust and caring. After the streaming exercise, sometimes in their personal journals, clients have reported feelings of both fear and emancipation as they have allowed themselves to share their inner life with me. I have been deeply touched by the honor of having a window at their heart, and I have been changed by that honor.

The therapeutic relationship is often changed by process work. This is particularly true at the depth represented by streaming. The helping relationship is not an abstraction. It is a lived and developing connection between human beings. Although my clients' relationships with me have unfolded through this kind of work, however, even more fascinating is how their relationships with themselves have often deepened and developed. Beyond noticing the sheer level of activity and complexity inside themselves, many clients come to sense something that opens remarkable possibilities for their explorations of new ways of being. They sense that there is more than one of them. They begin to appreciate the power and mystery of that which is glibly called a "self." Their relationship to that power and mystery is our next topic.

NOTES

1. I strongly recommend Les Greenberg's (2002) *Emotion-Focused Psychotherapy.*
2. Moreno (1946, 1959, 1962).
3. Moreno (1946, p. 351).
4. Stewart and Berry (1991).
5. Kelly (1973).
6. Kelly (1973, p. 403).
7. Kelly (1973, p. 401).
8. Kelly (1973, p. 418).
9. Kurtz (1986, 1990).
10. Person (1995, p. 9).
11. For a scholarly review of dream research, see Strauch and Meier (1996).
12. Strauch and Meier (1996, pp. 241–242).
13. Palombo (1999).
14. See, for example, Baars's (1997) work on the "theater of consciousness." Boundary issues are at the heart of the constructivist emphasis on contrasts in self-organization (e.g., the two kinds of people in the world). It was long thought that there were two kinds of sleep: rapid eye movement (REM) sleep, in which we dream, and non-REM sleep, in which we do not. It is now apparent that dreaming can take place in both sleep states and some waking states. Some researchers are even entertaining the possibility that we are always dreaming while asleep (Strauch & Meier, 1996).
15. Foulkes (1985, 1999).
16. In gestalt dream work, one is asked to take the perspective of different parts of the dream (see Hill, 1996).
17. LaBerge (1985); LaBerge and Kahan (1994).
18. Brown (2000); Rea (2001); Vaughan (1979, 1986).
19. A large proportion of dream contents are, in fact, conversations rather than images. Dream dictionaries may serve a useful function in stimulating suggested possibilities, but they should be used cautiously.
20. Exaptations are adaptations that may have originally emerged for one purpose but have come to serve other functions. Virtually all land-dwelling mammals sleep, and dreaming appears to be an important part of that process. As Foulkes's research shows, children's dreams are different from those of adults. Developments in dream activities generally accompany developments in waking consciousness (e.g., narrative structure and complexity).
21. Hill (1996); Taylor (1992).
22. James (1890).
23. Allen (1999).
24. For further readings on free association and stream of consciousness, see Ishai (2002); Klinger (1971); Kris (1996); Natsoulas (1996–1997); Pope and Singer (1978); Stern (1983); and Velmans (2000).
25. Petitot, Varela, Pachoud, and Roy (1999); Varela and Shear (1999); Velmans (2000).
26. Mahoney (1983, 1991); *www.constructivism123.com.*
27. Bugental (1978).

28. Drawing a blank at the beginning of a first streaming session is common. I use a three-sequence strategy in response: (a) Ask about bodily sensations, (b) ask the client to choose a word and repeat it rhythmically until it changes, and (c) give the client an in-the-moment illustration of my own stream of consciousness. These are explained and illustrated in a streaming video (Mahoney, 1983; *www.constructivism123.com*).
29. In general, I do not speak much during a client's streaming. Otherwise, it can become a closed-eyes form of conversation rather than a self-exploratory exercise.
30. Bowlby (1985, 1988). See also his brilliant reconstruction of Charles Darwin's life (1990).
31. Cushman (1995).
32. Wachtel (1987).

CHAPTER 9

SELF-RELATIONSHIP AND SPIRITUAL SKILLS

The self is a central mystery in consciousness. Fascinations with the sense of self have been apparent for centuries.[1] Even during the half-century when the self was deemed an unscientific topic in a psychology dominated by behaviorism (ca. 1913–1963), the self remained a strong interest of the reading public. It has become so entwined with popular psychology that bookstores often grant a shared display space to psychology and self-improvement.

The first formal psychological treatment of the self is often credited to William James. Just as consciousness can be viewed as a complex and changing stream, James found the self to be a multifaceted mystery with remarkable malleability. He noted, for example, the difference between the self being observed (which he called the objective self, or "me") and the self that is observing (a subjective "I"). He struggled to understand this second, knowing self, which is more like a witness and moves closer to a spiritual perspective. Are you the same person you were as a child? Yes and no. Has your body changed? Yes and no. Has your self changed? Yes and no. Are you the same person in different relationships? Yes and no. Will you be the same person with the same self a year from now?

A self is itself constantly under construction. Indeed, one of the paradoxes of the self is its changing stability. The self is not a fixed entity or a blueprint that resides within the person. As Ernst Cassirer liked to note, one of the primary functions of words and other symbols is to pull things out of the flow of time and "fix" (stabilize) them for examination or exchange. Words may be used to describe a river, but even the most moving words cannot capture its flow. The same is true with consciousness and the self. Both are ongoing processes whose dynamic complexities cannot be contained by even our most accommodating concepts. We must resign ourselves to very crude approximations. Still, what we are struggling to understand and express is central to our own experiencing.

Self psychology and consciousness research have begun a fascinating dialogue. James was onto some promising tracks. New technologies in neuroscience have also encouraged creative integrations of views drawn from phenomenology, consciousness studies, and spiritual wisdom traditions.[2] Constructivism has been encouraging many of these dialogues and integrations. Constructive psychotherapy views each individual as being engaged in activity that organizes and makes sense of his or her experience. The experience of self is a recurrent theme. No matter where you go, there you are.[3] You are the only person you have to be with all the time. You are the only one who needs to be present when you die. A large part of your quality of life depends on the quality of your relationship with yourself. Indeed, your relationships with others—which powerfully influence your self-relationship—are themselves affected by who and how you experience yourself to be. We are relational beings. As Stephen Gilligan points out, this applies as much to our inner as to our outer life.[4] Much that we experience is in parts or kinds. "There is a part of me that" is an important statement. We are all naturally multiples. We contain multitudes, as Whitman intimated and James affirmed. Our "multiversity" can be both agonizing and inspiring. The war among the selves has claimed many lives. The transformation of inner wars into weddings has saved lives and propagated well-being.

Self-relationships are often a central theme in psychotherapy. Self-relationship is not simply self-image or self-esteem.[5] It is more than body image, self-concept, or the distance between a real and ideal self. What I mean by self-relationship is much more protean and process-oriented. It includes how one relates to particular dimensions of experience—thoughts, emotions, memories, sensations, images, dreams, fantasy, and so on. Self-relationship also refers to the processes by which we create and combine parts. Differentiation and transcendence processes will shift our discussion from the local self to the larger self and spirituality. Focusing for the moment on the local self, my practical emphasis is on self-compassion.

Self-compassion is among the most important skills that can be taught in psychotherapy. Rare is the client who could not benefit from some self-directed mercy or forgiveness. Self-criticism, self-blame, and self-rejection are frequent components of many dysfunctional patterns. They are themes that often emerge in therapeutic discourse. These themes are also common in stream of consciousness reports. But years ago, I stumbled onto a technique that offers a remarkably clear and simple picture of a person's relationship with himself. It requires only that he stand or sit in front of a mirror and pay attention to what he thinks and feels. "Mirror time," as I call it, is now one of my favorite exercises for assessing and assisting self-relational skills.

MIRROR TIME

Many years ago, I was seeing a man named Adam, who had presented with a variety of problems that included anxiety disorders, anorexia, bulimia, depression, obsessive–compulsive disorder, and personality disorder. I was his eighth psychotherapist in a course of treatment that spanned 22 years.[6] Adam and I were involved in intensive, long-term work together, and we were nearing the completion of his life review project. At the time, I was also seeing a 13-year-old client named Gary. Gary's mother had found a small amount of marijuana hidden in his room. Thinking she would give him a good (educational) scare, she phoned the police. Gary was arrested, and the juvenile court referred him to me for four sessions of therapy. Needless to say, Gary was not an enthusiastic client, and he had understandable concerns about trust. In our first two sessions, he was silent and sullen. I found myself telling him stories (much like Milton Erickson had done with me so many years earlier). Gary surprised me with a gift of appreciation at our third session: a small mirror with a Harley-Davidson motorcycles logo across the top. It was a prize he had won at a local carnival the previous weekend. I was delighted with what his gift might mean about our alliance and immediately put it up on the bookcase next to my desk. Gary and I had a productive session, and I spent considerable time after he left making notes about things I wanted to say to him in our final meeting.

That was when Adam arrived for his weekly appointment. As was often the case, Adam was in a "crisis mode": agitated, feeling irritated and urgent, sure that his life was on the brink of disaster. Adam sat down and began describing his crisis, but I noticed that he kept making these sharp turns of his head toward my bookcase. Finally, pointing to the new mirror, he asked, "Is that new? I don't remember seeing it before." I replied that it was indeed new.

Adam then asked, "Would you mind moving it? I keep catching a glimpse of myself in it, and I lose my train of thought."

I said, "Of course," and reached for the mirror. I do not know why, but instead of moving it out of sight I put it on my desk directly in front of Adam.

His reaction was one of alarm. Adam literally jumped up from his chair and began pacing around my office. "No!" he shouted several times. "No way!" His agitation was palpable. He seemed frightened and offended.

"I can't believe that you would *do this* to me!"

"Do what, Adam?" I asked.

In an explosion of anger, he pointed his finger at me and said, "If I have to look into a mirror to be in therapy with you, *then I am out of here*! I'll find another therapist!" It was an ultimatum.

I leaned forward, picked up the mirror, and placed it face down on my desk. "Adam," I said, "you don't have to look in the mirror. I apologize. I did not mean to provoke you." His face softened and his pacing slowed. "Can you help me understand what you are feeling right now?"

After a few minutes, Adam was able to explain to me that he hated his reflection, that he had spent countless hours of his life poking at pimples and lamenting his unattractive features, and that "he was not about to spend good money doing it in therapy." I again apologized for the distress I had caused him. We finished the session, talking about a current dilemma he was experiencing at work.

When Adam left my office that day, I spent a lot of time in front of that mirror myself. I began to imagine how a mirror might become a tool in my work with clients. In the following weeks, I experimented with myself and some willing colleagues and graduate students. Both in private and in pairs, we simply explored how we responded to this novel situation of looking at ourselves in a mirror without a cosmetic or personal hygiene task to organize the experience. No hairbrush, toothbrush, cosmetics, or moisturizers—just ourselves with ourselves. Most of us noticed that our attention was first drawn to superficial features—wrinkles, fat, hair, and the like. What some of us also noticed—and this was later corroborated by clients and laboratory volunteers—was that eye contact with oneself had a special quality. It was difficult to describe, but it was also powerfully intimate. As one colleague said, "I can fool most of the people a lot of the time, but I can't fool him (meaning himself)." This accidental discovery opened up a whole new avenue of research on self-relations, which I have pursued now for more than 20 years. In addition, it encouraged me to introduce mirror time to more and more clients, and I have learned invaluable lessons about the complexities of self-relationship in the process.

Adam and I continued our work together as before. Then one session, a few weeks later, he asked if I still had that mirror. I said, "Yes," and asked him why. He said, "I don't know. I just can't stop thinking about my reaction to it, and I think that maybe I am supposed to look in a mirror." I was impressed with his clarity and courage, and I explained to him that I now had a full-length mirror if he wanted to try it. He was again visibly shaken, but he said that he thought it was what he needed to do. We meditated briefly, emphasizing his centering skills and setting positive intentions for the experiment he was about to conduct. I then led Adam to another room where there was now a large mirror. When we entered the room, he hesitated, his steps faltering like those of a frightened child about to encounter a huge monster in a dark place. I stood in a corner and let Adam approach the mirror in his own way, at his own pace. He literally crept toward it, shuffling his feet sideways until he was on the edge of his own reflection. There he paused for several seconds, his hands visibly trembling. "Shit!" he said, then "I'm going in!" With a large deliberate step, he placed himself directly in front of the mirror and stood there staring at his reflection. It was such an intense encounter that I took a deep breath, preparing myself for the unknown next moment in this very intimate drama.

He stood there silently for some time. The look on his face slowly changed from trepidation to puzzlement. After a while, I asked him what he was feeling. He grinned slightly and said, "The guy in the mirror doesn't look as fucked up as I feel." He sighed. Taking a step closer to the mirror, Adam smiled and said, "In fact, I wouldn't mind *being him*!" The man in the mirror, he said, seemed more real than he felt. That session was a turning point in our work together—a turning point that led to more process work and some significant shifts in Adam's patterns of relating to himself. It was not a magical transformation, but it was the beginning of some hard and productive work on how he experienced himself. As I elaborate in a later section, entering the self through a mirror can also initiate a leaving of the self and the surface.

I have invited many individuals to explore the possibilities and challenges of mirror time, and I continue to consider it a valuable tool in both the assessment and facilitation of self-relations. There is, of course, no one "right" way to conduct mirror time. I tend to rely on a protocol that has evolved for me over years of practice. I present a simple rationale along the lines of "This may help me to understand you better, and it may help you to improve your ways of relating to yourself." A handout for mirror time as homework is offered in Appendix H. I emphasize the importance of setting intentions (1) to explore within boundaries that feel safe; (2) to open to a broad spectrum of thoughts, feelings, and images; and (3) to incorporate the experience, whatever it may be, into one's personal development. I often precede the mirror exercise with about 5 minutes of centering meditation, focusing on breathing, relaxation, trust in process, a sense of safety, and a commitment to self-care that gives clients permission to stop or redirect the experience at any points they choose.

Clients look into a mirror. They see themselves as they do—sad, ugly, old, fat, sensitive, and so on. It is common for individuals to be initially preoccupied with their appearance. They may note their wrinkles or blemishes, their weight, their hair, and so on. An interesting difference among clients is the length of time it takes them to move beyond these cosmetic surface features to more substantial themes. The shift from the surface to their interior is often marked by their looking directly into their own eyes. If they do not spontaneously engage their own gaze after a few minutes, I may encourage this through a questioning suggestion (e.g., "And when you look into your eyes?"). I may encourage them to alternate between having their eyes open and closed. This invites them to integrate what they are feeling with what they are seeing, and it creates opportunities for new experiences of the image in the mirror.

I use a variety of mirrors for different clients at different phases. Some are handheld. Others are portrait size and sit on a table or desk. Still others are full-length and encourage a standing posture. With some clients, I encourage an alternation between periods of having their eyes open and closed. With closed eyes, it is much easier to focus on bodily sensations, emotional processes, and mental images. With eyes open, there is an almost-automatic process of "externalization," and experiencing "from" is overshadowed by experiencing "toward." The alternation between these modes seems to encourage the emergence of a more integrative balance that embraces the inner and outer realms. Some clients prefer to do their mirror time exercises in the privacy of their own home. I recommend dim or gentle lighting, and many find the presence of a live flame helpful (e.g., candles, an oil lamp, or a fireplace).

Like all techniques, I tend to introduce mirror time early in a session and allow plenty of time for processing. My advice is don't press. Don't expect it to work miracles. Just let it unfold as it does (or doesn't) for each individual. Treat it as an exploration or an experiment (which it is). Any and all results are informative and navigationally relevant. If it isn't helping, discontinue it. Some clients will ask to come back to mirror time when they feel ready. Others may be better served by not exploring this dimension at all.

Mirror-time exercises can be very powerful adjuncts to psychotherapies that emphasize self-relationships.[7] When a person really begins to experience herself, not only as the image in the mirror but also as the human being looking into that mirror, this can create a whole new realm of experiencing and communicating. It is not unusual for clients to assume different voices and phenomenological "positions" during mirror time. Reminiscent of the dominant–submissive polarities popularized in some forms of Gestalt psychotherapy, Transactional Analysis, and a range of other approaches, clients who begin to dialogue with their mirror image are often initially attracted to clear contrasts: the "good" me and the "bad" me, the "critic" and the "wimp," the "true" and the "false," and so on. I have witnessed processes in which these dichotomies have literally evolved in front of my (and my clients') eyes. For example, one client liked to do mirror time standing up, and he moved to the left or right when he was speaking from different parts of himself. The critical and relentless judge stood to the left of center and spoke with a harsh voice. The alternate voice was quiet and vulnerable, reminiscent of a victimized self. This voice was spoken from a position about 6 inches right of center. After dozens of exchanges between these poles, the client suddenly stepped back from this two-dimensional pendulum. With a voice tone that was startlingly close to my own, he said, "OK, you two. This can't go on forever. We won't be in psychotherapy forever. I will have to be Michael, and we will need to work together!"

I encourage dialogues among the parts of themselves that clients may feel (e.g., the neglected child, the angry rebel, the victim of abuse, the saintly sage, and so on). This is where I most often "coach" my clients in their self-relating. A typical scenario is that a client, looking into the mirror, becomes self-critical and begins attacking not only her appearance but also her personality—her character. To condense it into a stereotype, the client says to her mirror image, "You are nothing but a sniveling, neurotic imposter who pretends to be one way to other people when you are truly the opposite: a despicable and pitiful failure of an attempt to be a real human being."

In a person who has a well-developed dialectical balance, such a statement evokes a strong counterresponse. But many clients do not have such a balance, and that is why they are seeking our services. The "bully" of self-criticism and self-negation has the upper hand in their developmental dialectic. There is no possible response except submission and guilt. "I am a guilty shit; I should be treated like shit; shit is my specialty." It is here that the insights and methods of the cognitive therapies can be helpful.[8] This is where I intervene, whether my client is working with a mirror or not. If she is working with a mirror, I may sit behind her and serve as a "whispering coach" who suggests responses to her self-critical attacks. I may tap her on one shoulder or the other and suggest possible responses, often framed in terms of a compassionate balance. If some part of her has maligned her character or attacked a particular action, I may try to counterbalance the negativity with either an emotional reaction (e.g., "That makes me feel . . . ") or a more proactive response (e.g., "But that also means that . . . "). My primary goal is to encourage a response, whatever its form. Otherwise, the negative message is left hanging, as if it were the final word.

Consider an excerpt from one client's sessions. It was the second time we had used the mirror to explore his self-relating. I sat behind him. He began with a sigh.

"I feel tired. I *look* tired. And old. Old."

"Close your eyes for a moment, Samuel. Where do you feel the tiredness and the oldness?" [pause]

"In my eyes." [pause]

"Anywhere else?" [pause]

"My shoulders. My chest. My heart. My heart is heavy and tired and old."

"Can the tired part of you say something?" [At this he spontaneously opened his eyes.]

"You're a stupid old fool, Samuel. [pause] You've lost your chance."

(I presumed that he was here referring to his divorce, which was a current theme in our work) [pause] "And you let people think that you're contented when you're just an empty shell going through the motions of being alive." [At this point he closed his eyes again and his head dropped slightly forward; I put my hand on his shoulder.]

"Is there a part of you that can say something kind to that stupid old fool? [long pause] Perhaps something you might wish for him?" [pause; he opened his eyes]

"I wish I could hold you, old fool. [pause; his eyes began to look watery] I wish I could fill your emptiness and let you rest." [I squeezed his shoulder gently and then removed my hand.]

"A very loving wish," I said. I slowly moved from my position behind him and sat in the chair in front of him, and then continued, "That tired old heart of yours is also pretty tender." [A slight smile passed briefly over his lips, and he turned away from the mirror to face me.]

"Yeah, I guess I am tender, [pause] just not often enough with myself."

This brief exchange illustrates how coaching can be implemented. When a client cannot think of something kind or positive to say to himself, we sometimes pursue that incapacity. I may describe my own feelings in witnessing his dilemma (e.g., "I find myself feeling sad at the thought that you have such difficulty being gentle or caring with yourself"). Or I may role-play this missing element in his self-relating. We teach self-relationship to our clients not only in how we coach them in mirror time, but also in how we express our own relationship with self.

The mirror is a physical tool for emphasizing and amplifying self-perception and self-awareness. It is useful as a means of highlighting this dimension, but it can also become a distraction when the focus is on the tool rather than the process. The potential power of mirror time is to open a process of self-relating in such a way that more adaptive patterns can be developed. Besides mirror time, I use a range of exercises that encourage my clients to explore and refine their self-relating (Appendices I, J).

It is worth emphasizing that the experience of self is fundamentally a relational experience. We first learn to see ourselves through the eyes, actions, and words of others. When we come to see ourselves differently, it is often through the help of others seeing us differently. This is one of the important roles for psychotherapy. I am using the word "see" both literally and figuratively here, and there is an advanced form of mirror time that can sometimes bridge both senses of meaning. The *trespasso* is something I first learned in workshops on spirituality and consciousness, and I have since incorporated it into my own practice.[9] After testing the waters with preliminary mirror-time exercises, a client can be encouraged to focus her gaze on a spot midway between the eyes (e.g., either the bridge or tip of the nose or the middle of the forehead). At close range (a few inches), there will be a strong urge to move the focus to either eye (an attentional shift that is often unconsciously made after blinking). Suppression of blinking will, of course, result in the formation of tears. If the urge to blink is resisted and focus is fixed on a middle point, however, there is often an experience of the face changing or moving (even when it is motionless). The individual may have flashes of herself as older or younger, or as if gesturing (e.g., smiling, winking). It can be a bit unsettling until the client realizes that the standard and stable view is always accessible by a quick shift of focus back to one of the eyes or the whole face. One client compared it to a brief and voluntarily altered state of consciousness: "This is wonderfully weird! When I don't blink, it is as if the features of my cheeks get wavy or something! It is like having fast frames of film flashing through—me when I was a kid . . . me as a gaunt old man—all just shuttling through at warp speed unless I move my eyes." Another client commented that it was both the opposite of and similar to night vision in pilots. To double-check their glimpse of a faint light at night, pilots are instructed to scan back and forth past the region of sky where they thought they might have seen something. Because of the blind spot at the back of the retina, looking directly at a faint point of light will actually make it harder to see. "With this, I have to keep my gaze fixed. I can only see my other selves by not looking at them."

For clients who are ready to explore realms of experiencing that are less dominated by visual stability, the trespasso exercise offers valuable possibilities. In this procedure, it is easy to sense that the self is not located in one position (e.g., in the mirror or inside the body looking into the mirror). One can choose to see and feel it from either location, or one can witness the oscillations and images made possible by a simple shift of focus.

This more advanced form of excursion into self-relationship also creates "transpersonal" options.[10] The self emerges from capacities and quests for self-consciousness, which in turn require experiences of "otherness" and "individuation." For some clients, self-relational and social skills may be among the most important results of psychotherapy. People often need to learn skills in centering, emotional regulation, and self-comforting. Skills developments in these domains are valuable. Regardless of where they begin, however, lessons of skillful self-relation often lead toward explorations of larger meanings. Whatever the technique, in process-level work, there are often moments of ambiguity, losses of balance, and glimpses of possibilities. These are often strongly emotional episodes in which an old framework is shaken or a new option is briefly sensed. They are signs of personal revolutions in progress. I have seen it manifest in multiple ways during mirror time. Clients may move "into" themselves (usually via one of their eyes) or otherwise develop a "felt sense" that there is something "more" or "deeper" calling to them. They may note a similarity between their momentary facial expression and one they have seen in a parent, grandparents, their children, or significant others. Tears may flow. Tiny muscles may twitch. Pupils may dilate. Anger, sadness, fear, disgust, compassion, love, hate, tranquility, disorientation, and joy are common, often in waves and mixtures. This is why it is important for therapists to be experienced in working with the full spectrum of emotionality.

It is also important for therapists to be open to expressions of religiosity and spirituality. Many clients are not just talking to themselves. Others are talking to a personal deity or a spiritual realm. Some get responses that surprise them. William James noted that normal, waking consciousness is separated from other expanses by the thinnest of veils. The same is true of the isolated self of Western individualism. Clients who move deeply into self-relational work often find that they are exploring a range of relationships that they had ignored or compartmentalized. More than a few of my clients have reported that their "work on themselves" made them more aware of such things as spiritual emptiness, their longings for a sense of the sacred, and relationships or communities in which they would feel encouraged to explore their spirituality.

SPIRITUAL SKILLS AND PERSONAL DEVELOPMENT

Exercises such as mirror time, centering, and meditation begin with self-focus, yet they often lead far beyond the self. Just as "the way out" of a problematic pattern may be "the way in" of self-relationship, so it is that the way in (toward self-understanding) often leads again toward an outward shift of interests. I do not view this developmental progression as simple or linear; that is, I don't believe that everyone who begins with a personal problem ultimately develops an interest in spiritual practices. Nor do spiritual practices automatically circumvent very hard work on self-relationship. The kind of focus I am talking about is not an either–or split between self and spirit. Rather, it is an enlargement of focus that embraces the very important realm of personal identity (a local, embodied, emotional, and transient locus of "selfhood") within a much larger and equally important realm of levels of relationship (with family, friends, community, humanity, the biosphere, and, ultimately, the infinite and eternal). A client presents for therapy preoccupied with a personal problem. The presenting problem is often part of a repeating pattern, and the meanings of problems and patterns are forged in relationships. Clients who pursue process-level work may find themselves wrestling with their core ordering processes (COPs)—what is "really real" and possible or impossible? How do their feelings reflect their values? Who are they? How should they live?

Once again, the way in blends with the way out. Viktor Frankl liked to say that the healthy eye does not see itself. It does the seeing. His point, I believe, was that outer directedness is natural and healthy. He believed that excessive self-focus can be dysfunctional, and it can. But the healthy eye does see itself in a mirror, and I believe that eye-to-eye and I-to-I exercises can create a valuable path leading into and then beyond self-focus. Self-relationship skills are important in well-being. Such skills include capacities for gentle witnessing, nonjudgmental acceptance, and fluid movement through the changing contents of experiencing. Some clients become frustrated with phases of their own skills development. It is not uncommon, for example, for clients exploring mirror time to express frustration at being unable to "see" anything remarkable—either in the mirror or inside themselves. Some try very hard to see things differently, or to see something in themselves that they believe I am capable of seeing. "What am I looking for?" is a frequent question. "What you are looking for is what is doing the looking." This simple response, attributed to St. Francis of Assisi, emphasizes the importance of how one is looking rather than what one sees.

Consider an illustration from the recent integration of mindfulness meditation and cognitive therapy. Cognitive therapy was originally developed and evaluated as a treatment for depression. Beyond the pain and dysfunction associated with an episode of depression, it is also a pattern with strong gravitational pull. With the help of therapy, and perhaps medication, people can often improve their mood and functioning. However, relapse is a high probability. After a second or third episode of serious depression, people become even more vulnerable to relapse. Cognitive therapy researchers had developed a therapy that helped people recover from periods of depression, but they were faced with a serious challenge in preventing relapse.

It was first thought that cognitive therapy achieved its effects by changing the content of what people said to themselves. This is no longer a tenable explanation. In the courageous and creative inquiry of Zindel Segal, Mark Williams, and John Teasdale, a more process-oriented and relational model has emerged:

> Although the explicit emphasis in cognitive therapy is on changing thought content, we realized that it was equally possible that when successful, this treatment led implicitly to changes in patients' *relationships* to their negative thoughts and feelings. Specifically, as a result of repeatedly identifying negative thoughts as they arose and standing back from them to evaluate the accuracy of their content, patients often made a more general shift in their *perspective* on negative thoughts and feelings. Rather than regarding thoughts as necessarily true or as an aspect of the self, patients switched to a perspective within which negative thoughts and feelings could be seen as passing events in the mind that were neither necessarily valid reflections of reality nor central aspects of the self.[11]

In a series of studies, these researchers incorporated a meditation component into a program designed to reduce relapse in people recovering from a recent depressive episode. Jon Kabat-Zinn helped them develop a mindfulness (*vipassana*) meditation course that emphasized skills in gentle (nonjudgmental) awareness, breathing meditation, body awareness, and a flowing style of consciousness. Individuals who went through this meditation training were much less likely to suffer from later depression. Relapse was reduced by "cultivating a different relationship to life more generally. Central to these attempts is the development of a different relationship to experience."[12] Interestingly, capacities for "centering" and "decentering" were central to success. Also associated with positive results was a shift from "predicting and controlling" life particulars to "welcoming and accepting" them. Note the shifts from "self as center" to a multicentric perspective, and from absolute power to gentleness and flexibility. These are axes of oscillations that often lead toward interest in spiritual issues and practices.

The word "spiritual" is one whose meaning is rapidly changing. To be spiritual once meant that one was "religious," that is, a member of an organized church with explicit creeds and an identified community of members. But the meaning of the term "spirituality" began to change dramatically in the 20th century, particularly with the spread of Buddhism, Taoism, and the planetary popularization of secular spiritual practices.[13] For decades now, trade books on spirituality and self-help have blended together to dominate lists of best-sellers. Ongoing studies of its changing meanings suggest that spirituality is a much broader and more abstract dimension for contemporary humans, and that it is not closely linked to deism, theism, or particular views about life after death.[14] Indeed, the word "spiritual" is now being used as a synonym for "wise," such that the world's spiritual traditions have come to be viewed as vast and invaluable resources of wisdom about life. Cultural and historical processes have also reflected the recent surge in global spiritual seeking. This seeking is reflected diversely (e.g., in word use, book sales, popular rituals, and everyday practices). The collective consciousness of the planet appears to be in the midst of an unprecedented growth spurt. It is not just the rate of the change that is unprecedented. It is its quality. Never before in human history has there been such a global expression of the simultaneous sense of both emptiness and saturation, the awful and the awesome, or alienation and heartfelt connection. Human rights concerns have matured into a more integral consciousness of ecological ethics, and the virtues of health have converged with practices of wholeness and balance.

The word "spirit" literally means breath. We associate life with breathing. When a dying person breathes his last breath, it is sometimes said that his spirit has left his body. We inspire until we expire. And the term "spirit" has taken on subtly complex connotations over time and across cultures. When we "conspire," we literally breathe together. When a person is tired or depressed, we say that her spirits are low. Jerome Frank contends that the essence of psychotherapy is the "restoration of morale"—the restoration of spirit. In this sense, at least, psychotherapy is a form of spiritual service and a context for spiritual skills development. What are such spiritual skills, and how do they connect the realms of inner life with outward action? These are questions I continue to explore in my research and clinical work.[15] For many people, the term "spirituality" includes six basic themes:

1. *Connectedness* (e.g., a sense of relationship, healthy interdependence).
2. *Timelessness* (embracing the ever-present moment of "now," flowing with impermanence, respecting a timeless infinity).
3. *Meaningfulness* (the presence of connecting patterns, even if those patterns remain mysteries).
4. *Gratefulness* (appreciation, joy, love, good will).
5. *Peace* (patience, forgiveness, acceptance, compassion).
6. *Hope* (active engagement in the process of living).

Although it is increasingly common for clients to come into therapy with interests in spiritual issues and practices, it is also common for such interests to develop in the course of therapy. My studies of the personal lives and development of therapists also suggest that career therapists often develop deeper appreciations for spiritual traditions as scaffoldings for meaning systems and sources of healthy ritual practices (Chapter 11).

What are the spiritual skills I recommend to my clients? Many have already been mentioned in previous chapters: centering skills, breathing meditation, body balance exercises, and so on. As Segal, Williams, and Teasdale have noted, the essence of spiritual practice is not so much what is done as it is the manner of doing it. Interestingly, these authors also report that their effectiveness in teaching these skills was dramatically improved when they personally began practicing them. This resonates with my own experience. I can recommend books and describe spiritual skills to clients, but they learn those skills best when I practice them in their presence. And I practice them well in sessions when I practice them frequently in the rest of my life.

Clients may ask how to do it: "How can I be more spiritual? What can I do?" These are charmingly simple questions. Over the years, I have developed some simple responses.

> Learn to pause. [I often do this by taking a deep release breath.] Stop for just a few moments. Listen. Pay attention. Savor what you are sensing. [release breath] Be grateful. [You could be insensible or in pain.] There is preciousness in *this* moment. And this one. [pause] And this one. If there is pain or frustration as well, be compassionate. Have mercy. [pause] Accept what is there. Accept how you are. [pause breath] Trust.

> There are reasons. Let them be. [pause] Let your actions reflect your ideals.

"There you go," I said, after sharing this sequence with a client. With a magician's gesture of the hands, I said, "Poof! You're spiritual!" We laughed. Bringing spirituality into psychotherapy is a lot like bringing the body into psychotherapy. They are both already there. For clients who like tangible reminders and notes, Appendix K is an option. One client summarized the five themes as Pause, Witness, Appreciate, Yield, Serve. She pointed out that they fit the acronym PWAYS, and she liked the idea that it rhymes with "praise." Whatever helps. I make no claims for the adequacy of this simple list. The literatures on spiritual practice are vast and valuable. Mnemonics and maps can be helpful. But don't mistake them for the territory.[16]

It is also important to emphasize that spiritual skills are neither easy nor assured paths to happiness. Despite popular marketing ploys, personal happiness is not the primary goal of most spiritual traditions. This fact is often overlooked or diminished in modern, industrialized cultures that feed and breed on pragmatic bottom lines. If happiness is not the product of such practices, why pursue them? If they are not accountable to a metric of pain and pleasure or "bang for the buck," what is their possible relevance or utility? There are many possible responses to such questions, and the most meaningful responses question those questions themselves. Happiness is not purchased, and pain is a necessary part of sentient life. These statements fly in the face of a common myth in our culture. I call it "the myth of arrival." It could also be called "the illusion of cure," "the myth of completion," or "the fairy tale of living happily ever after." It is a deep and pervasive theme in our lives, a formative message to our children, and a formidable seduction in the marketplace of self-help and self-improvement books.

The myth of arrival is a primitive theme in legends and fairy tales across many cultures and eras. These are stories that encourage hope and perseverance in the face of adversity and evil. They have served important roles in our survival. At the heart of the myth of arrival is a turning point or moment of arrival, after which "the worst is over," suffering has ended, and bliss is bountiful. In the usual form of the story, the central character—through grace, courage, cleverness, good fortune, hard work, supernatural intervention, or some other means—finally achieves lasting happiness. He or she has overcome the central challenge of life and can stand triumphant atop that achievement. Embedded in the myth of arrival, of course, is a personal message for each of us, namely, that for us, too, there will come a day when our struggles and suffering will be finished. Depression, anxiety, anger, and all manner of "ill-being" (dis-ease) will finally end. We will wake up one morning and clearly recognize that we have "arrived": We have gotten ourselves and our lives "together" in a way that can never be undone.

We will be healthy and happy. We will be in the job, the home, and the relationship that we have always wanted, financially comfortable and fundamentally at peace with ourselves. From that point on, we will enjoy calm seas and smooth sailing. Our most dangerous and painful trials will then be over, and we can thereafter coast peacefully through the remainder of our happy life.

It is a seductive myth, and not a fundamentally malicious one. It offers hope, which is essential in human existence. The myth of arrival may be most tempting to believe when we are enduring our most challenging life episodes. But it is also paradoxically maladaptive, because it promotes an impatient and impractical grasping toward an unattainable goal. It encourages us to expect "arrival," and to feel frustrated and unsuccessful until we have reached that mythical destination. Partly out of faith in its message, we may strive to be finished—to be perfect, enlightened, and otherwise living in a past tense of accomplishment. Such striving is itself a formidable burden, and we see references to it throughout the literatures of existentialism and spirituality.[17] The arrival myth encourages us to deny the fact that "the next problem is always in the mail."[18] Whether it is a flat tire, a tax audit, a lump in the breast or on the prostate, or the illness or death of someone we love, there will be another challenge. Life keeps coming at us. There is no path without pain; there is no life without suffering. This is a central message in the teachings of all major religions.[19] The paths of spiritual enlightenment do not avoid or deny that pain. Indeed, they often embrace it as a powerful vehicle of personal development. To paraphrase Thomas Merton, one does not become a monk in order to suffer more or less than other human beings, but in order to suffer more efficiently.

The so-called "good life" is not the same as "feeling good" all the time, as some popular self-help books imply. The good life is one that acknowledges pain in ways that make it more meaningful. The goal of such a life is to remain open, engaged, and developing in the full spectrum of life. In this sense, at least, one is "already there" when one is most engaged. That engagement may feel like a desperate attempt to get somewhere else until one pauses to appreciate. The destination becomes a journey. Just being present becomes a welcome achievement. This message has been taught to me repeatedly, but my favorite lesson came from a 6-year-old philosopher.

When my son Sean wanted to play "pee wee" (beginner's) baseball, I ended up being a coach for his team. I was supposed to teach a group of boys and girls the basics of the game—rules, throwing, catching, batting, and running the bases in the proper direction. My goal was for them to have fun and to feel good about themselves and what they could do with their bodies. In the process, I thought they might learn some important early lessons about life—the nature of rules, fair and foul territories, and the inevitable challenges of both winning and losing. I was right, I think, about everything except this last lesson. I allowed everyone to play, regardless of their current athletic skills, and the other teams went all out for winning. My policy did not make me popular with some of the parents, who wanted me to put only our talented tykes on the field.

We arrived for the final game of the season with a 0-16 record. But in that final game, a miracle seemed to be imminent. Our players hit and fielded well, and the other team (which had beat us twice before) just could not put bat or glove on the ball. In the final inning, we were seven runs ahead. The excitement was almost uncontainable, and I heard whispers throughout the infield: "We're gonna win! We're gonna win!" The other team had the last opportunity at bat, with a seven run deficit. Still, as luck and life would have it, the tide began to turn. They started hitting, and our miniature infielders and outfielders began to miss catches, drop balls, and throw wildly. Before we knew what had happened, the other team had scored eight runs and won the game.

As their parents sulked in waiting, my kids gathered around for hugs and good wishes (as well as their coupons for free hot dogs and sodas). I gathered up the equipment and walked to the car with Sean and his good friend, Robbie. They climbed in the backseat and we set out for home. That was really when the lesson began for me. Robbie was inconsolable. He pulled his red baseball cap down over his face and muttered, "We're losers, Sean. We're losers. Even the Bad News Bears won *one* game!" I heard Sean try to console his friend: "It's OK, Robbie—it's just a game," to which Robbie snapped, "It's NOT a game—it's BASEBALL!!!" After a few moments of silence, Sean came back with another therapeutic attempt: "Well, it's OK, Robbie; we're all winners anyway." Robbie yanked the baseball cap off his face and, fighting back tears, he shouted, "Face it, Sean! It was 24 to 23. We lost. We're losers!"

There was an awkward silence in the car, and I dared not even look in the rearview mirror at these two Lilliputian characters in their Philadelphia Phillies uniforms. I wasn't sure if they were aware of my listening, and I didn't know if Sean was saying things for both Robbie's and my benefit. After several blocks of silence, however, Sean asked a question that I have never heard before or since. He said, "Robbie, do you know how many sperm were trying to be you?" I was so shocked by the question that I had to pull over to the curb, and I leaned forward to open the glove compartment, as if I were looking for something. As mystified as I was, Robbie said, "What are you talking about, Sean?" And Sean then voiced one of the most profound philosophical lessons I have ever heard: "I saw this thing on television, and there were these millions and millions of sperm trying to get to the Mommy's egg . . . and they're all in this big race . . . and the only ones who get to be persons are the ones who win the race . . . so everybody who is a person is a winner." Robbie and I were both silent, probably for different reasons. In that moment, I realized that Sean was right. The most important competition of our lives is always behind us. Along with birth certificates, every newborn child should be awarded a gold medal to signify that fact.

A POSTSCRIPT ON TECHNIQUES

In this and previous chapters I have described techniques that can be used in the practice of constructive therapy. Constructive practice is not defined by techniques, but by an overall view of human beings and the processes by which we organize and reorganize our lives. I have tried to communicate a view of techniques that both respects and challenges traditional portrayals. The art of human helping will not be found in specific words or meticulously repeated rituals, unless those words and rituals reflect something deeper than their own surface structure. In discussing techniques, I have moved from the concrete to the abstract and back again, connecting, I hope, the centrality of meaning to the practice of both life and psychotherapy. Let me now turn to some concluding reflections on the experience of change and the challenges of being a life mentor.

NOTES

1. Anderson (1997); Bermúdez et al. (1995); Csordas (1994); Cushman (1995); Epstein (1993); Ferrari and Sternberg (1998); Ford (1987); Gallagher and Shear (1999); Gergen (1991); Gilligan (1997); Guidano (1987, 1991); Heidrich, Forsthoff, and Ward (1994); Hermans and Hermans-Jansen (1995); Hoshmand (1993); Keats (2003); Kegan (1982); Kohut (1971, 1977); Lewis (1992); McAdams (1993); Rosenberg (1979); Schore (1994); Schwartz (2000); Wheeler (2000).
2. Austin (1998); see also the *Journal of Consciousness Studies* and *Constructivism in the Human Sciences*.
3. Kabat-Zinn (1994).
4. Gilligan (1997).
5. An innovator of this concept, James believed self-esteem to be the simple ratio of personal achievements to personal aspirations. One could feel better about oneself by increasing the numerator or reducing the denominator. Studies of self-relationships have made it clear that there is far more complexity involved.
6. Mahoney (1991).
7. For discussions of the use of mirrors in therapist training, see Beskow and Palm (1998). Research on mirrors and self-awareness is reviewed in Ferrari and Sternberg (1998); Mahoney (1991); Selby and Mahoney (2002); Williams, Diehl, and Mahoney (2002). For self-relational emphases in therapy, see Gilligan (1997), Stone and Winkelman, (1985), and Keats (2003).
8. Alford and Beck (1997); A. T. Beck (1976); J. S. Beck (1995); Beck et al.

(1979); Ellis (1962, 1998); Greenberger and Padesky (1995); Salkovskis (1996).

9. The term "trespasso" comes from the intimacy of looking into another person's eye. In some cultures, the left eye is believed to be a portal to the soul. When this eye is entered without permission, it is considered trespassing. The trespasso can be done in a trusting dyad (e.g., teacher and student, therapist and client) rather than a mirror.
10. The term "transpersonal" was chosen by Abraham Maslow (1968, 1971) and Anthony Sutich when they were searching for a word to describe the realms encountered by self-actualizing individuals, particularly during their peak experiences. They found that word in the writings of Carl Jung. See Hunt (1995), Vaughan (1979, 1986, 1995), Wade (1996), Walsh (1976), and Walsh and Vaughan (1980, 1993).
11. Segal et al. (2002, p. 38; italics in original).
12. Segal et al. (2002, p. 219).
13. Batchelor (1994 (1997); Garvey (1985); Hunt (1995); Kapleau (1980); Lesser (1999); Roof (1993); Russell (1992); Schwartz (1995); Steindl-Rast (1983, 1984); Taylor (1999); Tillich (1952); Woodruff (2001).
14. The term "spiritual" has only recently begun to appear in scientific writings and in psychological research. ("Spiritualism" is quite different from spirituality. For historical and cultural discussions, see Washington, 1993, and E. Taylor, 1999.) For a long time, it was thought that a person had to be *either* scientific *or* spiritual (yet another example of our "two kinds" mentalities). Psychology's courtship of the prestige enjoyed by the physical sciences led many of its pioneering figures either to ignore spiritual experiences or to dichotomize science and spirituality. William James was a courageous exception. He and a few other brave souls pioneered challenges to the traditional segregation of the secular, the scientific, and the spiritual (Shafraanske, 1996; Taylor, 1999; Vaughan, 1995; Walsh, 1999; Wilber, 1998, 1999). They opened not only doors but also dialogues. And dialogue is ultimately dialectical, contrast-generated—a process that inherently invites developmental unfolding that is infinitely creative. For other discussions of the meanings of spirituality, see Brussat and Brussat (1996); Emmons (1999); Garvey (1985); Graci, O'Rourke, and Mahoney (2003); Kovel (1991); Lash (1990); Mahoney and Graci (1999); McCullough, Pargament, and Thoresen (1999); Miller (1999); Roof (1993); Smith (1988); see also periodicals such as *Spirituality and Health*, *Body and Soul*, and *What Is Enlightenment?*
15. Mahoney and Graci (1999); Graci et al. (2003).
16. Caro (1993, 1994); Caro and Read (2002); Korzybski (1937).
17. Becker (1973); Miller (1999); Muller (1992); Ram Dass (1970); Vaughan (1995); F. Walsh (1999); R. Walsh (1999); Walsh and Vaughan (1980, 1983); Wilber (1998).
18. Kopp (1972).
19. Kornfield (1993, 2000); Smith (1958); R. Walsh (1999); Watts (1963).

CHAPTER 10

THE EXPERIENCE OF CHANGE

There are two kinds of people in the world: those who change and those who don't. This tacit assumption can be found at the base of many debates in theoretical psychology. Some geneticists suggest no one changes beyond a mold that is set at conception. For them, we are nothing more than programmed expressions of genetic blueprints. Freud did not think people changed much after early childhood. We are neurotic expressions of our past. Watson and Skinner believed that human behavior was quite pliable. We are our environmental contingencies. Maslow argued that the potential for human transformation is remarkable. We are limitless.

Who was right? Scientific evidence suggests that all of them grasped a piece of truth, but none of them embraced its complexity. People do express their genetic inheritance, but they do it in highly contextual and individualized ways.[1] Early experiences make big differences in developmental trajectories, yet many people transcend them.[2] Environments do select behavior patterns, yet we select and change our environments.[3] Human potential may not be limitless, but it is much greater than most psychological models have yet appreciated. So where does that leave us? This is not simply an abstract, theoretical question. Its concreteness was brought home to me by a client.

Karen first consulted me for help in losing weight. It turned out that her husband wanted her to lose the weight and to resume sexual interactions with him. They had not been sexually intimate for more than 7 years, and this had become a sensitive theme in their ongoing martial difficulties. During the course of her work with me, Karen was introduced to the stream of consciousness technique. We were both unprepared for her central discovery, namely, that she had been repeatedly abused by her drunken father and several of his military friends, some of whom made 8-mm "home movies" of their violations of her. Neither of us really believed that this series of heinous events actually happened, until she recovered her childhood medical records and heard her mother confess that it was regrettably true.

Karen went through 6 months of the most intense, soul-searching depression I have ever seen. She often thought about suicide, which was an understandable fantasy given what she had just learned. She felt that she could not trust her own memory, her own perception, and, hence, her own personal reality. What kept her going, I think, was the love of her two children, the support of several close friends, her strong nurturing bond with her dogs, and perhaps an occasional hug from me.

One day, Karen opened our session with the question, "How much can people change?" I must have looked puzzled as she elaborated. "How much can I change? I mean, I was raped by my 'daddy.' . . . He was supposed to be my protector, and he let other men use me. It was cruel, and I was just a kid, and it happened again and again. Can I get over that? Can I really hope to ever have a normal, happy sex life after that?" (I was speechless as she said this.) "Maybe I should just give up on that and invest my energies in my kids and dogs and work."

She bowed her head with her elbows on her knees, her hands covering her face. She was asking me, I believe, whether she had warrant for hope. I didn't know what to say. She was so direct and self-aware, and the question she asked was not abstract. My first tendency was to avoid the gravity and directness of her question.

"Karen," I said, "you *have been* through a lot. You were cruelly violated, and it has had its effects on you." I could feel the tension in my voice, perhaps because I was distancing from the pain that was at the core of her question. She did not move. "There *are* some experts in the field who would say that you might be better off investing your energies in other dimensions of your life, that your abuse was so early and cruel and repetitive that you will never be able to overcome it." Hearing myself say these words was almost surrealistic, and I paused at their gravity. During my pause, I heard a sound I shall never forget: a quiet but heavy sound, unmistakable in its signature. It was the sound of a tear hitting the carpet. Underneath her hands, her eyes were swollen with the tears of her suffering. I could hardly bear it, so I quickly added.

"On the other hand, there *is* another group of experts who say that we should never foreclose on the possibilities of human resilience." The words sounded too technical to me. I tried to translate. "People have survived cruelties and tragedies that we can barely imagine. Indeed, some have "harvested" their traumas in ways that allowed them to lead fuller and more satisfying lives." I was on a hopeful trend, and I wanted to make sure that she felt both sides of her possibilities. I continued, "And there is at least a possibility that *if*—and I know that it is a big *if*—you ever choose to be sexually intimate again, because of its special meaning to you, it could be an experience far more precious than might be imagined by people who have never been abused."

Several seconds passed in silence. I could still feel the tension inside myself. Then Karen lifted her head and lowered her hands. Her face was covered with tears. And she asked me the most difficult question I could have imagined: "Mike, . . . which camp are *you* in?" I felt my heart racing and a strong temptation to avoid the question. Karen sensed that. She held my eyes in her gaze, and I felt so awkward. She repeated her question, slowly and with emphasis, "Which camp are you in?"

I fumbled for words and began with an apologetic "Well, I could be doing you a big disservice . . . " Karen confronted my evasiveness. "Mike, just level with me. What do you think?" And, with heart racing, I said, "Karen, I refuse to foreclose on human resilience. I don't know why. . . . [I stumbled] I have just seen too much and learned too much not to side with hope."

She mustered a halfhearted smile and sighed deeply. It wasn't so much a sigh of relief as of recognition. "I thought that's what you would say," she said. We continued working together for several more months; then I moved thousands of miles away to another job. We kept in touch, primarily through holiday cards. Karen's life changed in fits and starts. She filed for divorce. She changed jobs. She went to night school. She saw another therapist. She quit therapy. She moved several times. Every New Year's, Karen would send me a picture of herself, her kids, and her dogs, along with a note about what had happened in their lives in the previous year. Then, one year, her holiday card had a special "P.S." at the bottom: "Remember the time I asked you how much I could change? You were right! Thank you for keeping the faith."

Not all life stories end happily, and we must remain sensitive to this fact. Karen did not change overnight, nor was it easy. But she did change. Personal revolutions do occur. I have had the privilege of witnessing their emergence more often than I had expected. What brings them on? How do people change? And what is going on when people don't change? These questions turn out to be connected, as are their answers.

STATIC CLING: A COMPASSIONATE LOOK AT PEOPLE WHO DON'T CHANGE

There is little warrant for dividing people into absolute categories of those who change and those who do not. But some hard facts should be acknowledged:

- Many people don't change.
- Of those who do change, many change very little.
- Many people don't change until they have to.
- Changing is often difficult and painful.

At first glance, these facts may seem to suggest a futility or pessimism. But other facts need to be considered:

- Many people do change.
- Dramatic changes (personal revolutions) are becoming more common.
- Intentional change is possible.
- Many changes bring greater engagement with life.

These facts reflect a bigger picture, that of a dynamic complexity that embraces the puzzle of essential tensions and emergence. This is the puzzle addressed by constructivism and complexity studies.[4] The same person is both changing and remaining the same at different levels. A synopsis is presented in Appendix L.

Many people do not change, or do not change much, because we are fundamentally conservative creatures. This is not our fault. It is our life form. Coherence and continuity are built into life support, and it should not be surprising that these themes are expressed in our psychological life as well. Constructivism emphasizes the human tendency toward structure. We not only seek order but we also need it. We are organized by systems of activities and are often very protective of our own patterns. Our core ordering processes resist changing. They become our habitual ways of being. Habits become homes. Like a familiar easy chair or a well-worn path to the bathroom or kitchen, habits become ruts of being. The power of repetition is formidable. It is more than simple inertia or the shift from conscious to unconscious activity. Old patterns become family. Their familiarity adds an appealing quality. Even when their consequences are predictably painful, old habits offer comfort. Repeatedly returning to old patterns is a frequent and frustrating reality for many people who are trying to change. I am often struck by a parallel phenomenon studied in attachment behavior in humans and other primates. The "secure base" is clung to most vigilantly during episodes of distress. It can be the arms of a parent or lover, a place to hide or escape, or the proximity of an alpha member. Even if the safety they provide is an illusion, an illusion is preferred over the alternatives. In a similar fashion, old habits often become sanctuaries. Familiarity breeds more than contempt. It breeds its own perpetuation.

Failure to change is often termed "resistance," and that concept has a long history in psychotherapy. Freud came to believe that resistance was where the work lay. One of the issues still being debated is whether people act in ways that sabotage their own well-being.[5] Freud was not an optimist when it came to human nature and human potential. He saw resistance to change everywhere, and he viewed such resistance as expressing self-destructive tendencies related to a death wish.

Resistance is often viewed only as opposition. But there are essential tensions in all phenomena, and such tensions are central to both life and development. There is a tension between what is changing and what is not. There is a kind of basic logic in not changing. It is not the symbolic logic of Aristotle.[6] It is more of a "being logic" expressing primitive and powerful needs for order, sometimes at any price. Many clients and therapists are so preoccupied with change—with solving a personal problem—that they often overlook the fact that the problem is often a solution. It may be a painful and costly one, but problems often develop as solutions to previous problems. Look at almost any form of chronic psychological distress and dysfunction: addiction, agoraphobia, anorexia, anxious avoidance, bulimia, depression, obesity, paranoia, obsession, compulsion, and even schizophrenia. All can be viewed as costly and painful solutions.[7] They tend to be short-term solutions to problems of pain and meaning. The solution becomes a pattern—a well-entrenched pattern—and immediate benefits are offset by long-range costs (see Figure 5.1). Acts of avoidance, protest, and withdrawal are often motivated by their felt protectiveness. We are wise to honor these felt needs, even when they may not seem necessary. In other words, we are wise to work *with*—rather than against—resistance. How?

Years ago I was supervising an apprentice therapist. He was seeing a client in a training clinic. The client, a young woman in her late 20s, had experienced a puzzling episode of anxiety when she was asked to stand next to her father for a family photograph at a recent holiday reunion. Her sister, who was already in therapy, encouraged the client to seek counseling about her experience. The student therapist had taken several seminars with me. In his third meeting with this client, he decided that it might be helpful to encourage her to learn how to center and relax herself before she began to explore the possible meanings of her perplexity.

He said, "Well, perhaps this would be a good time to explore an exercise in relaxation. Please assume a comfortable position in your chair and close your eyes." Much to his surprise and consternation, she defiantly said, "No."

"No?" he asked awkwardly.

She repeated with firmness, "No. I didn't *do* childhood, and I don't *do* fantasy."

My supervisee did the best that he could with the remainder of their session, and then he rushed to my office with the videotape. "What did I do wrong?" he asked. "Why is she being resistant?" "What did she mean about not doing childhood or fantasy?"

I reviewed the videotape with him and tried to reassure him that what had happened was actually a valuable lesson, not a personal tragedy. He asked what I might have done differently, and I was painfully aware of how easy it is to be a historical consultant rather than an agent in the moment. I told him that what I would like to think I would have done was to honor and align myself with her so-called "resistance." As soon as she said the word "no," I hope that I would have had the presence to leap into that moment of surprise and say something like "That is wonderful! Thank you for being so clear on your limits. You said 'no' because some part of you does not feel safe or ready to explore an exercise like that. The part of you that said 'no' is taking care of you—protecting you—and it should be respected. I want to develop an alliance with that part of you. I want to encourage its expression."

Compassion is central both to understanding and comforting the difficulties of change. Lack of change is too often equated with failure. Sometimes lack of change reflects hard work. I once worked with a man who was obsessed with developing a new personality. Half-jokingly, he said he wanted to transform from a caterpillar into a butterfly. One session, he reported a fascinating dream. We had been doing mirror time as part of his work on self-relationship. In the dream, he found himself inside a cocoon, cramped in a small space and growing uncomfortably large. He was struggling to break his way out. His voice conveyed the intensity of the struggle. But then he paused.

"What happened? I asked.

"I finally made it," he said. "And there was a mirror on the wall nearby. So I rushed over to see my new self." He paused again.

"I was still a caterpillar." He sounded both sad and angry. "The same wormy, segmented, unfinished being."

I sat there for a long time without moving or saying anything. I felt the weight of his resignation. He was sure that his dream meant that he would always be as he was. Although there were parts of me that were eager to offer other interpretations and somehow lift his spirits, I also felt a deep respect for the courage needed to recount that dream. We sat in silence for several minutes.

"You have gone through hell, time and again, only to find yourself the same." He looked up at me, and his eyes glistened with tears.

"I don't know what to tell you. You try as hard as anyone I know. And you suffer deeply." His eyes dropped at those words.

"I don't know if you are supposed to learn to love yourself as the klutzy caterpillar you feel yourself to be." (There were ripples of almost a smile.)

"But, Tomas," I said slowly, "I *don't* think you are supposed to try harder."

I am reminded of an incident in 19th-century biology, when scientists were fascinated with the details and processes of metamorphosis—the transformation of a life form. The time spent transforming was studied closely. Some clever biologist wondered if he might accelerate the transformation. Because metamorphosis is a metabolic process, he reasoned that anything that would elevate metabolism would also accelerate development. He knew that heat tended to raise metabolic rates, so he thought it might be a useful way to accelerate this phase of development. It took him a while to identify the delicate range of temperatures involved, but he was finally able to demonstrate that he could accelerate the metamorphosis of moths by slowly and gently heating their cocoons. His results were repeated several times by himself and by other biologists. There were rumors of a major scientific breakthrough. Then one of his colleagues recognized something that had been overlooked. The moths that were accelerated had emerged with incomplete wing structures. They couldn't fly. Their wings never fully developed.

Pushing too hard can create not only unnecessary pain but also additional resistance to change. One of the lessons learned in self-relational work (Chapter 9) is that an old view of the self often remains in power so long as it is resisted or rejected. Like any other life form, it fights for its own survival—even when its fighting is self-destructive.

Tomas was pushing to replace an ugly view of himself with a totally different and beautiful one. But his caterpillar parts were not permitting it. If one looks closely at the transformation process, the butterfly retains quite a bit of its caterpillar being. Old parts serve new functions, and there is an emergence of new structures and skills. But they are part of the same being. The individual who goes through psychological transformation is the same being. Old habits or tendencies are not eradicated. We need to appreciate that fact.

Tomas did eventually change. He met someone who saw in him neither a caterpillar nor a butterfly. She saw only a sweet and sensitive man who tried very hard. With her support, Tomas began to appreciate his strengths and forgive his shortcomings. The less he pushed himself to be different, the more he changed. They eventually moved to a small, rural town, where the pace of life was slower and appearances were less important. I don't doubt that Tomas continued to face both new and old challenges, but he faced them with a larger sense of who he was.

Most people do not turn their lives around, shift their identities, and adopt entirely new patterns of life activities in a matter of days.[8] Core ordering processes are generally resistant to such rapid and extensive transformations. Core change is more often hard work requiring patience, persistence, and devoted practice that spans years, if not a lifetime. Helping clients who are not changing can be very difficult. Their pain is palpable. The experience of being stuck is seldom pleasant, and both therapist and client may feel disappointed, impatient, or angry. I remember a conversation with a good friend in which I was expressing my frustrations over the slow progress of some of my clients. My friend was Vittorio Guidano, the Italian psychiatrist who helped pioneer constructivist therapy.[9] Vittorio was fascinated with the similarities exhibited by people with common problems (e.g., eating disorders, anxiety, obsessive–compulsive patterns, and depression). I was more interested in the uniqueness of my clients and the processes by which new patterns emerged in their development. One evening after dinner, Vittorio said, "Michele [pronounced softly in Italian as Mee *kay* lay], I think that you are more of an optimist when it comes to people. I am more of a pessimist. You are fascinated with how people change; I am struck by how they remain the same." His comment had an impact on me. I returned to my work wondering whether he was right. Was I encouraging my clients to hope and work toward changes that were out of their developmental reach?

Over the course of the next year, Vittorio and I continued our pattern of weekly phone conversations, but we did not return to that topic. Then, we met again at a conference. At our first dinner, I told him how often I had thought about his comments about my optimism. During the intervening year, I had felt repeatedly humbled by my clients' difficulties. So many of them worked so hard, yet made so little apparent progress in overcoming or transforming lifetimes of trauma and dysfunction. I said, "Perhaps, you are right, my friend. Perhaps I should be less optimistic."

After patiently listening to me, Vittorio said, "Michele, this is so interesting. I came here tonight with the same conversation on my mind. It was the first thing I wanted to talk with you about. And I came here to tell you about my surprise at what has been happening in my practice. In the last year, I have seen clients change in ways that I did not think were possible. Several were clients I have seen for many years, and we were resigned to their patterns of personal organization. And yet, somehow, they changed. It was a mystery to me and to them. I am not just talking about simple changes. I am talking about dramatic changes in their sense of themselves, in their work, in their relationships. They went through personal revolutions. I have no explanation for why they changed so much and so suddenly after so many years without progress. I came here tonight to tell you that you were right."

CORE CHANGE: PERSONAL REVOLUTIONS

The particulars are unique to each individual, but experiences of change reflect basic patterns and processes.[10] Gregory Bateson talked about two kinds of change. First-order change is a relatively minor adjustment of the system. It could be compared to fine-tuning or pruning. Second-order change is major transformation. It involves a shift in overall organization and functioning. Such dramatic change is stressful. Magai and McFadden express it as a sequence of "surprise/shock, emotional disequilibrium, appraisal, reflection, and, at least potentially, personality change."[11]

The surprise or shock phase is not essential. Sometimes change processes are initiated by what Baumeister calls "the crystallization of discontent"[12]; that is, the person endures a prolonged period of "disquiet,"[13] which may intensify or ultimately coalesce into a critical need for change. Interestingly, the Greek origin of the word "crisis" has the double meaning of danger and opportunity. Many personal accounts of life change reflect a feeling of "hitting bottom" or "being trapped" in a way that somehow alerts the individual to the need for action—the need to do something.

Whether inaugurated by some unexpected surprise or by an incubation of disquiet, life change is often characterized by waves or oscillations that reverberate throughout the entire being and life patterns of the individual. Oscillations are virtually universal in dynamic systems. But the oscillations experienced just before and during a major life change are much more intense and extreme than usual. In technical terms, these are the "critical fluctuations" that reflect the collapsing dominance of an old order. They precede a "phase shift" to a new order. The variability expressed in these fluctuations makes the individual extremely sensitive to influences that might otherwise be insignificant.

It is not unusual for clients (or therapists, for that matter) to be frightened by the phenomenology of transformational change. "Derealization," or the sense of an unstable or changing reality, is common. Partly because of the intense emotional processes involved, everyday perceptions may be altered.[14] One's spouse, children, or coworkers may somehow "look different"; night sounds may seem strange and suddenly distressing; smells and tastes may seem unfamiliar. This can be terrifying. Bodily rhythms may be disrupted, and somatic stress reactions may be triggered: insomnia, headaches, gastrointestinal distress, dermatological problems, and so on.

"Depersonalization," losing one's sense of identity, is also common and distressing. It is understandably disconcerting when the person you see in the mirror begins to look like a stranger. Such experiences are all the more terrifying when the individual has no understanding of why they are happening or what they mean. It is not surprising that individuals in the throes of major life changes are often concerned that they are "going crazy" or otherwise "losing it" (i.e., their grasp of or contact with reality).

There is a sense, of course, in which they *are* losing something, namely, their former life order. Constructive therapists do not automatically pathologize such phenomenology. With rare exceptions, a constructivist is more likely to "normalize" clients' experiences in the process of significant life change. When my clients are struggling to understand what is happening to them, I try to explain—in words and metaphors to which they can relate—that they are undergoing an important developmental transition. I try to build on their own descriptions of their phenomenology to illustrate and make sense of their experience. Most clients are aware that "something is happening," for example. That is a good place to start—to affirm or validate their experience that something significant is happening to them. I go on to explain that it is happening *within* them, and that it is apparently a major "renovation" or "personal revolution" that may have sweeping effects on how they experience themselves and their worlds. With compassion and generous reassurance, I try to explain that they are going through a natural and healthy developmental process.

It may not *feel* natural or healthy to them, of course, particularly if their personal emotional organization has been one that has discouraged a trust in their feelings or in their capacities to endure difficult challenges. This is a phase in therapy (and development) at which many people want to turn back. It reminds me of the experiences of some women in the late stages of childbirth, when the pain and the fear may be so overwhelming that they just want it to be over. As one woman said to her obstetrician, "All right! I quit! I don't want to be pregnant anymore!" But there are points beyond which one cannot ignore the process. Helping someone through the labor of core personal reorganization is like skilled midwifery.[15] Knowing when to rest and when to push is critical. The presence of a trusted and caring other is invaluable. Therapists, like midwives, have valuable experience with the labor of contractions, expansions, and the emergence of new life.

Helping someone through a personal revolution is challenging. Some clients may become more dependent on the relationship and on their therapists. This is often a period when attachment to the therapist (or "transference") is intensified and occasionally romanticized. Some clients may become angry and withdraw from therapy. It is also during a personal revolution that many clients struggle with significant issues and changes in their everyday lives—relationships (old and new), roles, meanings, and shifts in their values. I try to remain attuned to their changing needs and to offer as much support as I can. Overall, I encourage them to "trust in their process" (whether they understand it or not) and to focus their energies and attention on immediate priorities and short-term goals that lie in the direction they hope to develop. Regular practice of centering skills is critical. When they are ready (and their readiness will oscillate as well), I encourage them to engage in exploratory behavior and responsible experimentation with new patterns. These are sometimes structured via techniques such as those described in the preceding chapters.

From the variability provided by core order oscillations, new forms—new patterns of activity—compete with one another (and with older patterns) for selection and "promotion" to the status of an "established" (everyday) way of being. It is as if—in the process of biological evolution—we have replicated inside ourselves a microcosm of the same processes by which our ancestry was selected and shaped. Variation, selection, and retention are the essential processes of both biological evolution and personal development. The competition gets fierce (and sometimes ugly). Even after having been repeatedly shown to serve the system less well than newer alternatives, old patterns still find their way back into the body's "driver's seat." These setbacks can be very frustrating, particularly if they are viewed as total relapse into old habits. Navigating these developmental cycles—and avoiding their pull toward downward spirals—is a challenge. This is when professional help can be particularly valuable.

Equilibrium emerges in cycles as a new systemic organization takes form and new patterns of activity become familiar. These new patterns—and the overall systemic organization that they comprise—are selected not only by their consequences but also by their degree of coherence with individuals' past and unfolding sense of themselves and their life narrative.[16] The new sense of self and world is more likely to be viable when it incorporates the old sense of self and world into a larger, more complex, and more elaborated system. The matrix enlarges, and with it the meanings and actions that it can permit. If clients have changed their interpersonal relations during the preceding (chaotic) phase (and this is common), their new relationships may influence the selection and maintenance of new activity patterns.[17] New patterns of attention and perception also lend themselves to the stabilization of the emergent organization, which is on its way to becoming "tacitized" as an unconscious personal reality. Finally, practice—enactment—contributes to the cohesion of emerging form. New patterns require not only stepping into new roles but also practicing them to the point that they become second nature.

EMOTIONALITY AND CHANGE

One of the primary facts about change is that it is emotional. Our feelings are not simply vestiges of our animal legacy. They are also foundations and filters for much of our consciousness.[18] Constructive neuroscience has amply documented that embodiment and emotionality are the crucibles for our "higher" mental processes.[19] Our thinking, our attention, and our endless activity are all embedded in seas of emotions. Emotionality is an essential expression of how we are organized and how we function. Throughout the lifespan, humans of all ages continue to operate out of emotional patternings. Indeed, as recent integrations of personality theory and research have begun to suggest, much of what we mean by the term "personality" involves styles of feeling and activity that express the individual reality of the person.[20] What and how clients are feeling (or not feeling) *is reality* for them, and it has developed out of a personal history in which they have done their best to learn survival strategies. The therapist—through training, experience, and continuing personal development—strives to respond in ways that serve to comfort and challenge. This striving is part of what makes psychotherapy such a demanding profession (Chapter 11).

With regard to the role of emotional communication in psychotherapy, John Bowlby wrote:

> There are, in fact, no more important communications between one human being and another than those expressed emotionally, and no information more vital for constructing and reconstructing working models of self and other than information about how each feels toward the other. During the earliest years of our lives, indeed, emotional expression and its reception are the only means of communication we have. . . . Small wonder therefore, if, in reviewing his attachment relationships during the course of psychotherapy and restructuring his working models, it is the emotional communications between a patient and his therapist that play the crucial part.[21]

Working with emotions is itself an emotional challenge. One does not work with emotions in some abstract sense. One works with human beings who are feeling, and what they are feeling is often intense, heavy, painful, or frightening. Given the power and primacy of emotions in organizing and disorganizing our personal lives, it is important that therapists be familiar with more than theory and research on this topic. It is not just the client who is feeling, or who will be changed. We, too, will be feeling our way through the therapy process. I believe it is imperative that we honor emotions (our own and our clients') in that process. In order to work constructively with the spectrum and intensity of human emotions, we must learn to appreciate their role in our lives and to experience them. This is more easily said than done, of course, and clients often stretch us in our own emotional development. An experiential familiarity with feelings is a must for constructive practice. There are now excellent resources on emotional intelligence and emotion-focused psychotherapy.[22] But written and audiovisual resources are not the same as lived experiencing. Professional workshops and supervision are crucial to such learning, and personal therapy is often an invaluable option. I return to that option in the final chapter of this volume.

COURAGE AND CREATIVITY

Personal revolutions require considerable courage and a willingness to take risks. "Waiting it out," or waiting for others to decide our fate, often results in more pain and struggle. Not choosing is a choice. Not acting is an act. In 1874, Fitz-James Stephen put this fact much more eloquently:

> We stand on a mountain pass in the midst of whirling snow and blinding mist, through which we get glimpses now and then of paths which may be deceptive. If we stand still we shall be frozen to death. If we take the wrong road we shall be dashed to pieces. We do not certainly know whether there is any right one. What must we do? "Be strong of a good courage." Act for the best, hope for the best, and take what comes. . . . If death ends all, we cannot meet death better.[23]

Courage is not the absence of fear. Courage is intentional action in the intimate presence of fear. It requires "heart" (in Latin, *cor*). We thus "en-courage" (literally, "en-hearten") clients in their commitments and life choices, and much of our encouragement takes the form of our exhibiting courage and creativity in our work with them.

Knowing how to comfort, how to challenge, and when to do how much of either is an essential and complex skill of the constructive therapist. In earlier chapters, I have described techniques that might be useful. But what most techniques leave out is the act of creation—the spontaneous generation of a novel expression of life activity; hence, my cautionary remarks about the potential tyranny of technique. Human interactions are heavily scripted by social and cultural processes and role definitions. Life itself is not so tightly or neatly ordered. Many clients are in therapy because they feel that life has "thrown them a curve" or otherwise challenged them with something they did not expect. Part of what they hope to learn in therapy is how to respond to the unexpected. I believe that part of our responsibility as therapists is to teach them, as best we can, how to respond not only to their current life challenge but also to future challenges that neither they nor we can anticipate.

Creativity on the part of the therapist is a crucial element in constructive therapy.[24] Each client is unique. Although a client's experience and development may be reflected in the same abstract principles as that of any other client, the particulars of each life are never the same. Besides allowing the therapist to be more flexible in responding to these inevitable individual differences, creativity is an important element in the creation of novelty. And novelty, once again, is necessary for all learning and development.[25] The best way to teach clients how to risk new experience is for the therapist to do just that—in front of their clients' very eyes, and when they may least expect it! I am *not*, of course, saying that "anything goes," nor am I denying that clients sometimes need more familiarity (confirmation, affirmation) than novelty. But I believe that responsible and judiciously chosen excursions into the unexpected are invaluable ways of teaching clients to venture risks in their own patterns of being. Two illustrations from my clinical practice come to mind.

The first involved a man who had been struggling with chronic and intense depression. Seeing him was always difficult and draining, because his pain and hopelessness hung heavy in the room when he was there. On this particular day, he was even more despondent than usual, and I was already tired from a long day. His face was always sad and hollow. When I met him in the waiting area, he hardly acknowledged my greeting. He shuffled silently down the hall behind me, then painstakingly lowered himself into his usual position in the chair next to my desk. His frame was bent forward, as if he were in an advanced stage of osteoporosis, and his head drooped toward his knees.

"How are you, John?" I asked.

Almost a minute went by before he responded. "I am getting worse," he whispered.

I waited for him to elaborate, but there was only silence. (Meanwhile, inside me, there were the voices of my very human self saying, "Oh, God! Why me? Why tonight? He is my last client. I just want to go home.") Finally, to break the silence and foster some movement, I said, "How so?"

He was silent for perhaps half a minute, and then he said, "I used to be depressed. [long pause] Now I can't feel anything. . . . " His words and voice died off in weakness as he uttered this.

Quietly, unconsciously assuming his voice tone, I said, "*Nothing*?" (Inside me the voices continued, "Damn! This is going to be a long hour!")

[short pause] "Nothing."

We continued in silence for several minutes. Finally, without looking up, he said, "You don't say anything . . . just like my analyst."

Perhaps his words struck an old sensitivity. I don't know. But I heard myself say, "John, would you mind standing up?" When I heard myself voicing these words, my immediate internal reaction was one of panic ("Michael, what the hell are you doing? Where are you going with this?").

John looked at me for the first time in the session. His puzzlement was obvious as he said, "What? . . . What did you say?"

Almost mechanically, I repeated, "Would you mind standing up?" Again, my insides echoed disbelief. ("Jesus Christ, Michael! What are you going to do if he *does* stand up? What are you going to do if he *doesn't*?")

"You want me to stand up?" he asked incredulously.

"Yes," I said, despite the disharmony inside me. My heart was pounding nervously.

He shook his head and then—with great effort—slowly pushed himself up to a crouched but standing position. He stuffed his hands in his front pockets, looked down at me, and said, "O . . . K, . . . now what?"

That was where I got stuck. I had no idea where I was going with this little venture. I felt embarrassed, and I'm sure I looked it.

He repeated, "Now what?"

[brief pause] I said sheepishly, "I don't know."

His brow furrowed and his eyes squinted. Looking down at me, in a slightly stronger voice, he said, "You don't know!?"

I timidly said, "No."

He began to sway a bit as some inner tension built. His mouth tightened, and he shook his head.

"You asked me to stand up and now you don't know why!!!????"

I nodded.

"Good God!" he said with disgust. "I don't know how you make a living at this! You're pathetic," he grumbled. "How do you live with yourself?"

At a loss for words, I simply looked at him. His face was alive with contempt. Suddenly, I said, "John, are you *still* not feeling anything?"

His face went from ashen to red in a flash, and his mouth fell open. "You son of a bitch!" he said with a half-smile, and dropped back into the chair. "You tricked me!" The rest of the session went well.

Of course, John thought I had planned it that way: He wrote in his diary that night that I was some strategic genius in the emotional realm. I think I was clever and lucky, for the most part, and willing to risk doing something different (even when many parts of me were protesting the risk).

The second clinical illustration may sound equally bizarre, but, again, it illustrates my point about risking to teach by doing. I was in a small country for some invited lectures, and it was my first time there. I knew nothing of the language, and my audience was too reticent to ask questions even though its members seemed to understand my English. The only exception to the reticence was a very bright and extremely well-read young man. When I finished a morning lecture on the history of constructivism in European philosophy, he asked a very detailed question about Vico's relationship to the disciplines of history, philosophy, and the social sciences. That afternoon, when I closed with an emphasis on the importance of respecting our clients' phenomenological realities, he asked me to compare Heidegger's later writings with those of Cioran, Foucault, and Merleau-Ponty. On a third occasion, after my cautioning about the tyranny of technique, he asked me to compare William Barrett's works, *The Illusion of Technique* and *Irrational Man*. These daunting questions were asked in a manner that I construed as being challenges to the thoroughness of my scholarship.

It turned out that he would challenge more than my scholarship. At lunch that day, I informed my hosts that I would need a volunteer from the audience for my scheduled afternoon demonstration of constructive psychotherapy. Immediately, several of their assistants spread out to look for volunteers. Perhaps half an hour later, an assistant nervously informed me that they had found a volunteer. Something about the way he said that made me ask who the volunteer was, and he reluctantly informed me that it was the young man who had asked all the difficult questions. Overhearing this, my host said, "Don't worry, we can get a student to play a role with you."

I said, "No, don't ask a student; just tell me what you know about this volunteer."

My host proceeded to tell me that this brilliantly challenging young man was a professor in another field at a small college in a nearby country. No one seemed to know him. I said, "OK, please tell him that I appreciate his willingness to role-play a client." I said that I would invite him forward during the afternoon session, and that he should feel free to change his mind both before and during his explorations with me. In the afternoon, I lectured on assessment, technique, and process. Thinking that I might demonstrate the use of a mirror in assessing and fostering self-relationships, I asked my volunteer to step forward. He was fitted with a lapel microphone, and we sat facing each other, as if in a first encounter. I introduced myself and I asked how I might help. What happened thereafter came close to being one of my worst nightmares about public demonstrations of my skills as a therapist. My pseudoclient described himself with great conviction as a postgraduate failure who had never finished his master's degree. Two years earlier, he had suffered the breakup of his only significant romantic relationship. Since then, he said, he had been unable to work. He had lost his job in a bank and was living on loans from his parents, while he spent most of his waking hours sitting in front of his computer screen without ever touching a key.

As he described this scenario, my mysterious volunteer also began to show signs of "decompensation." There, in front of me and hundreds of people, he appeared to "deteriorate" or "regress." His speech became progressively more disjointed, and he began to rock back and forth in his chair. As he rocked, he used one hand to trace figure eight's on his knee. I was not the only therapist in the room who was wondering whether this was well-acted drama or genuine momentary disorder. It was an eerie and palpable ambiguity. If he was role-playing a client, he was doing a better job than hundreds of other volunteers I had seen. If he wasn't role-playing—if this was something real in this moment—how was I to handle it?

His speech deteriorated into a repetition of phrases and partial sentences, and his gaze seemed to be focused on the floor, just above the movements of his index finger on his knee. I tried to forget about the audience and the mirror I had hoped to use. He looked like some clients I have seen who were rapidly withdrawing, contracting inward. As he spiraled down, I struggled for something to say or do. Without knowing where I was going with it, I reached over to touch his knee and called him by his first name. His movements stopped for a moment and he looked at me. I said, "I do not know how best to help you, but I have an idea. [pause] Perhaps you would like to try it." His eyes stayed with mine, but his right hand began to move again in slow figure-eights on his knee.

Using my own right hand to demonstrate, I said, "You might want to see what it feels like when you touch yourself here (I touched the center of my forehead with the middle finger of my right hand and then paused; his right hand slowly moved from his knee to his forehead). We were entering into a synchrony. After a brief pause, I moved my hand from my forehead to my abdomen (about halfway between my diaphragm and my navel) and I said "And here." His hand glided down to his abdomen. Very slowly, I said, "And back to here" (placing my middle finger again on my forehead) and "Back to here" (moving my hand again to my abdomen). We did this a third time, slowly and intently. Then I said, "I don't know if this will be helpful or not, but I would encourage you to practice it whenever you begin to feel distressed." He looked at me and nodded an "OK," his hands now at rest on the arms of his chair.

"And I wonder if this might not be enough work for one day?" I said. He nodded, stood up, shook my hand, and returned to his seat in the audience. I asked if there were any questions or comments. My audience was silent, perhaps as stunned as I was. I returned to my lecture notes. The volunteer waited until my afternoon lecture was finished to thank me again personally. I asked if he felt all right about our interaction, and he said that he was "most grateful."

That night, I shared dinner with a group of people who had been at my workshop both days. Speaking in their own language, I could not follow the topics of their conversations. Finally, my host asked if I knew what people were talking about. "No," I said, and I was curious, because they seemed to be unusually animated. She said, "They are wondering where they can read about this technique of touching the forehead and the abdomen three times slowly. In what book can it be found?" I smiled, and she continued, "They are wondering how you knew to do just this, and what it means?

I looked at her and said, "I have never done that before today." She looked incredulous. "I don't know why I did it,[26] or what it means. I just knew that I needed to do something and that is what emerged." We both laughed. What was funniest, I think, was the fact that my colleagues thought I knew what I was doing and where I was going. They presumed that I had good reasons for doing what I did, and what better proof did they need than such a grateful response from my volunteer client? Looking back from the perspective of several years, it may have been clever of me to have engaged this man's attention and to redirect his need to move his hand in a way that changed the pattern. But that was hardly my plan or a conscious strategy. I was taking a risk. It could have turned out differently.

Much of what we call creativity is intuitive and tacit. I encourage my clients to trust that much of their life navigation is under the direction of processes well outside the limits of their consciousness. They may struggle desperately to "figure out" the most rational or reasonable path of action, and this is an adaptive strategy. The left (reasoning) hemisphere is a wonderful tool: Don't leave home without it. But many life choices are much more complex than logical computation, and we are fortunate to be the evolutionary inheritors of much more than we know.

TRANSITION AND TERMINATION

When all goes well, clients emerge from therapy with greater self-awareness, more openness to experience (particularly emotional experience), improved self-relations (increased capacities to self-accept, self-forgive, self-affirm, and self-comfort), and a greater sense of personal agency. Some emerge with better communication skills and new options for relating to others, intimately and otherwise. Many feel better about the world, more involved in projects other than their own development, and more appreciative of everyday particulars. Most importantly, perhaps, many clients emerge with a more hopeful engagement with their own life and the lives of others. With hard work, courage, and good fortune, there comes a time when the client is ready to move on. This is technically called "termination," although I wish we would substitute a term that is more appropriate to the transition involved. With John Bowlby and others,[27] I believe that termination is one of the most important phases of the therapeutic transaction. I like to use the metaphor of a journey, because it captures so many of the particulars of a temporary movement together. Each person is under his or her own power, the pace may be adjusted, there may be pauses and vistas, and there is often a sharing of dialogues. Dialogues about choice points. Acts of courage. And always an awareness that there will come a point where the paths will part and the travelers will each go their own way.

I make it a point to talk explicitly about the process of separation and how my clients are feeling as they prepare for our last session. I always ask them to write a brief synopsis of our work together,[28] and I often write something for them to take with them. I also give them a small gift, often an unusual pebble or a shell I have found on the beach, something that I give uniquely personal meaning when I present it to them. These symbolic "transition objects" are gestures of caring and good will, of course, and they are often treasured by clients (as I have learned in much later contacts).

One of my all-time favorite portrayals of the entire process of psychotherapy came from a client named Patricia, whom I had asked to write a brief synopsis of our work together as part of our preparations for our final session. When she arrived for that session, she greeted me with a very bright smile and handed me an envelope. I asked her if I should read it now and, after the first few lines, I handed it to her and asked her to please read it to me. She was reluctant at first, but then she read her own words, at first haltingly, and later with fullness and accentuation:

I didn't want to do this exercise. I sat down several times to start it, but nothing came except tears, and I had to stop because I was crying. It is still hard for me to believe that we won't see one another every Tuesday morning.

Anyway, the only thing I could come up with to summarize my experience of psychotherapy is an image that came to me while I was crying. I was a little girl, maybe 4 or 5 years old, and you were my father. You were teaching me how to ride a bicycle without training wheels. I had on long pants and a long-sleeve shirt, and we were on the playground behind my old school. It must have been a weekend, because there were no other people there. You began by putting one hand next to mine on the handlebars and the other on the bicycle seat. As I tried to keep my feet on the pedals and get them going in smooth cycles, you ran along with me, just fast enough to help me balance, but not so fast that I was too scared.

After a while, you relaxed your grip on the handlebars and just touched them lightly with your finger. When you took your hand off, I screamed, "No! No! Not yet!" The front wheel began to wobble sideways. You grabbed hold again and helped me straighten it out. I think you said something reassuring, but I don't know what it was. I also think you smiled at me, but I wasn't looking at your face.

It seemed a long time before you took your hand all the way off the handlebars, and I kept looking over to see that it was still there if I needed it. You were always there, running along with me and saying nice things that I can't remember. My next "scare" was when I realized that you had begun to relax you grip on the bicycle seat. I didn't know you had done that until I wobbled so badly that I almost fell. You caught me around the waist and the bicycle just leaned to the side, rolling along underneath us at a very silly angle. I think I laughed or you laughed, but now I am crying.

Sometime later, you let go of the seat entirely. I think I said, "I can't do it!" And you said I could: "You can steer for yourself and you can keep your balance." "But I will fall!" I said, and I did. This time you didn't catch me, and I hit the pavement with my shoulder. You were right there, lifting the bike off me and picking me up. You held me and you let me cry. You helped me learn that the hurt goes away. Then you said, "Let's try again." I did. I kept falling, of course, and you kept picking me up.

Somewhere in all of that you started dropping back. I was making bigger and bigger circles around the playground, and you were slowing to a walk around the center. Even though you were more distant, your voice stayed close to me. I was so excited about my own power to move that I began to get up from my falls and back on my bike before you could reach me. Later you just walked slowly around the middle and smiled encouragement at me. Sometimes you said, "Don't watch me. Watch where you're going."

That is how it felt. I will always remember your voice and your smile. Thank you for being so patient with me. Thank you for teaching me to keep trying.[29]

When she finished reading and handed it back to me, we both had tears in our eyes.

I close this chapter with a poem I wrote many years ago. It was inspired by an early Kris Kristofferson song, and it began as a gift for a client. Over the years, the poem has come to mean even more than I realized when I wrote it. I believe it speaks to many of us involved in the mysteries of change:

Pilgrim in Process[30]

It's a season of transition and you're on the move again
On a path toward something you cannot disown;
Searching for your being in the labyrinths of heart
And sensing all the while you're not alone.

Yes, you seem to keep on changing for the better and the worse
And you dream about the shrines you've yet to find;
And you recognize your longing as a blessing and a curse
While you puzzle at the prisons of your mind.

For as much as you seek freedom from your agonies and fears
And as often as you've tried to see the light,
There is still a trembling terror that your liberation nears
As you struggle with the edges of your night.

For your Reason is a skeptic and rejects what it desires,
Playing hard to get with miracles and signs;
Till a Witness gains momentum and emerges from within
To disclose the patterns well *above* the lines.

Then a window has been opened and you've let yourself observe
How the fabric of your Being lies in wait;
And you want to scream in anger and you want to cry for joy
And you worry that it still may be too late.

For the roller coaster plummets with a force that drives you sane
As you tightly grasp for truths that will abide;
Never fully understanding that your need to feel secure
Is the very thing that keeps you on the ride.

You survive the oscillations and begin to sense their role
In a process whose direction is more clear
And you marvel as your balance point becomes a frequent home,
And your lifelong destination feels like "here."

So with gentleness and wonder, with questions and with quests
You continue on the path that is your way;
Knowing now that you have touched upon the shores of inner life,
And excursions deeper can't be far away.

There will be so many moments when an old view seems so strong
And you question whether you can really change;
And yet, from deep within you, there's a sense of more to come
And your old view is the one that now seems strange.

Take good care, my friend, and listen to the whispers of your heart
As it beats its precious rhythm through your days;
My warm thoughts and hopes are with you on your journeys through it all . . .
And the paths of life in process find their ways.

Do be gentle, Process Pilgrim; *learn to trust that trust is dear*,
And the same is true of laughter and of rest;
Please remember that *the living is a loving in itself*,
And the secret is to ever be in quest . . .

NOTES

1. Bateson and Martin (2000); Oyama (2000); Schwartz and Begley (2002).
2. Lewis (1997); Mahoney (1991).
3. Bandura (1986); Rychlak (2003).
4. Arciero et al. (2003); Beck and Cowan (1996); Chamberlain and Bütz (1998); Combs (1996); Gleick (1987); Haken (1996); Hayek (1964); Kauffman (1993, 1995); Kelso (1995); Krippner (1994); Mahoney (1991); Mahoney and Moes (1997); Masterpasqua and Perna (1997); Pagels (1988); Palombo (2000); Pattee (1973); Prigogine (1980); Prigogine and Stengers (1984); Robertson and Combs (1995); Schiepek et al. (2003); Weimer (1982, 1987); Wilber (1999).
5. Davis and Hollon (1999); Dowd (1999); Duncan, Hubble, Miller, and Coleman (1998); Eagle (1999); Heatherton and Weinberger (1994); Kegan and Lahey (2001); Lyddon (1993); McAdams (1994); Pervin (1994); Prochaska and Prochaska (1999); Reid (1999); Snyder and Ingram (2000); Spence (1987); Wachtel (1982, 1999).
6. One can, however, sense intuitive parallels. Aristotle's logic hinges on the law of identity ($a = a$). Likewise, the integer—which plays such a central role in mathematics and science—is literally that which remains "untouched" and whole.
7. Arciero (1999); Arciero and Guidano (2000); Ecker and Hulley (2000); Mahoney (2000b); Neimeyer and Raskin (2000); Sass (1992).
8. There are, however, important exceptions. Rapid personality transformations do occur. William James acknowledged this in his classic studies of religious conversions, and others have documented them as "spiritual emergencies." In recent studies of "quantum change," some of the characteristics of such transformations have become more clear (Grof, 1975; James, 1902; Loder, 1981; Miller, 1999; Miller & C'de Baca, 1994, 2000; Vaughan, 1979, 1986; Wade, 1996). The majority of "quantum changers" report that their change experience was surprisingly sudden and accompanied by strong emotions or an altered state of consciousness. Mystical or spiritual experiences are common but

not essential. Another kind of shift is an insightful one in which the particulars of life take on new meanings. Note that we are again looking at two kinds. Both mystical and insightful forms of quantum change involve enduring shifts in people's sense of themselves and their perceptions of the world. The phenomenon of quantum change or rapid transformation deserves our continuing theoretical and research attention. It appears to be more common than psychologists had assumed. Moreover, we are wise to acknowledge the implications of such transformations for our ideas about human possibilities. There may be much more flexibility and resilience in human core ordering processes than we have yet begun to imagine.

9. Arciero and Guidano (2000); Guidano (1987, 1991, 1995a, 1995b); Mahoney (1999).
10. Arciero (1999); Arciero and Guidano, 2000); Baumeister (1991); Debats (1999); Dollinger (1986); Duncan et al. (1998); Freedland and Berenthal (1994); Gibson (1988); Greenberg and Paivio (1997); Guidano (1987, 1991); Masterpasqua and Perna (1997); Orlinsky and Howard (1975); Magai and McFadden (1995); Prigogine and Stengers (1984); Soldz and McCullough (1999).
11. Magai and McFadden (1995, p. 311).
12. Baumeister (1994).
13. A term powerfully illustrated in the writings of the Portuguese poet Fernando Pessoa (1974, 1991).
14. Bruner (1994); Lewis and Haviland (1993); Magai and McFadden (1995); Niedenthal and Kitayama (1994); Oberst (1999); Schiepek et al. (2003); West and Schlesinger (1990).
15. Socrates spoke of philosophical mentoring as midwifery, technically termed "maieutics" (Scott, 2002). His mother, coincidentally, was a midwife. Freud also used the analogy for psychoanalysis.
16. See Arciero (1999); Arciero and Guidano (2000).
17. Baumeister (1991).
18. Barrett and Russell (1999); Beiser (1974); Carstensen, Pasupathi, Mayr, and Nesselrode (2000); Cassidy and Mohr (2001); Cervone and Shoda (1999); Chamberlain and Bütz (1998); Diener (2000); Diener and Larsen (1993); Feldman-Barrett and Russell (1999); Flack and Laird (1998); Gilbert and Bailey (2000); Kitayama and Markus (1994); Lewis (1992); Lewis and Granic (2000); Lutz (1999); Niedenthal and Kitayama (1994); Panksepp (1998); Salovey, Rothman, Detweiler, and Steward (2000); Schaie and Lawton (1997); Tellegen, Watson, and Clark (1999).
19. Damasio (1995, 1999); Lakoff and Johnson (1999); Panksepp (1998).
20. Bohart and Tallman (1999); Heatherton and Weinberger (1994); Lamiell (1987); Magai and McFadden (1995).
21. Bowlby (1988, pp. 155–156).
22. Fosha (2000, 2001); Goleman (1995); Greenberg (2002).
23. Stephen (1874, cited in James, 1897).
24. Bohart and Tallman (1999); Leitner and Faidley (1999); Lyddon (1993).
25. For further readings on creativity and the crucial role of fluctuation and variation in development, see Haken (1984, 1996), Kelso (1995), Nachmanovitch

(1990), Schiepek et al. (2003), Siegler (1994), Thelen (1992), Thelen and Smith (1994), Thompson, Thompson, and Gallagher-Thompson (1995), Van Geert (1998, 2000), and Varela and Singer (1987).

26. I had watched Steve Gilligan (1997) do something like that a few months earlier.
27. Bowlby (1988); Quintana (1993).
28. See Kühnlein (1999) for related work.
29. Mahoney (1991, p. 274).
30. Mahoney (2003).

CHAPTER 11

BEING HUMAN AND A THERAPIST

I had not planned to be a psychotherapist. My decision to study psychology was shaped by a single session of unexpected therapy. I had suffered a trauma in adolescence that shook my world. I left home without finishing high school, and I pursued some dangerous adventures. My adventures were cut short by the sudden development of serious respiratory problems. At age 18, a physician told me that my condition was untreatable, and that I would die young and incapacitated. In the meantime, he recommended that I quit construction work, stop traveling, move to a warm dry climate, and go back to school. He mentioned Arizona.

I had not planned to go to college, and I lacked a high school diploma. A local community college was kind enough to let me take courses on a probationary basis. My health continued to deteriorate. I learned at the library that there were two universities in Arizona. I chose between them by tossing a coin. When I arrived for summer school, the woman in the registrar's office was amused by my naivete. I did not know that an application was required. Reviewing my transcript, she said that I was acceptable, but I needed to declare a major. I had not thought about a major, and it felt like an overwhelming choice at the moment. I said I didn't know what I wanted to be. She said, "That's OK. You have until Monday to decide." It was Friday morning. I drove to Encanto Park in downtown Phoenix and had a panic attack. My heart was racing and my head was spinning. I went to a phone booth. I looked up "psych" in the Yellow Pages. I needed some help. I knew virtually nothing about psychotherapy, but I was desperate. There were hundreds of names. I called one that listed several specializations. I explained that I had only $60 in life savings and I needed to make an important decision by Monday. Some cancelled appointments created a window of opportunity. I wrote down the directions to the office.

The therapist was a gaunt old man in a wheelchair. He seemed wise and gentle and spirited. When he learned that I was new to the area, he told me stories about the local Superstition Mountains. The Lost Dutchman's Mine was hidden in them somewhere. He told me stories of his children's adventures in uncharted areas of those mountains, where bandits lay in wait. Before I realized it, my 2-hour session was almost up. I nervously told him why I was there. I needed to declare a major. I said, "I have always wanted to be a writer, but I don't think there would be much job security with an English major." He nodded. "And the only other thing is . . . well, I took a psychology course in night school and the teacher encouraged me to consider it as an area . . . and the things I like to write about *are* what goes on inside people . . . but . . . but . . . " He waited. My heart was racing again. "But I get anxious and depressed . . . and what right would I have to tell other people what to do with their lives when I don't know what to do in my own?"

He lifted himself up on his arms to shift his weight, then tilted his head to the side. A long silence lingered. I can still remember the sound of the back of one hand rubbing slowly against the stubble along the side of his jaw. Finally, he said, "You know, Michael, some of the best football coaches in this country have never played the game." I don't remember whether either of us said anything else other than "good-bye." I remember feeling greatly relieved. I declared psychology as a major on Monday. Over the next 2 years, I had to work extra hard to make up course deficiencies in that area. My senior year, the honor society in psychology invited a local therapist to come talk to us about our career choice. My therapist was the featured speaker. I had no idea he was well known for his wit and wisdom. By chance, it seems, I had chosen Milton Erickson to be my first therapist.

The question that I asked him was itself a protean one. It has to do with expectations and roles, authenticity and responsibility. I would come back to it again and again in my career. I would eventually come to study the personal lives of therapists and the impact of their work on their lives. I would become a therapist for therapists—another development that I could hardly have anticipated. But before all of this, there were many other chance events that shaped my personal and professional life. That Monday, when I declared psychology as a major, I was assigned to an advisor. He was in his first year of teaching, and he generously took me under his wing. His name was Dave Rimm, and he patiently mentored me toward applying to graduate school. Arizona State University was an enclave of Skinnerian behaviorism at the time, but Dave was also interested in the works of Albert Ellis, Joseph Wolpe, and Arnold Lazarus. He invited one of his former professors to give a colloquium to the department. That was how I met Albert Bandura, who became my mentor in graduate school. Chance encounters in life paths. The chances and the encounters multiplied, and my paths continued to differentiate.[1]

I learned to practice behavior therapy and became involved in the cognitive revolution when it swept through both clinical and experimental psychology. But the shifts in my theoretical allegiance were far less significant than the shifts in my experience of what it means to be a psychotherapist. My first clients quickly taught me that I had a lot to learn. I was well versed in the theories, the research, and empirically evaluated techniques. But I was not prepared for much of what I encountered. My clients were not like the clients in the textbooks. They didn't change as quickly or as easily as the texts said they should. The problems they came in with were not simple, or they didn't stay simple. Their progress wasn't as linear or consistent as I had expected. And it was hard work. The emotional demands were sometimes overwhelming. I don't know what I had expected, but clinical practice asked much of me. Each in his or her own way, clients pressed me for more than I knew. "Trauma" used to be a word on a page. So were "life" and "death." They were abstractions. I thought I knew their meanings until I sat heart to heart with people. What do you say to someone who has accidentally killed his or her own child? How do you help someone die? What about the ones who are beaten or raped? I saw great human strength and courage, but I also heard much that scarred my own heart.

I decided to enter personal therapy again, this time for support and a closer look at myself. I began taking workshops that allowed me to meet other therapists and explore different methods and approaches to the work I was doing. I began to work with even more challenging clients and, eventually, to serve as a therapist for other therapists. I continue to feel humbled and privileged by the demands of this profession. I am convinced that these demands merit our appreciation. That is the focus of this final chapter.

VICARIOUS SUFFERING: THE WOUNDS OF HELPING

Milton Erickson used to say, "My voice will go with you." His voice did. What he did not say was that our clients' voices also go with us. Their stories become part of us—part of our daily lives and our nightly dreams. Not all such stories are negative—indeed, a good many are inspiring. The point is that they change us.

Professions have come to be defined in part by the distance maintained between the professed expert and his or her clients. In becoming a profession, psychotherapy has followed this same pattern. We are warned to distance ourselves from our clients. Be conservative, maintain objectivity, watch everything you say, don't care too much (or, at least, don't show it), and follow the book (whichever one is currently in force). Play it safe. A professional is a technician, not a friend. Take good notes. Be prepared for forensics and litigation. Always inform the state or its agencies. Don't let the client reach your heart. These are central messages in many programs for training psychotherapists.

Still—with all these boundaries and bureaucratic protocols for our interactions—isn't it interesting that our clients so often and so powerfully make it through to us? They touch us, and they ask us to touch their lives with our comfort, compassion, and counsel. Rather than just being "cases," names on manila folders that require stacks of insurance forms and paper trails, they become real human beings struggling with multiple and endless crises in worlds where their options are often significantly limited. We think of them in between meetings. They make their way into our daily consciousness, our dreams, and sometimes our life reflections.

We are changed by our work. Do we become desensitized to the suffering? This may happen to a few who prefer a more detached style of therapy, but career therapists often report becoming more compassionate as a result of all the suffering they have witnessed.[2] Indeed, those who open themselves enough to the emotional interactions that permeate psychotherapy also seem to develop greater emotional flexibility and an increased level of comfort with the full spectrum of emotions. The latter may be among the benefits derived from a career in psychotherapy.

But there is also a paradox involved in our vicarious suffering. It could be called the paradox of wrestling "hope from hell." That is often what it feels like. Because of our training and licensing, we are given special privileges and responsibilities. The privilege of confidential communication permits us to invite our clients to share the secrets of their hearts. The process of that sharing is often central to their coping and development. But the secrets that they share with us are often painful to hear, difficult to imagine, and hard to forget. Many of their stories tell of the worst kinds of human capacities: intentional cruelty, deception, greed, hate, insensitivity, irresponsibility, violations of human decency. We are repeatedly exposed to stories of hell: tragedy, heartlessness, and the willful infliction of pain. This can be a challenge to our own faith in human nature.

The paradox comes from what we are asked to do as helpers. While listening to such stories from clients, we therapists are expected to pull hope out of their hell. Along with the clergy and our colleagues in medicine, *we are socially sanctioned protectors of hope*. We are professionally charged with the responsibility of encouraging our clients to keep the very faith that, in us, may be under constant challenge by our work. We are supposed to help our clients to endure their personal hell, to trust that their suffering will diminish, to believe that they are valued and viable beings, and that their lives are worth living. So we are protectors of hope, while also being frequent witnesses to daunting insults to human decency and dignity. I believe this paradox is a significant one. Therapists with strong religious convictions may have less difficulty coping with it, just as clients who experience a deep faith in their religion are often thereby aided in navigating their lives.[3] But no one is immune to such affronts, and the therapist who lacks a hope-protecting philosophy of life may be particularly vulnerable to the challenges presented by the "hope from hell" paradox. This may be why nonreligious therapists so often find themselves interested in the world's spiritual and wisdom traditions.

THE PERSON AND PERSONAL LIFE OF THE THERAPIST

There are many myths about what therapists are really like as persons.[4] In the most negative portrayal, a therapist is a fundamentally neurotic voyeur who delves into other people's private lives in order to avoid dealing with his own problems. He is assumed to have come from an unhappy childhood and a dysfunctional family. This "pseudoshrink" has extensive personal problems and a dark and sinister side. He is, of course, the opposite of the stereotype of the therapist as guru, the "supershrink." She is a warm and wise oracle who can read minds and heal hearts. Her energy is boundless, and she is never at a loss for words or wisdom. In between these two extreme stereotypes lies the "wounded healer," an image common to healers and shamans in diverse indigenous cultures.[5]

Hippocrates, the father of Western medicine, was following the inspiration of the mythical figure Asklepios (also Aesculapius), who was raised by the centaur Chiron. Asklepios developed unusual healing powers despite the fact that he suffered from a personal wound that would not heal. There have been many interpretations of the myth, and I have addressed it repeatedly in working with therapists as clients. Healers are often assumed to be veterans of developmental difficulties. They may be survivors of trauma and often feel themselves to be "different." Healers in aboriginal cultures often live at the boundaries between their community and natural wilderness. Their difference is sensed by both them and their community. Many healers identify with paths of healing and service very early in their lives; others are shocked into such service by a later life event. What is "wounded" about the "wounded healer" is a matter of interpretation. In some cultures, "wounded" means little more than a veteran of life experience. To be wounded in such cultures means to be experienced in life, and life experience is a sacred source of wisdom. In some spiritual traditions, love is described as a permanently open wound—an ever-flowing aperture on life that works to keep itself open. The term "wounded" tends to have more negative connotations in industrialized cultures, where "vulnerability" (literally, the capacity to be wounded) is equated with death. In the latter, the wounded healer is more likely to be viewed as a pathetic figure—one who can heal despite a grave wound, or who can influentially preach what he cannot effectively practice.

Negative stereotypes about psychotherapists have not been corroborated by research findings.[6] Most therapists have not come from troubled childhoods or dysfunctional families. Most report having had happy childhoods. The majority are healthy and satisfied with their lives. Comparisons across professions have been rare, but they render a positive portrayal of therapists.[7] The dimension with which therapists are least satisfied is their bodies,[8] and that may be a common cultural phenomenon. But let us not gloss over some facts that merit attention, namely, that some therapists are impaired by personal difficulties and others, though technically unimpaired, are seldom helpful to their clients. In an ideal world, impaired therapists would seek and easily receive help, and ineffective therapists would find another line of work. But ours is not an ideal world, and our profession is just beginning to serve its servers. Many of the therapists I have counseled have been worried about personal impairment and inadequacy. The vast majority of them were very competent professionals who served their clients well.

Quite frankly, I have come to worry more about therapists who are overconfident about their competence. There are distinguished "diplomates" in psychotherapy who are appallingly poor therapists, and sometimes bona fide assholes. How these individuals got licensed, and how they maintain their licenses, is mystifying. We have probably all met therapists we didn't like. We may be embarrassed to share professional categorization with them. They are challenges to our identity.[9] If we focus only on them, we will surely be disheartened. Fortunately, one also meets some authentic *menschen* who embody the spirit of authenticity and compassionate wisdom.[10] They, too, struggle, and they develop because of this.

The average, well-functioning therapist suffers most of the same problems as any other human being. Anxiety is common, and acute anxiety may predominate in early years of practice. Depression is not unusual, especially after personal losses and in the midst of chronic physical and emotional depletion. Feelings of isolation are common, perhaps because of being sequestered in privacy for large parts of the day. Health problems run the full gamut, without any apparent exceptions from the general population. Relationship difficulties seem to be a frequent source of personal concern for psychotherapists. The reasons for this are a matter of speculation, of course. Is it more difficult to relate to therapists? Do they practice communication all day and then fail to communicate in their private lives? Do their learned styles of being therapeutic interfere with their abilities to be authentically present to a life partner? In response to such questions, I have sometimes joked about my impression that we therapists develop unusual skills in appearing to be paying attention when we are not. Such skills might serve us well in a long day of therapy, yet serve us poorly if they permeate our intimate life. But relationship difficulties are seldom as simple as this, and I question whether any speculations have yet captured the likely complexity involved. Moreover, I believe that the challenges encountered in therapeutic work often demand development on the part of the therapist, and different rates and directions of development are common sources of difficulty in human relationships.

Clients sometimes want to believe that therapists live personal lives that follow a Hollywood script of confident well-being; structured support from/to family and friends; leisure time that is fulfilling and enriching; a healthy regimen of nutrition, exercise, and prayer or meditation; and restful sleep filled with sweet dreams of past treasures and future enjoyments. It is perhaps "human, all too human"[11] for our clients to want to believe such things. It may be a corollary of the myth of arrival. The real danger of such beliefs is that they may encourage therapists to actually believe that their personal lives are supposed to be perfect. When they are not, they may be inclined to think and feel that "something is wrong" (often with them, but also with their relationships, therapeutic work, or the world itself). In the face of a personal life challenge or some chronic theme of unhappiness, they are inclined to fault themselves. This is often associated with painful and unwarranted inferences (e.g., that they are poor therapists [because they don't have their personal life fully "together"], that they are imposters [playing the role of an expert on life when their own lives are in a mess], or that they suffer from the "Moses complex," meaning that they can lead others to the "promised land" of expanded well-being, but they cannot enter themselves because of a prior sin).[12]

The recent increase in research on the personal life of the therapist may well reflect our personal and collective fascination with who we are as professionals. It also reflects a deepening appreciation of the "human factor" in helping relationships. This appreciation has only recently gained ascendance in theory and research on psychotherapy. Those approaches that initially minimized the role of the therapist or the therapeutic relationship have been forced to accommodate the evidence. Therapists do not just bring theory, knowledge, or technique to the therapeutic process; they also bring their own style of being, their presence, and their hearts. We should therefore not be surprised that the person of the therapist is second only to client variables in predicting the outcome of psychotherapy.[13]

A THERAPIST'S PERSONAL LIFE

I have had the privilege of working with many therapists as they navigated their lives as professional helpers. I do not feel comfortable discussing "case histories," even in the abstract, because of my concerns about privacy and trust. More often than I can recount, I have witnessed both intentional and unintentional "leaks" about clients. In casual conversations, I have heard someone disclosing details that led to a likely identification of the client from whose life they came. One does not have to live in a small town to have experienced such "synchronous" revelations. And many therapists—particularly therapists in personal therapy—are aware of how delicate their privacy may be. In my own experiences as a client, I have felt the pain of learning that my own privacy had been violated. Therefore, when I began focusing my private practice on therapists, I decided to fortify and more closely monitor my commitment not to discuss detailed case material with anyone.[14] But, just before he died, one man not only gave me permission to discuss his life as a therapist, he also urged me to do so. He hoped that parts of his story would serve others in the profession.

Apollo, a very private man, had been practicing psychotherapy for more than 40 years when I met him. It was his stream of consciousness that I excerpted in Chapter 8. His orientation and life circumstances are less important here than are his courageous self-awareness and complexity. He lived in a large metropolitan area where I had been invited to speak. I was giving a workshop on the topic "The Personal Life of the Psychotherapist." There, as in this chapter, I tried to emphasize five things:

1. Psychotherapy is a very difficult and complex challenge for both therapist and client.
2. Therapists are changed at least as much as clients in the process of psychotherapy.
3. Many therapists bear heavy burdens of expectations that they/we must be unusually happy, enlightened, or wise in order to be legitimate professionals.
4. Self-care—enactive compassion for oneself—is essential for the personal well-being and professional responsibilities of psychotherapists.
5. Personal therapy and spiritual practices can be invaluable resources in our development.

I was speaking to a group of 200 practitioners and felt deeply affirmed by their reactions.

That night in my hotel room, I received a call from one of the participants in my workshop. I call him "Apollo." He was one of the oldest and most experienced therapists in the metropolitan area. We had been briefly introduced earlier in the day, and he had made a point of thanking me before he left that afternoon. That evening, he phoned me to ask if I might have time for breakfast before my plane departed the next day. I agreed.

He met me in the hotel lobby the following morning, and we drove to a small coffee shop on the outskirts of the city. As we began breakfast, he complimented me on my remarks during the workshop I had just completed. I felt more than flattered. He was a seasoned therapist. Moreover, several of my friends who lived in the area had already pointed him out as "their personal therapist." They were glad that I was endorsing the merits of personal therapy for therapists, and they sang his praises. He was, in that area, the primary "therapists' therapist." One friend estimated that perhaps as many as half of the people who had participated in my workshop had, at one time or another, consulted Apollo for personal help.

Apollo and I went for a walk in a nearby park after breakfast and there, on a park bench, we talked. He was cautious and reflective at first; then, he began to move toward a more personal tone. He asked me why my workshop had not included any details of my private practice with therapists as clients. I had discussed the results of several large surveys, but I had not mentioned any particulars. I told him that I did not feel comfortable discussing therapists' "case histories" because of my concerns about their privacy and our trust. "We make connections without knowing how we made them," I said, "and I have come to view confidentiality as sacred."

Apollo nodded his head slowly as we sat on the park bench. A period of silence followed, and my attention was drawn to the sounds of some children playing in the distance. Somewhere in those seconds, Apollo had begun to weep quietly into his hands, which now covered his face. A large man of composure and dignity sat next to me weeping, and I was moved by his tears. He had no one to talk to, he said. On his broad shoulders and in his big heart, he carried the secrets of many years of service to a large community of therapists—who carried on their own shoulders and in their own hearts the struggles and tragedies of thousands of individuals, families, and groups in their shared community. He wiped away his tears with his hands, then—looking directly and deeply into my eyes—asked me if I would consider seeing him as my client. I was surprised by his request, perhaps because I could have as easily asked him the same question. Without breaking our gaze, I unconsciously put my hand on his knee and said, "Yes." There was a part of me that felt intimidated by his far greater life experience, but I also sensed that I might have something to offer this seasoned caregiver.

We agreed to meet face-to-face at least four times per year and to be otherwise in contact by phone and mail. Sometimes we met in his city, other times in mine, and occasionally elsewhere. There were times when we used half-day sessions, and other times when we spent weekends together. I had conducted some long-distance "episodic" therapy with clients before meeting Apollo, and I knew that this form of work could have its advantages and disadvantages.

We worked together in this manner until his death, almost a decade later. He taught me much about life, about psychotherapy, and about both living and dying consciously. I feel very privileged to have known him, let alone to have served him as a therapist. Given my personal coda about not discussing "case material" from therapists, I would not be discussing Apollo here had he not both authorized and requested that I do so. In the final months of his life, Apollo gave me a key to a storage space. There, among his personal effects, I found three large boxes that contained almost 50 years of episodic and very personal diaries. He had told me about these diaries during our work together, but I had never seen them. When it became clear to him that his remaining time was very limited, Apollo asked me if I would consider keeping them, reading them, and rendering from them what I felt to be worthwhile from his personal and professional life. Part of his request was that I destroy his diaries before my own death—a request aimed more at protecting his clients and friends than himself. I accepted. When the dark shadow of death appeared to loom over my own life a short time later, I hurriedly reread his diaries and then ceremonially burned them.

Why do I call him "Apollo"? Primarily because of his passionate interests in astronomy. He was particularly enthralled by the Apollo 13 mission because of its human and technological heroics. He mentioned it several times over the years of our work together, but I came to a deeper appreciation of its significance for him only when I read his diaries after his death. There—in a series of scattered thoughts and rough, artistic sketches that spanned many years of personal and professional experience—he had laid out some gems that resonate deeply with themes in this book, particularly the delicate and dynamic relationship between order and disorder.

The Apollo 13 mission was intended to "repeat" prior explorations—to land humans on the moon, to collect soil samples, and to conduct experiments. Moon landings had so quickly become "routine" to the earthly public that little television attention was given to this mission, until those now-famous words were uttered: "Houston, we have a problem." The problem was acute and critical, involving the explosion of oxygen and fuel tanks, and it created a poignant life-and-death crisis. Like so many life crises, it was totally unexpected and stretched the coping skills and creativity of the crew and their terrestrial network. There was chaos, both aboard the space module and at NASA headquarters in Houston. Some experts recommended that the astronauts immediately reverse their direction—which amounted to an "about face" of 180 degrees, spending their little remaining fuel in what would have been a futile attempt to return "home" (to earth's gravitational field). Other experts (correctly) calculated that this would amount to suicide, because their remaining energies—if reversed—would bring them only part of the way home, and then they would drift off into lifeless limbo.

What my client Apollo realized and utilized (in his own life and in that of many of his clients) was that the energy and inertia of an accidental tragedy could force a system into a delicate and life-saving resonance with other forces that could be harnessed to serve its survival and development. Clear and guaranteed solutions are rarely apparent in life or in space. The Apollo 13 crew was in "new territory," and there were constant reminders that they were on the edge. However, and importantly, with close and trusting communication with their "ground crew," who meticulously struggled at both abstract and phenomenological levels to simulate the situation, a microscopic slit of hope was elaborated. The moon's gravitational field could be strategically used to "slingshot" the crippled vehicle back toward earth. *But* the main navigational computers had to be shut down to conserve energy, and the three-man crew had to emigrate from their center of power—the "command module"—into their parasite, the "lunar landing module," which they had intended to use and then abandon on the surface of the moon. What they had intended to abandon now became their sole means of life support.

The functions of the lunar landing module were transformed in this crisis. It went from a peripheral to a central role. The landing module's life support resources became critical, as did its energy sources. Its engines had been designed to permit a soft landing on the moon. But these engines were instead harnessed in the midst of this crisis to adjust the trajectory of the crippled spacecraft. Without computers, these adjustments were calculated from Houston but executed by the seat of the crew's existential space pants. For the remainder of their trip, it was not clear whether their "strategic intervention" would allow them to survive. A mistake of less than one tenth of 1%—in either direction—would have sent them either skimming off the earth's atmosphere into oblivion or entering that atmosphere so directly that they would incinerate within a few minutes. Neither the crew nor their "secure base" in Houston knew which it would be when radio contact was lost at their reentry into earth's atmosphere. They all suffered, but they survived. The Apollo 13 mission became a modern epic of heroism.

Apollo had many diary entries with sketches of the Apollo 13 trajectory—an elongated and lopsided figure "8." He kept notes on his own developmental trajectories, which he depicted as loops of gravitational attraction among personal issues. His drawings reminded me of the sketches of a theoretical physicist. Some would have the names of people who had been important in his life: his parents, a brother who had died when they were teenagers, a college sweetheart, his wife and their two young children (all killed by a drunk driver years earlier), his first client to commit suicide, a client whose stalking and lawsuits had haunted him for years, his primary mentor, a first and second therapist, a married woman friend whom he secretly loved, and, in the final diaries, me. Some of his drawings were time lines with dominant emotions drawn as larger circles. He read works of popular science and science fiction, and elements of these also made their appearance in his diaries: chaos theory, black holes, virtual realities, utopias, holocausts, multiple universes, synchronicity. Besides the drawings there were diary entries that resembled outlines of never-written articles on life and therapy. Notes to himself. Ideas. Worries about different clients. Memories. Single words or lines marking recent experiences. An opera, a dream, resolutions, epiphanies, nightmares, reflections on the profession.

Our conversations were often just that—conversations. He struggled with many of the same issues with which his therapist clients struggled. Loneliness. Disillusionment. Despair. Guilt. Cycles of exhaustion. Feelings of being an imposter. Desire, envy, regret. It was not all negative, of course. Apollo often felt richly rewarded by his work, and he enjoyed a number of hobbies that helped him relax. Over the years, our conversations began to move toward a mixture of mentoring, reflections, and recommendations. I offered my support and affection. I comforted and challenged. But Apollo often took the lead and urged me to write what he could not. At times, I felt like a young journalist interviewing a sage veteran about the labyrinths of life and its counsel.

I knew and worked with Apollo for over 8 years. Some of our interests and characteristics were eerily similar. Working with him was unlike any other work I had done before, and it changed me in ways that I am still only beginning to appreciate. He was a sweet, strong, and wise man. I was the designated guide in our relationship, but our interactions were fluid. I did not reveal much of my personal life to him, but he was keenly aware of fluctuations in my energy and attention. We often sat or walked in silence. When we walked, I was particularly aware of subtleties. Our pace. Pauses. Shared gazes at a vista, clouds, wildlife. We often gravitated toward a park bench (reminiscent of our first meeting) and simply watched the lives that moved past.

When he developed his illness, Apollo became even sweeter and more crystalline. He enjoyed his last 3 years perhaps more than any others in his life. He continued his practice, even when he was visibly weak and pained. Toward the end, he began physically to remind me of Milton Erickson—a gaunt spirit with a radiance of being that was unmistakable. Our conversations became more frequently focused on "the work," by which he meant our shared profession. He revealed even more to me then, and I think he did some of his best therapeutic work in those final years. I had more difficulty with his imminent death than he did, and I felt guilty when he comforted me about his dying. I had just begun work on this book. He encouraged me to make it a "work of heart."

"Tell them," he said. "Tell them what it can be like. Tell them how hard it is to be a helper . . . and how sweet it is, too. Give them a taste." That is what I am trying to do.

THERAPIST SELF-CARE

Let there be no doubt: Being a therapist is not easy. You name it, and we probably have to deal with it. Abuse, anger, anguish, argumentativeness, anxiety, assholes, attorneys, bureaucracy, cruelty, denial, dependence, despair, dysfunctional families, embarrassment, grief, guilt, hope, injustice, love, meanings, policies, politics, prejudice, racism, sexism, and downright stupidity. The range of challenges directed toward us should be appreciated by agencies that influence the selection, training, and licensing of mental health practitioners. Trainees should know, up front, that they are entering a life path of considerable developmental challenge. Those psychotherapists who come from happy families and scarless childhoods should be informed that they will hear true-life stories that will stretch their abilities to imagine. Those trainees coming from dysfunctional families should be cautioned that they will hear stories that may revive old memories and deep issues within them.

Our work constantly demands that we develop, often in ways and at moments that we could not have anticipated and do not prefer. Like our clients, we too need rest, encouragement, recreation, emotional support, laughter, love, meaning, and communities of kindred spirits. Psychotherapists—perhaps like many other health care professionals—are often more comfortable giving care than receiving it. This may be a factor in career choices. The most consistent lesson to be learned in a career of caregiving is that balance and circulation are essential. We need to take care of ourselves. This is not just to protect the quality of our services to our clients. We need to take care of ourselves because we, too, deserve to enjoy our personal lives. I have summarized my recommendations for therapist self-care in Appendix M. If you are a therapist, I urge you to take a few moments to read those recommendations.

Self-care is a tricky matter. It sounds good and it makes sense. But there are so many things that need to be done, so many responsibilities. If you are not careful, self-care can become another item on a long daily "to do" list. One more thing to monitor. But self-care is not something you can do first thing in the morning and then check it off (like a workout or medication). Self-care is a skillful attitude that needs practice throughout the day. It is the release breath taken when you notice muscle tension. It is a welcome tear or smile at the sight of a flower or squirrel. It is the indulgence of an impulse to relax and enjoy. Over the years, I have become more and more convinced of how important this message is. At workshops such as the one where I met Apollo, I have carried this message to many health care professionals. I have given and received many hugs in the process, and I am grateful. But the lessons are endless, and I am still a student. Several years ago, after a grueling schedule of workshops on therapist self-care, I was suddenly hospitalized for exhaustion and pneumonia. I lay in bed for what seemed like an eternity, listening to the darkness and the sounds of the instruments that were maintaining my life functions. The phone rang. I thought it was one of my children. Instead, it was a therapist friend from another country who had heard that I was dying. "You *can't* die!" she yelled. "We need you! We need you to remind us to take care of ourselves!" I removed my oxygen mask just long enough to hoarsely shout a few choice words.

My own practice of self-care is improving, bit by bit. These days, I travel less for work and more for pleasure. I have the faithful companionship of my Lhasa Apso, Baby, who goes to work with me daily. She is ever ready for play and affection, and she is a welcome reminder of trust. I now pause for more playgrounds and sunsets. I balance better. But I am only human, and I make mistakes. If I do work too hard and end up exhausted again, though, please do me a favor: Let me rest.

PERSONAL AND SPIRITUAL DEVELOPMENT

When asked how being a therapist has affected their lives, most therapists emphasize enrichment rather than impairment.[15] Therapists frequently report that their work has made them more respectful of individual differences and the importance of human relationships. They believe that a career in helping has made them wiser, more self-aware, more tolerant of ambiguity, and more capable of enjoying life. Negative responses are significantly less common (e.g., feelings of cynicism, helplessness, premature aging). Moreover, the ratio of positive to negative effects generally increases with years of experience as a psychotherapist. Theoretical orientations do not seem to matter.

Two other findings from survey research have intrigued me. Therapists commonly report that their own psychological development has been accelerated by their work and—regardless of their own religious background or beliefs—that their work often feels like a form of spiritual service. Both of these findings make good sense. Of course our lives are accelerated. One cannot be intimately involved in so many other lives without being challenged in the process. Career therapists would be fascinating "objects" of longitudinal studies in human development. I learned much more in a few hundred hours with Apollo than I learned from thousands of college sophomores completing questionnaires. If human change processes are accelerated and amplified in therapists, shouldn't we be studying them?

The spiritual service response has also begun to make more and more sense. Psychotherapists are, after all, akin to modern confessors and clerics. We listen, we witness, we nurture the human heart. We respond to the shocks of existence—life and death, good and evil, voids and virtues. We help people mourn and celebrate, forgive and move on with life. Our clients have faith in our faith in them. Atheists and mystics alike make leaps of faith. Faith is the essence of hope, of continued engagement in the mystery. As Huston Smith says, the mystery of life is not like a murder mystery—a "whodunit" that will be resolved in the final chapter.[16] Life is itself a sacred mystery whose relentless elusiveness is central to its sanctity. Psychotherapy is a form of spiritual service. Practicing psychotherapy can be a form of spiritual practice.

THE CHALLENGES OF PRACTICING CONSTRUCTIVELY

Being a psychotherapist is a complex challenge. Being a *constructive* psychotherapist is all the more so. I believe that constructive psychotherapy places unique and unusual demands on the therapist—demands that are above and beyond those that fall on the shoulders of just any psychotherapist:

> The psychological demands of constructive metatheory are unsurpassed by those of any other contemporary perspective. No other family of modern theories asks its adherents to maintain such a degree of self-examining openness, to so painstakingly tolerate and harvest (rather than eliminate) ambiguity, or to so thoroughly question both the answers and the questions by which they inquire. It is not easy to be a constructivist—a point that may help explain why, until recently, it has also been less popular than other approaches. Popular or not, however, it continues to appeal to a sizeable and growing minority of both theorists and therapists—a minority, I might add (with conscious bias), whose products are disproportionately represented at the frontiers of modern inquiry. Whatever developments emerge in our next century of study and service, many will have been offered or influenced by those who have accorded the human knower a proactive role in the knowing and the known.[17]

These are strong assertions, of course, but I believe they are warranted in light of the conceptual and practical demands of a constructive approach to mental health services. Challenges and rewards apply to all approaches to therapy, of course. Those challenges are amplified considerably when therapy is practiced in a constructive manner.

The challenges are many. Constructivism is a nonauthoritarian approach in which openness and "connected knowing" are primary.[18] Constructive practice requires honoring individuality and diversity, without sliding down a slippery slope of "anything goes" relativism.[19] There is no fixed, linear algorithm that can be applied to every person. Choices must be made with an awareness of limited knowledge and existential responsibilities. A constructive therapist realizes that she cannot be neutral, objective, passive, or unaffected.

The constructive therapist is also aware of his own limited awareness. He appreciates the extent to which the most basic and important processes of organizing our moment-to-moment experience operate at levels far beyond what we consider conscious awareness. Among other things, this means that both client and therapist are always communicating far more than they are explicitly verbalizing to themselves or each other. Likewise, the learning that takes places in the context of therapeutic interaction is always more profound than either the client or therapist consciously realize. These acknowledgments encourage the constructive therapist to balance his attention between relatively more and less conscious aspects of his work with a person, that is, to attend to both his explicit formulations of a given client's situation and resources, as well as to a multitude of less specifiable impressions and inclinations (intuitions, "feeling tones," personal dreams, etc.).

The list of challenges involved in practicing constructively is a long one. I have summarized some recommendations for such practice in Appendix N. Rather than here attempt to elaborate these challenges in words, I am drawn to a visual image. Imagine, if you will, that life is an unfolding landscape, and that the psychotherapy client is a traveler in trouble. Frightened, tired, and often feeling lost, she witnesses the movement of humanity all around. She sees other travelers moving in different directions, some racing with haste, and others crawling in pain. Most of these individuals travel well-worn paths that are common to other travelers. A few travel alone and on more isolated paths, some of which they are creating as they walk them. Some individuals are not moving at all. It can be a bewildering panorama.

Along the way, there are many people asking for help and many others offering assistance. Among the latter are psychotherapists, many of whom establish themselves at choice points along the most frequently used paths. And it is here that therapists begin to exhibit some of their most important differences in strategies of helping. Some of them are essentially selling maps or information about the terrain ahead. They claim to know the best route for traveling to the destinations sought by their clients. They may offer advice and opinions on the merits of the destinations themselves. They are, in a sense, life path travel agents.

Those therapists who practice from a constructivist metatheory, however, are seldom seen selling maps or advocating particular destinations. What distinguishes constructivists from other kinds of therapists is their willingness to join temporarily their clients' processes of travel. Such a counselor is willing to walk in the moccasins of those being served and to take turns leading and following. A constructive therapist respects her clients' needs to rest as well as their occasional needs to run. She is compassionate and comforting when clients feel frightened or despairing. If a client feels that he cannot move on his own, she is willing to wait, or she offers to carry some of the client's burden for a while. But the power for movement and the responsibility for choices of direction always return to the client. Indeed, a large part of what gets discussed and otherwise exchanged in this moveable dialogue has to do with choices, agency, and the meanings that are constructed around them.

When there are dangers or falls along the path, which are inevitable, the counselor remains focused on the safety and well-being of the client. Some choices are painful to make; other choices result in additional pain, at least temporarily. The constructive therapist strives to reduce the dangers when she can and to minimize the damage of movements that have brought the client pain. Lessons about life—lessons that are always unfinished—are harvested as they occur in exchanges between these travelers and in interactions with other travelers. And, when it is time, the constructive therapist and client take their separate life paths, both having been enriched by their time and travel together. This is, at least, my image of what it means to counsel constructively.

Training for the profession of psychotherapy often emphasizes the importance of boundaries. The emphasis is on the distance and difference between therapists and clients, and their roles. But boundaries are also areas of connection. When therapists are my clients, I feel that connection all the more deeply. We are family. We serve the human spirit. Let me therefore close with a poem written from one therapist to another. I hope that it reflects a few of the crystals I have been polishing in this and previous chapters. I thank you for your companionship through these pages, and I wish you well on your pilgrimage.

Healer Healing[20]

Can I help but feel the pulling
    of my heart between the poles?
You are hurting, seeking healing
    Who or what has cast our roles?

I am healer by profession
    I am holder of the heart,
I sell time and clever counsel . . .
    hybrid science, sacred art.

We are beings, both becoming
We are pilgrims, you and I
Help me help you in our process
Let us laugh as well as cry.

Wisdom licks the heart that's longing
    giving trust through healing rite
Smiling gently, softly humming
    Serve and See . . . Love, Life, and Light.

NOTES

1. Bandura (1982); Mahoney (2000a).
2. Guy (1987); Radeke and Mahoney (2000).
3. Brown (1994); Pargament (1997); Shafranske (1996).
4. Geller and Spector (1987).
5. Harner (1982); Walsh (1990).
6. Elliott and Guy (1993); Guy (1987); Mahoney (1991, 1997b); Mahoney and Fernandez-Alvarez (1998); Orlinsky, Ambühl, et al. (1999); Orlinsky, Rønnestad, et al. (1999); Radeke and Mahoney (2000); Skovholt and Rønnestad (1992).
7. Elliott and Guy (1993).
8. Radeke and Mahoney (2000).
9. And, in my personal experience, what I find most distasteful or distressing about such colleagues is often an important lesson about myself and my own limitations.
10. For me, Jim Bugental has been one of those people (Mahoney, 1996).
11. The title of Friedrich Nietzsche's 1878 book.
12. The flip side of the Moses complex is the *bodhisattva* phenomenon, illustrated by Gautama Buddha. This conveys the image of a being who has actually touched into genuine enlightenment and could remain there but, instead, chooses to reenter the realm of human suffering in order to help others work their way through it.
13. Hubble, Duncan, and Miller (1999); Lambert (1989).
14. This commitment has not prevented me from seeking expert advice and peer counsel from colleagues—which has been invaluable. But it *has* amplified my cautiousness in how I ask for such advice and counsel, and it has deepened my sense of privilege in shared privacy. I have heard countless stories I will never repeat, even though it might "unburden" me emotionally. I have come to believe that confidentiality is not simply an ethical and legal responsibility, but a sacred one.
15. Mahoney (1991); Mahoney and Fernandez-Alvarez (1998); Radeke and Mahoney (2000).
16. H. Smith (1958).
17. Mahoney (1988, pp. 312–313).
18. Goldberger et al. (1996); Mahoney and Mahoney (2001).
19. Doherty (1995); Raskin (2001); B. H. Smith (1988).
20. Mahoney (2003).

APPENDIX A

Constructivism

History and Current Relevance

The meanings and history of constructivism are still emerging. They are, so to speak, "under construction," and this is congruent with the essence of the perspective itself. The verb "to construct" comes from the Latin *con struere*, which means to arrange or give structure.[1] The ongoing nature of structuring (organizing) processes is the developmental heart of constructivism. There is intentional emphasis on the present participle—the "ing"—form of verbs and the dynamic-process nature of reality and human experience. This dynamic, developmental, and evolutionary aspect of constructivism turns out to be pivotal in its role in the history of ideas. Even though it can trace a legacy far back into written and oral history, "constructivism" is a term that is just now making its way into the vocabulary of psychology. It does not yet appear in most dictionaries of psychology. If one looks at the psychological literature over the past quarter-century, "constructivism" is a relatively rare term but one that is being used with increasing frequency. Figure A.1 shows that the words "constructive" and "constructivism" are becoming more common in the titles or abstracts of psychological articles. Interestingly, it is a term that has become popular across theoretical boundaries. "Constructive" and "constructivist" are being used, for example, to describe developing perspectives in domains ranging from biology and brain science to cognitive-behavioral, humanistic, and psychoanalytic psychotherapies.[2] This broad popularity suggests that constructivism has considerable potential as an integrative framework.[3] It can incorporate the wisdom embedded in traditions that have been considered incompatible. As Thomas Kuhn pointed out, revolutionary developments in sci-

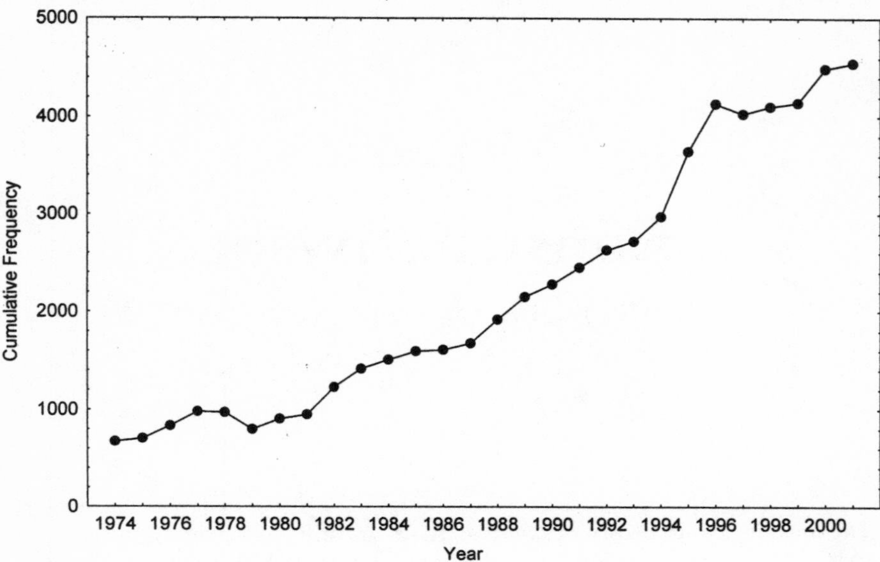

FIGURE A.1. Cumulative frequency of titles and abstracts using terms like "constructive, constructivism, constructivist" in the psychological literature.

entific paradigms often require and reflect changes in words and their meanings.[4]

Attempts to organize the history of constructivism continue to unfold, and they reflect emerging appreciations of multiple legacies.[5] Constructivism is a perennial in the history of ideas. Themes of constructivism can be heard in ancient voices. Among the earliest recorded proponents of some form of constructivism, for example, are Lao Tzu (6th century BC), Buddha (560–477 BC), and the philosopher of endless change, Heraclitus (540–475 BC). Lao Tzu was the Chinese philosopher whose writings form the basis of Taoism. He was supposedly visited by the younger Confucius, who was impressed with Lao Tzu's emphasis on a receptive and fluid frame of mind. Believing that there is an inherent rhythm to all things, Lao Tzu recommended living in harmony with the flow. Like Heraclitus, he also believed that opposites coexist and, in fact, require one another. This idea is expressed in the visual symbol of the Tao, which depicts two enfolded opposites (yin and yang), each of which contains as its center the source of the other.[6]

There are also claims that the aged Lao Tzu may have encountered and influenced a younger man named Prince Siddhartha, who later came to be called Buddha.[7] Parallels between these traditions are significant. The constructivism of the Buddha is clear. The book of his spiritual reflections (*Damapada*) opens with:

> We are what we think.
> All that we are arises with our thoughts.
> With our thoughts we make the world.[8]

The resonance between many Buddhist teachings and aspects of contemporary constructivism are becoming increasingly apparent.[9] Buddhist teachings begin with four fundamental truths:

> Life is full of dissatisfaction (suffering).
> Suffering is caused by clinging, craving, or grasping (these actions are primarily aimed at creating permanence, controlling things, and making distinctions or separations).
> The cessation of suffering is possible by ceasing these actions.
> The way to achieve freedom from suffering involves a path of actions (the Eightfold Path).

From a Buddhist perspective, human suffering results from our desperate resistance to change (impermanence), our persistent grasping for more than we already have, and a deep and illusory sense of separation from one another and our worlds. Among its practical recommendations for the reduction of suffering, Buddhism has encouraged the regular practice of skills that include mindfulness (conscious present focus), compassionate relationship (with self and others), flexibility, flow, and balance.

The insights of the pre-Socratic philosopher Heraclitus (540–475 BC) also had a constructivist tone in their emphasis on change processes and development. Heraclitus is famous for his saying that one "cannot step into the same river twice." Is the river ever the same? Is a person the same at any two points in time? Heraclitus was a "process philosopher," as reflected in his central statement that "all is becoming." This emphasis on process is a central aspect of constructivism. He was also a pioneer in dialectical thinking and the role of interacting contrasts or tensions in the very heart of existence. Heraclitus believed that there is a "tension of opposites" in all things, and that the music of life reflects ever-changing vibrations in the dynamic dance of contrasts. His insights have fared well in light of scientific research. Life systems are now known to express essential tensions between stable and variable patterns of activity.

Besides Lao Tzu, Buddha, and Heraclitus, many other individuals have contributed to what is now being called "constructivism." In the last three centuries, however, the contributions of several individuals have been pivotal in the development of constructivism as a major perspective in western cultures: Giambattista Vico (1668–1744), Immanuel Kant (1724–1804), Arthur Schopenhauer (1788–1860), and Hans Vaihinger (1852–1933). Vico said that human knowing involves an imaginative construction of order in experience, thus implying that the knower cannot be separated from what is presumed to be known. Living and teaching in Naples, Vico was a Renaissance humanist whose writings challenged the emerging dichotomy between rationalism and empiricism.[10] He saw the flaws in René Descartes's separation of the mind from the body and the Cartesian quest for absolute certainty via disembodied reason. Vico also criticized Francis Bacon's dismissal of universities and the ancients.

In place of these extremes, Vico argued that human knowing must be understood as a process of construction that takes place in social and historical contexts. He maintained that our thinking expresses metaphors of the body, and he suggested that fantasy, imagination, mythology, and etymology (word origins) are important resources for understanding ourselves. Vico was a lonely voice in the revolution taking place in views of human knowing. He maintained that modernity had "enshrined the cult of power and of self, and this cult leads to divisive, disintegrative practices, of which war is the epitome."[11]

Immanuel Kant was a philosopher who lived in Königsberg. His writings were complex and extensive, and he revolutionized philosophy in much the same way that Copernicus revolutionized astronomy. He noted that Copernicus's suggested shift from an earth-based to a sun-centered model of the heavens was also an invitation to an even more revolutionary shift in human thinking. Copernicus did not see the heavens differently until he caught a glimpse of our shifting position as an observer. His novel perspective emerged only as he included us as observers on an earth that might be moving. What he saw did not change so much as how he saw. Distinguishing between *noumena* (things in themselves) and *phenomena* (our personal experiencing), Kant argued that we can never completely extricate ourselves from our own experiencing processes. He described the mind as an active organ, "which transforms the chaotic multiplicity of experience into the orderly unity of thought."[12] Kant emphasized the power of patterns in our thinking, and he regarded ideas as regulative principles. Although these patterns place limits on our knowing, Kant did not view us as prisoners of our minds. He had faith in an autonomous will, and he related that faith as an ethics of action. Kant believed that we participate in the construction of a universal lawfulness, and that integrity and good will are categorical acts. Kant suggested that we know much more than we realize; and that we endlessly classify. A philosopher of astronomy as well, Kant offered an argument for the evolution of solar systems and galaxies.

Arthur Schopenhauer (1788–1860) also deserves credit in the philosophical heritage of constructivism. I had not appreciated this until recently. Some philosophical historians—such as Bryan Magee—argue convincingly that Schopenhauer has been both misunderstood and underrecognized as a significant influence on later developments in philosophy and psychology.[13] He noted, for example, that "the world of experience is something in the construction of which the observer is actively involved; that it is of its nature permanently shifting and, this being so, evanescent and insubstantial."[14]

> Among other things, it was his perception, before Darwin, that the human mind was the product of a biological process of evolution that helped him develop an understanding of the role played by unconscious motivations, and the importance among those of sex, in a way that prefigured Freud. In addition to being one of the first Europeans to acquire an intellectually serious grasp of Hindu and Buddhist thought he was able to relate this in a Kantian metaphysics which, long before twentieth-century physics, held that all matter was reducible to energy.

Through his writings, Schopenhauer influenced Freud, Jung, Vaihinger, Wittgenstein, and Heidegger. An outspoken atheist, Schopenhauer praised the quests of spiritual seekers, many of whom came closest to seeing that "we are there already / But not aware of it."[16]

In 1876, Hans Vaihinger elaborated some of Kant's ideas about phenomenology (subjective experience) and possibility. In his *Critique of Pure Reason*, 1781, Kant had discussed the provocative dimension of "as if." Vaihinger focused on this dimension in his studies. In the *The Philosophy of "As If,"* Vaihinger argued that the primary purpose of mind and mental processes is not to portray or mirror reality, but to serve individuals in their navigations through life circumstances. Vico had emphasized the role of fantasy and myth in human adaptation. Vaihinger said that we live our lives via "functional fictions." He described the mind as "an organic formative force" that is reciprocally adaptive; that is, the mind adapts itself to its changing environment and also adapts its patterns of experiencing (including perception and thought) to serve its own needs. "The mind is not merely appropriative, it is also assimilative and constructive."[17] Vaihinger's principle of functional fictions would form the cornerstone of Alfred Adler's theory of individual psychology. Although Adler is often classified as a neo-Freudian, he was clearly an important contributor to constructivist thinking.[18] Wilhelm Wundt was a contemporary of Vaihinger, and his perspective (which he called "voluntarism") included constructive dimensions.[19]

William James also explored several constructivist themes, and he and several colleagues carried the curiosity of constructivism across the transition from the 19th to the 20th centuries. James was one of the few pioneers of psychology to respect and reflect its multiple relationships to biology, medicine, philosophy, physiology, social systems, and spirituality. Recent biographical studies of James illuminate his courage and creative complexity.[20] He was truly a visionary, and many of his insights and intuitions continue to pulse throughout contemporary inquiries into cognition, consciousness, and wisdom. But William James was not the only bearer of constructivism into 20th century thought. James M. Baldwin, Charles H. Cooley, Mary Whiton Caulkins, George H.

Mead, Charles S. Peirce, and Benjamin Whorf also examined and documented the active contribution of the knower and social–symbolic processes to the experience and particulars of knowing.

Later developments in constructivism included Frederic Bartlett's classic work on reconstructive processes in memory.[21] Bartlett's research clearly demonstrated that remembering is not a simple process of retrieving "copies" of experience from some mental filing cabinet. He showed that we tend to organize and simplify our memories, and that we often embellish and elaborate on particular details, so that they fit an emerging story. At about the same time that Bartlett was inviting us to forget our old models of memory, Jean Piaget was beginning a series of influential studies on children's cognitive development.[22] Drawing on the dynamic view of learning described by Johann Herbart (1776–1841), Piaget described knowing as a quest for a dynamic balance between what is familiar and what is novel. This balancing act is accomplished by the coordination of processes of assimilation and accommodation. Assimilation is essentially the incorporation of new experience into old (already existing) structures for knowing. Accommodation is the modification of the old (dynamic) structures when new experiences are too different to be handled. All learning and development hinge on the sensitive coordination of this balance. We are always changing our experience to fit our assumptions, and ourselves to accommodate challenges to our past ways of experiencing. Piaget emphasized that we organize our worlds by organizing ourselves, and this theme of self-organization pervades constructive views of human experience.

A powerful theoretical presentation of constructivism was offered in Friedrich A. Hayek's book *The Sensory Order.* In this treatise, Hayek showed that "much that we believe to know about the external world is, in fact, knowledge about ourselves."[23] He was awarded a Nobel Prize in economics in 1974. When I met him in 1977, I was intrigued by his views on how our nervous systems reflect the same principled processes evident in biological and cultural evolution. Hayek believed that we are not only active participants in our own experiencing, but also that we are unaware of the vast majority of the processes by which we organize our lives. He cautioned against the assumption that we are capable of fully understanding and controlling such processes. It is not always possible or desirable to make the tacit explicit (i.e., to know how we do what we do). Moreover, Hayek argued that we are always more developed than we realize. When we come to recognize that we have achieved a certain level of development, for example, the very act of this recognition presumes the operation of still-tacit (unrecognized or implicit) processes. I shall not belabor this technical point, but it offers a reassuring reminder about our developmental complexity and the horizons of our current awareness.[24]

Another major event in the emergence of constructivism was the publication of George A. Kelly's *The Psychology of Personal Constructs* in 1955. Kelly's theory of "constructive alternativism," better known as "personal construct theory," emphasized both possibility and pattern in the self-organization of personality.

> The theory itself starts with the basic assumption, or postulate, that a person's processes are psychologically channelized by the ways in which he anticipates events. This is to say that human behavior may be viewed as basically anticipatory rather than reactive, and that new avenues of behavior open themselves to a person when he reconstrues the course of events surrounding him. Thus a thoughtful man is neither the prisoner of his environment nor the victim of his biography.[25]

Kelly went on to elaborate a truly original theory of personality built around the concept of constructs. For Kelly, constructs (organizing processes) were dichotomous (either–or) in structure and exhibited dynamic (ever-changing) aspects (e.g., in their permeability and relative tightness and looseness). Kelly translated his theory into a novel approach to psychotherapy, in which the role of the therapist is to challenge skillfully the client's ways of construing self, others, the world, and their possible relationships. Kelly's work has stimulated substantial research on personality and psychotherapy.[26]

Constructivism continued to grow throughout the second half of the 20th century and is now the focus of numerous books and two international journals.[27] The rapidity of its growth has sometimes made constructivism seem like a recent development, when, in fact, it has been emerging for centuries. As Paul Watzlawick put it, "As far as constructivism is concerned, only the name is modern."[28] Still, the visibility and growing popularity are new, as is the wider appeal to constructivist views in psychology. In 1996, the Society for Constructivism in the Human Sciences was formed to encourage and communicate developments in theory, research, and practices that reflect an appreciation for "human beings as actively complex, socially-embedded, and developmentally dynamic self-organizing systems."[29]

CONSTRUCTIVISM IN CURRENT AFFAIRS

Constructivism is playing an increasingly visible role in a diversity of dialogues. The range of that diversity is itself remarkable. One can find constructivist themes in contemporary work on neuroscience, human development, education, ethics, government, science, spirituality, and world peace. The expressions of constructivism in psychology and psychotherapy are only a part of the picture. I focus here on the role being played by constructivism in new views of science, but it is also important to note the relevance of constructive perspectives for ethics. Because constructivists challenge the idea of absolute objectivity, they are often mistakenly assumed to believe that "anything goes" or "one view is as good as another." Absolute justification is not a prerequisite for a moral stand.[30] Relativism is a "slippery slope" to those who presume to be the only ones standing on level ground. What we know of wisdom bids us caution in such presumptions.[31]

Values and ethics are often associated with subjectivity, and science, with objectivity. Constructivism is at the center of a very lively contemporary debate about science. This debate is being called—unwisely, I believe—the "science wars." This came about after science studies gained visibility and momentum in the 1970s. Science studies are literally that: studies of scientists and their institutions; the cognitive and emotional processes involved in discovery, hypothesis development, and data interpretation; the politics of publication; and so on. The journal *Social Studies of Science* was inaugurated in 1976 under the editorship of David Edge, and David Bloor led the Edinburgh School in developing the "strong programme" in science studies.[32] Bloor's term was intended to convey a contrast to the weakness he saw in Mertonian sociology of science, which had stopped short of challenging the knowledge claims of scientists. Far from being a strictly rational, linear, truth-grinding machine, science was shown to be a complex, nonlinear, dynamic process in which evidence, theory, and their interpretations were all quite fuzzy, pliable, and politically influenced. These assertions were extensively documented in field and laboratory studies across a range of scientific disciplines.

Challenges to the traditional, rationalist–objectivist view of science began to grow.[33] Facts—or at least expressions of consensus about what were facts—came to be cast as social constructions. This was consistent with Thomas Kuhn's ideas about the role of models and paradigms in shaping what was authorized as knowledge. Meanwhile, postmodern philosophy was finding its way into literary criticism and the humanities. If postmodernism were divided into only two parts, one could call them deconstructionism and constructivism. Deconstructionism maintains that all texts—indeed, all utterances—can be deconstructed into meaningless statements reflecting only the temporary "positionality" of their author. This is absolute relativism. It amounts to the pairing of "narcissism and nihilism as a postmodern tag team from hell."[34] Constructivism has a decidedly more positive tone. But constructivism and deconstructionism share the same word as their root, and they share some vocal proponents of social reform. Constructivists include many scholars in feminist theory and cultural studies (including cultural anthropology), as well as persons interested in environmental ethics, human rights, and social policy.

> While the new interdisciplinary field of social studies of science was slowly moving into an increasingly constructivist direction, emerging new fields such as cultural studies and women's studies quite independently also chose science as one of their primary objects of analysis. They were interested in studies of the Western bias of science or its inherent masculinity, usually with the implicit or explicit assumption that science as we know it could be otherwise. Students of rhetoric examined the rhetorical strategies of scientists, and the field of literary criticism, inspired by French postmodernism, started treating science as one of many "texts" to be "de-

> constructed." Also here we had a question of the traditional image of science, a downplaying of science as a rational pursuit, and an emphasis instead on science as power. Thus, there was one thing that seemingly united the new science studies and the new postmodernist humanist studies: they both veered away from the idea of science having an epistemologically privileged status.[35]

Throughout the 1970s and 1980s, there were increasing signs of conflict. Field studies made it clear that scientists were not "doing" science the way they (and the basic textbooks) said that science was done. Science, as actually practiced, was not a neat process of posing questions to nature, observing her unambiguous answers, and then respecting those answers by judiciously modifying the relevant theories. Observations of actual scientific conduct suggested perceptual biases, prejudices about what constituted data and what passed for an important question, emotional investments in which data to believe and how to interpret them, generous resort to "fuzzy logic," and large arational leaps from evidence to knowledge claims.

A war was officially declared in 1994 when Paul Gross and Norman Levitt published *Higher Superstition: The Academic Left and Its Quarrels with Science*. The rush to generalizations was striking. Critics of science were dubbed antirealists, relativists, and irrationalists. The conflict was said to involve two adversaries: (1) true scientists, who are objective realists, and (2) science analysts, mostly "social constructionists." The most recent major battle in the science wars has come to be called "the Sokal hoax." Inspired by the Gross and Levitt volume, physicist Alan Sokal wrote a piece intended to demonstrate that the postmodern constructivists could not distinguish sense from nonsense. He published an article, "Transformative Hermeneutics of Quantum Gravity," in *Social Text*, a leading cultural studies journal. Days later, he revealed in a different journal (*Lingua Franca*) that the first article was a hoax. He said that he wanted to show that nonsense would be published so long as it was phrased in postmodern lingo and espoused libertarian political views. The original articles are reprinted in Sokal and Bricmont's *Fashionable Nonsense: Postmodern Intellectuals' Abuse of Science*.[36] As Segerstråle points out, the aftermath of the Sokal hoax has included further polarization on the issue of who has the right to write about science.

At the heart of the science wars are issues of authority and power, and these issues have been central to human activity far longer than has science. Francis Bacon was first and foremost a politician. He equated knowledge with power. To the extent that knowledge becomes knowledge only after authorization, authority is also power. The essence of the science wars revolves around rights, powers, and turf. Who has the authority to question authority? Advocates of the science wars argue that only scientists are qualified to question science. But the separation of science from culture is itself impossible. Evolutionary biologist Stephen Jay Gould denounced the polarizing tendencies among both groups in this so-called war:

> We must reject the widespread belief that a science war now defines the public and scholarly analysis of this institution, with this supposed struggle depicted as a harsh conflict pitting realists engaged in the practice of science (and seeking an absolute external truth progressively reachable by universal and unbiased methods of observation and reason) against relativists pursuing the social analysis of science (and believing that all claims about external truth can only represent social constructions subject to constant change and unrelated to any movement toward genuine factual knowledge). The very concept of a science war only expresses a basically silly myth, rooted in our propensity for devising dichotomous schemes and supported by the invention of nonexistent, caricatured end-members to serve as straw men in a self-serving rhetorical ploy that can only generate heat without light.[37]

In defending a more balanced view of science as a "maximally reliable vehicle for this most adventurous of all improbable journeys,"[38] Gould concluded that

> all increments in the genuine "progress of science" must be won—by a complex and socially embedded construction of new modes for asking questions and attaining explanations. Science advances within a changing and contingent nexus of human relations, not outside the social order and despite its impediments.[39]

Observations cannot be separated from theories; Nature is seldom crystal clear in her answers; facts are seldom fixed and cumulative; and theory change is a complex social and psychological process. These were some of the insights laid bare by Kuhn's early work. In his treatise on essential tensions in the growth of knowledge, he considered the integration of "internal" and "external" accounts of science to be "perhaps the greatest challenge now faced by the profession."[40]

More promising than Bacon's rational objectivist account of science is a dialectical one in which discourse is a key process. The dialectical model posits a third factor, actually a community of characters that interpret the exchanges between Nature and her inquirers. As Marcello Pera notes, a dialectical model of science puts one

> in the best possible position for overcoming the tension between "internal" and "external," and between normative and descriptive philosophies of science. A dialectics *proper to* science . . . should be able to show how external factors become internal and how internal factors are conditioned by external ones.[41]

Science is a magnificent adventure enacted by human beings whose passions and talents are essential to the journeying. Science is learned by not only seeing it done well, but by also doing it under circumstances of well-paced challenge and masterful mentoring. Some of the most important skills learned and practiced in science are reflective and social in nature. How does one learn to recognize and challenge one's own assumptions? How does one engage in respectful dialogue with those with whom one disagrees? Skills such as these are at least as crucial to scientific inquiry as is the technical mastery of instruments and numbers.

Despite our limitations in transcending our own knowing processes, we need to engage in studies and conversations that can refine our inquiry. We also need to reimagine science as an inquiry process that collectively embraces the contrasts to which we are so prone as humans:

> It is better to think about the sciences as muddled rather than pure; to imagine the borders between the sciences and the worlds of language, culture, and politics as muddled rather than clear and distinct; to know scientists as complex hybrid figures rather than rarefied heroes; to see the work of the sciences as complicated interactions with a messy world . . . rather than a methodological, pristine encounter between mind and nature. . . . At their best, the sciences themselves put both the world, and their own processes of questioning that world, into the picture, the frame of inquiry.[42]

What we have learned about science—and psychology of science—should increase, rather than diminish, our fascination and respect for open inquiry constrained by pliable rules.

As a final comment on these alleged wars, I recommend that we stop using war metaphors. Albert Einstein liked to remind us that one does not end wars by continually preparing for them. Science is the last place we need warlike mentality. Differences—whether in belief systems, methods, or interpreted meanings—need not be dichotomized into adversarial confrontations. As the sciences of complexity are teaching us, variability and variation are the heart of both individual and collective development. Let us explore new metaphors and methods for fostering such development.

CONSTRUCTIVISM AND THE GUTS OF CONSCIOUSNESS

What is it about constructivism that is new or different? This question reflects an important assumption. We look for differences: two kinds of people, two kinds of experiences (novel and familiar), two kinds of theories (different and similar). Differentiation is a necessary and natural part of development. But too much emphasis on difference and differentiation can result in fragmentation. Separateness can come to be valued over synergy or symbiosis. There are phases in development that are better served by integrative shifts that unite. Perspectives on human development have long been divided by theoretical differences. Perhaps it is time that an integral shift be considered.

Despite differences in their methods and subject matter, it is tempting to draw a parallel to a quest in the physical sciences. For some time now, physicists have been searching for integral shifts in their models. Isaac Newton achieved the first grand unification in physics in 1687, when he integrated Galileo's theory of falling bodies with Kepler's theory of planetary motions. The result was the theory of gravity. In the 1860s, James Clerk Maxwell achieved the second great unification by summarizing the relationships between magnetism and electricity in four elegantly short equations. With the emergence of nuclear physics, the prospect of a "grand unifying theory" (GUT) became tantalizing. This perspective would show the integral relatedness of all the known forces (gravity, electromagnetism, and the weak and strong nuclear forces). Albert Einstein spent the better part of his life searching for his GUT. He made revolutionary contributions, of course, but died short of a GUT. In the 1960s, Abdus Salaam and Steven Weinberg unified the weak nuclear force and electromagnetism, and since the 1970s, there have been complex and highly abstract attempts to achieve the final GUT. The most popular family of such attempts in physics is now called "string theory."[43]

The emergence of chaos and fractal studies have diverted some attention and energy, and contemporary physicists do not expect the final GUT to emerge anytime soon. Many are, in fact, awed by what has already been placed in mutual relationship. Even as early as James Clerk Maxwell's second unification, it was clear that some remarkably powerful principles had been condensed. Speaking of Maxwell's equations, one of the pioneers in radiation physics said, "One cannot escape the feeling that these equations . . . are wiser than we are, wiser even then their discoverers."[34] Indeed, on his deathbed in 1879, Maxwell uttered something magnificently mystical: "What is done by what is called myself is, I feel, done by something greater than myself in me."[35]

Psychology deals with far greater levels of complexity than does physics. Until recently, however, psychology has been dominated by dualisms and differentiations. Considerable energy has been invested in isolating rather than integrating. Future historians will look back and marvel at what we assumed and what we overlooked. Suppose 30th-century historians were asked to summarize 20th-century psychology in a single, brief paragraph. I don't think it would be unfair of them to write:

> In the 20th century, psychologists were still dividing human experience. Among their favorite categories were behavior, cognition, and emotion. They argued over which of these was most important. Many assumed that mind and body were separate, that materialism was the only scientific platform, and that spirituality was superstition. Toward the end of the century, however, there were scattered signs of understanding the complexity and dynamic interdependence we have since come to appreciate.

Psychology is exhibiting the stirrings of an integral movement. This is apparent at many levels and in lines of development that stretch far beyond any single discipline. The works of Ken Wilber are an illustration, and they intertwine with those of Don Beck, Fritjof Capra, Robert Kegan, Arthur Koestler, and many others. In the words of Clare Graves, they reflect "an unfolding, emergent, oscillating spiral process marked by progressive subordination of older, lower-order behavior systems in newer, higher-order systems."[46]

Constructivism is part of this process. It is not just a new horse in the race. It is a perspective on horses, races, and much more. It is both old and new. Unity and diversity are being integrated in ways that speak to traditions of holism and hope. Dialogues are taking place that suggest an evolutionary leap in our understanding of what it means to be human and to be conscious. These dialogues are invaluable in these times, with our troubles, and in our professional helping roles. The emphasis is on connection rather than separation. The emphasis is on precious development, heart to heart. And spirit—in its marvelous spectrum of meanings—pervades. Let us hope that such a diverse, emergent, and embracing spirit finds continuing encouragement.

NOTES

1. To be etymologically correct, the Latin *struere* basically means "to pile" and the *con* signifies "together" (Partridge, 1983). This basic metaphor, along with its reference to building, may belie a vertical or hierarchical bias worth monitoring. As here interpreted, construction and constructivism refer to a never-ending process of organizing, disorganizing, and reorganizing.
2.. Arbib and Hesse (1986); Berger (1967); Berger and Luckman (1966); Bohart and Greenberg (1997); Bohart and Tallman (1999); Caro (1997); Carlsen (1988, 1995); Combs (1996); Ellis (1998); Epstein (1998); Ferreira and Nabuco (1998); Ford (1987); Freeman (1995); Friedman (1993); Freud (1988); Geertz (2000); Goldberger et al. (1996); Gonçalves (1994, 1995); Gonçalves et al. (2000); Gould (2000); Haken (1984, 1996); Ivey (1986); Ivey and Gonçalves (1988); Kauffman (1993 (1995); Kegan (1982, 1994); Kelso (1995); Luhmann (2002); Mahoney (1995a); Martin (1994); Mitchell (1988, 1997); Mitchell and Black (1995); Moore (2000); Nash and Merkert (1985); Oldfather, West, White, and Wilmarth (1999); Oyama (2000); Ronen (1997); Rosen and Kuehlwein (1996); Rosenbaum (1990, 1998); Rosenberg (1979); Scarr (1985); Schafer (1992); Snyder and Ingram (2000); Snyder and Lopez (2001); Spence (1982, 1987); Stolorow and Atwood (1992); Stolorow, Atwood, and Orange (2002).
3. Goldfried (1995); Norcross and Goldfried (1992); Wachtel (1987).
4. Kuhn (1962, 2000).
5. Anderson (1990, 2003); Davisson (1978); Jankowicz (1987); Mahoney (1988, 1991); Neimeyer (1985); Oberst (1998); Segal (1986); von Foerster (1984); von Glaserfeld (1984); Watzlawick (1984); Weimer (1977).
6. This idea would later be central to Wilhelm Wundt's theorizing (Blumenthal, 1975, 1980, 1985). For other discussions of polarity and dichotomy in human consciousness, see Lowen (1982) and Watts (1963).
7. For discussions of parallels among Buddhism, Confucianism, and Taoism, see Smith (1958).
8. R. Walsh (1999, p. 45). For discussions of Buddhist philosophy and its relevance for psychotherapy, see Batchelor (1994, 1997); Chödrön (1997); Epstein (1995); Harding (1961); Kabat-Zinn (1994); Kopp (1972); Kornfield (1993, 2000); and Merton (1968).
9. Mikulas (2002).

10. Berlin (1976); Combs (1996); Mahoney (1991); Mancuso (2001); Mazzotta (1999); Pompa (1975); Verene (1971); Vico (1710/1988, 1725/1948).
11. Mazzotta (1999, p. 211).
12. Durant (1926, p. 291).
13. Magee (1983, 1997).
14. Magee (1983, p. 342).
15. Magee (1983, pp. 432–433).
16. Magee (1983, p. 456).
17. Vaihinger (1911/1924, p. 2).
18. Carlson and Sperry (1998); Oberst (1998).
19. Blumenthal (1975, 1980, 1985). See also Sherrington (1906).
20. Simon (1998); Taylor (1996, 1999).
21. Bartlett (1932).
22. Piaget (1926, 1970, 1981, 1987a, 1987b); Piaget and Inhelder (1963).
23. Hayek (1952, pp. 6–7).
24. Hayek (1952, 1964); Mahoney (1991); Mahoney and Weimer (1994); Weimer (1977, 1982, 1987).
25. Kelly (1955, p. 560).
26. Davisson (1978); Feixas (1990a, 1990b, 1995); Feixas, Procter, and Neimeyer (1993); Jankowicz (1987); Kelly (1955, 1969a, 1969b, 1969c, 1969d, 1973); Leitner (1995); Leitner and Faidley (1999); Lyddon (1995); Maher (1969); Mancuso and Shaw (1988); Mischel (1980); Neimeyer (1985, 1995b); Neimeyer and Neimeyer (1987); Sewell (1995); Stewart and Berry (1991); Walker et al. (1996).
27. Bruner (1979, 1986, 1990, 1994); Bucci (1997); Cushman (1995); Efran et al. (1990); Faidley and Leitner (1993); Ford (1987); Ford and Urban (1998); Foster and Arvay (2003); Franklin and Nurius (1998); French (1985); Friedman (1993); Guidano (1987, 1991); Hermans and Hermans-Jansen (1995); Hoyt (1994, 1996, 1998, 2000); Joyce-Moniz (1985); Lyddon (1993); Maturana (1975); Maturana and Varela (1980, 1987); McAdams (1993); Neimeyer and Mahoney (1995); Neimeyer and Raskin (2000); Omer and Alon (1997); Raskin and Bridges (2002); Ronen (1997, 1999, 2003); Sewell (1997, 1998); Sexton and Griffin (1997); Thelen (1992); Thelen and Smith (1994); Varela (1979); Varela, Thompson, and Rosch (1991); Watzlawick (1984. The *Journal of Constructivist Psychology*, formerly the *Journal of Personal Construct Psychology*, is published by Taylor & Francis. *Constructivism in the Human Sciences* publishes multidisciplinary articles that reflect synergy across the humanities and sciences.
28. Watzlawick and Hoyt (1998, p. 190).
29. Honored contributors to this Society include Walter Truett Anderson, Albert Bandura, Jerome S. Bruner, James F. T. Bugental, Donald H. Ford, Viktor E. Frankl, Kenneth J. Gergen, Vittorio F. Guidano, Hermann Haken, Yutaka Haruki, Humberto R. Maturana, Joseph F. Rychlak, Francisco J. Varela, Heinz von Foerster, Ernst von Glasersfeld, and Walter B. Weimer. For information, contact Constructivism, Box 311280, Denton, TX 76203 or *www.constructivism123.com.*
30. Beck and Cowan (1996); Doherty (1995); Raskin (2001); Smith (1988); Taylor (1995); Varela (1999); Wilber (1998, 1999).
31. Brown (2000).
32. Bloor (1976).
33. Mahoney (1976/in press-b).
34. Wilber (1998, p. 140). For discussion of postmodernism, see Anderson (1995) and Melville (1986).
35. Segerstråle (2000, p. 5).

36. Sokol and Bricmont (1998).
37. Gould (2000, p. 259).
38. Gould (2000, p. 261).
39. Gould (2000, p. 258).
40. Kuhn (1977, p. 110). See also Mahoney (in press-b) and Weimer (1979, 1980).
41. Pera (1994, p. 11).
42. Fortun and Bernstein (1998, pp. xi–xiii).
43. Bloom (2000); Greene (1999); Nørrestranders (1998); Taubes (1999).
44. Nørrestranders (1998, p. 6).
45. Maxwell (cited in Nørrestranders, 1998, p. 6).
46. Beck and Cowan (1996, p. 28).

APPENDIX B

Consent Form

INFORMATION ABOUT CONSTRUCTIVE PSYCHOTHERAPY AND YOUR PERSONAL CONSENT TO PARTICIPATE

For best results and your own welfare, it is important that you understand what it means to be in psychotherapy. Please read the brief description below. If you have any questions or concerns, please feel free to discuss them with me. I would like you to sign this form and return it to me. You are welcome to a copy of it. Please be assured that your signature does not obligate you to anything or in any way reduce your rights. I ask for your signature simply as a way of ensuring that we both understand our roles and responsibilities in the work we will do together.

WHAT IS CONSTRUCTIVE PSYCHOTHERAPY?

Constructive life counseling, also called "constructive psychotherapy," is a special kind of human relationship offered as an educational health care service. Constructivism is an approach to life that derives from ancient wisdom traditions, and it reflects the lessons of continuing scholarship and science. The goals of constructive therapy are to help you better to understand and appreciate yourself and others, to help you to develop skills in solving problems and coping with challenges in your life, and to encourage your efforts to develop in directions that you find fulfilling and meaningful. It is "constructive" because it emphasizes your strengths and abilities. Challenges in your life repeatedly ask you to exercise and refine your *abilities*. These challenges emphasize the importance of your choices and actions, particularly in those periods of your life when you may see only *limited* or distressing options. I will do my best to understand and honor your distress. I may also suggest things that you might do. Developmental exercises may include our talking about your feelings, your problem(s), your experience of yourself, and your situation. I may ask you to keep personal notes about some of your experiences or to complete some self-report forms. I will honor your needs for privacy, and I will respect your decisions about what you choose to share with me. I encourage you to do the same. I may ask you to experiment with new or different ways of thinking, acting, or feeling. Your imagination, your honesty with yourself, and your commitment to your development will be important assets. We will work *together* during therapy sessions, and I will ask you to try some exercises at home or work.

HOW LONG WILL IT TAKE?

Timing will be important. Too much change or changing too quickly may feel overwhelming. Too little change or changing too slowly may feel discouraging or frustrating. I will try to pace my recommendations according to your needs. The length of our work together will depend on your personal goals, your energy, our abilities to communicate with one another, the challenges you face, and the unfolding of events in your immediate future. We can arrange to meet regularly or periodically. I will do my best to accommodate changes in our meeting schedule. If our work together continues for more than a month (and that is common), I may ask that we periodically review and jointly evaluate what we have done together. If you cannot come to a scheduled meeting, please let me know this at least 24 hours before our appointment. I bill for scheduled appointments that have not been cancelled.

WILL THERAPY HELP?

Most people benefit from psychotherapy, and I believe that these benefits are amplified when such therapy is conducted in a constructive manner. The most common benefits include improvements in self-awareness, self-esteem, self-confidence, hope, feeling understood, relationships with other people, emotional expressiveness, and taking an active and responsible role in one's life. There can also be risks associated with being in psychotherapy. You may already be in the midst of stressful changes or challenges in your life. My role is to help you to cope with these challenges in ways that serve your well-being and that of the people in your life. Periods of change are often stressful, and they are sometimes stormy. You may experience a range of emotions and changes in your relationship with yourself and others (including me). It is rare for people to be harmed by their experience in therapy. When clients are harmed, it is most often because of a violation of their boundaries or pushing too hard for dramatic change. I will honor your boundaries and your personal pacing.

You always have the right to choose whether or not to continue in therapy. If you feel that you might work better with another helping professional, I can offer information about possible referrals. With or without therapy, you may derive valuable benefits from self-help and social support groups, bibliotherapy (therapeutic reading), exercise, hobbies, music, nature, and religious or spiritual practices. I will be glad to help you explore possibilities in these areas.

HOW DOES THERAPY WORK?

Communication is essential to successful psychotherapy. I encourage you to ask me questions and to express your feelings and concerns as openly as possible. I will respect that the information you share with me is private (confidential). State law dictates some limits on your privacy, however, and you should be aware of these. I am legally obligated, for example, to report acts of child abuse or threats of violence. Please feel free to discuss the issue of your privacy with me. I am committed to serving you as best I can; honesty and trust between us are extremely important.

The most important factors contributing to success in therapy are persistence and patience, the quality of the relationship that we develop together, and the optimal pacing of exercises and experiences that encourage and strengthen new patterns of action, thought, and feeling.

WHAT WILL PSYCHOTHERAPY COST?

I will be clear about my fees and the arrangements for their payment. You should understand that payment by "third parties" (usually insurance companies or government agencies) often requires a diagnosis or treatment plan. These agencies sometimes limit how much they will pay in a given period of time. Please feel free to ask me questions about billing and how to obtain information about your health care benefits and options.

SUMMARY

Constructive psychotherapy is a special kind of human relationship in which I, as a professional helper, offer you confidential and personalized assistance. Our signatures below reflect our mutual understanding of this relationship, the fact that you have the right to expect professional conduct and competence from me, and that you always have the right to terminate your participation in therapy.

______________________	______________________
Therapist	Client
______________________	______________________
Date	Date

APPENDIX C

Personal Experience Report

PART 1: BACKGROUND AND CURRENT CONCERNS

Name: ________________________ Today's Date: ___________________

Age: __________________________ Occupation: ______________________

With whom do you now live? _______________________________________

This form is intended to help me understand you, your present concerns, and your needs in our work together. If you have questions or if you are not clear about any of these items, put a question mark (?) next to it and please discuss it with me.

Describe the primary problem or life concern that you would like help with. (If you need additional space, please use the back of the page.)

____

____

____

____

____

____

____

____

In a few words, how would you describe yourself as a person?

If your problem or concern involves other people (e.g., family members, friends, coworkers), briefly list them and their relationship to you.

What are you now doing to cope with or resolve the problem?

Have you tried any other solutions in the past?

____

____

____

____

____

____

____

____

____

____

____

Do you face any immediate challenges that we should deal with as soon as possible? Please note any concerns that feel urgent.

____

____

____

Check any of the following that accurately describe your present or recent experience. Check *all* that apply to you.

I am now feeling or I have recently been feeling . . .

______ depressed or sad
______ lonely
______ angry
______ guilty or ashamed
______ hopeless
______ exhausted
______ tearful or wanting to cry
______ confused
______ anxious
______ jealous
______ out of control
______ numb
______ sick to my stomach
______ aches and pains

I have been having experiences of . . .

______ painful headaches
______ blurred or poor vision
______ losing my balance
______ sleeping problems
______ strange body sensations
______ trembling
______ forgetfulness (memory loss)
______ violent impulses
______ hearing voices
______ chest pains

______	feeling unreal or empty	______	mood swings
______	dizziness	______	hearing problems
______	distressing dreams	______	unwanted thoughts
______	blackouts (unconsciousness)	______	wanting to hurt myself
______	seeing unreal things	______	wanting to hurt someone
______	drinking too much alcohol	______	using drugs too much
______	wishing I were dead	______	feeling desperate

Have you recently had any other feelings or experiences that you are concerned about or that might be important for me to know?

____

____

____

____

____

____

What medications or supplements (prescription and otherwise) are you now taking? Please specify the purpose of each.

Medication or supplement	Daily dose	Purpose
______________	______	______________
______________	______	______________
______________	______	______________
______________	______	______________
______________	______	______________
______________	______	______________
______________	______	______________
______________	______	______________
______________	______	______________
______________	______	______________
______________	______	______________
______________	______	______________

When was your last visit with your physician? ______________________

Have you ever been in psychotherapy or seen a mental health professional before? (Circle one) Yes No

If "yes," what were the approximate dates of your treatment?

from __________ to __________

What was the primary focus of your therapy?

____

How helpful was it?

____

What Are Your Sources of Strength?

Please circle any of the following that you consider to be sources of strength for you. Feel free to add your own in the blank spaces.

my sense of humor	my religious faith	my strong will
my patience	my family	my friends
my intelligence	my courage	my creativity
my stubbornness	my commitment to __________	

other: ____

How Do You Cope?

When you are challenged or distressed by events in your life, what do you do to cope or to comfort yourself?

____

____

____

How Can I Help You?

Please help me understand what you would like from me in therapy. Fill in any of the following that express your current interests.

"What I would like is . . . "

_____ information about __________________________

_____ help in understanding __________________________

_____ help in making a decision about __________________________

_____ training in skills, particularly __________________________

_____ support in __________________________

_____ suggestions for how to solve a problem of ____________________

_____ help with ____________________________________

_____ I don't know what I want help with.

PART 2: EMOTIONAL LIFE

Over the course of the last 90 days, to what extent have you experienced each of the following?

	Never				Often
Anger	0	0	0	0	0
Anxiety or fear	0	0	0	0	0
Enthusiasm or happiness	0	0	0	0	0
Envy or jealousy	0	0	0	0	0
Guilt	0	0	0	0	0
Hatred	0	0	0	0	0
Inner peace or tranquility	0	0	0	0	0
Joy	0	0	0	0	0
Love	0	0	0	0	0
Pride	0	0	0	0	0
Sadness or depression	0	0	0	0	0
Shame or embarrassment	0	0	0	0	0

When you were a child, which feelings or emotions were you taught to think of as "good" or "bad"?

"good": ____________________________________

"bad": ____________________________________

Which of the following expressions of emotions were *discouraged* when you were a child? (circle all that apply)

crying	whining	laughing	pouting
arguing	hitting	singing	nail biting
yelling	swearing	boasting	hiding
whistling	make believe	touching self	rocking

Which emotions do you *now* find most difficult or uncomfortable for you?

____

____

____

____

____

How well do you remember your childhood experiences? (Circle one)

Not very well — Very well

1 2 3 4 5 6 7 8 9 10

How would you describe your childhood in general? (Circle one)

Very unhappy — Very happy

1 2 3 4 5 6 7 8 9 10

Each of the following statements describes experiences you may have had as a child. Check all that apply to you and your childhood. Please add comments or questions in the margin. If you are not sure about an item, or if it feels too private, place a question mark next to it.

______	Our family life was happy.	______	I enjoyed school.
______	I made friends easily.	______	I felt loved and respected.
______	I trusted my parents.	______	I felt trusted by my parents.
______	My feelings were respected.	______	I felt good about myself.
______	My family moved often.	______	I was often sick.
______	I felt unlovable.	______	I was physically beaten.
______	I did poorly in school.	______	I didn't have many friends.
______	I was not allowed to cry.	______	I felt rejected or unwanted.
______	I tried to be perfect.	______	I had intense nightmares.

For the following, *underline* which words would make the statement true.

______ My mother/father was often or entirely absent.

______ My mother/father was often depressed/angry/anxious.

______ I was hospitalized for a serious illness/accident.

______ I was often ashamed of myself/my father/mother/family.

My mother . . .

______ was abused or abandoned as a child.

______ was sometimes violent.

______ suffered from physical illness.

______ suffered from alcoholism.

______ suffered from mental illness.

______ attempted or committed suicide.

______ suffered from a drug problem.

______ did not have any problems of which I was aware.

My father . . .

______ was abused or abandoned as a child.

______ was sometimes violent.

______ suffered from physical illness.

______ suffered from alcoholism.

______ suffered from mental illness.

______ attempted or committed suicide.

______ suffered from a drug problem.

______ did not have any problems of which I was aware.

When I was a child, I was sexually intimate with . .

______ a playmate

______ my father

______ my brother

______ another family member

______ someone outside my family

______ a friend

______ my mother

______ my sister

In their order of appearance in your life (from first to last), who were the people by whom you felt loved?

	Name	Relation to you
(1)	______________________________	______________________________
(2)	______________________________	______________________________
(3)	______________________________	______________________________
(4)	______________________________	______________________________
(5)	______________________________	______________________________
(6)	______________________________	______________________________

In their order of appearance in your life (from first to last), who were the people by whom you felt hurt or harmed?

	Name	Relation to you
(1)	______________	______________
(2)	______________	______________
(3)	______________	______________
(4)	______________	______________
(5)	______________	______________
(6)	______________	______________

What was your happiest experience as a child?

____

____

____

____

What was your most emotionally painful experience as a child?

____

____

____

____

PART 3: SPIRITUALITY

What were your parent's religions? How important was religion to them? _____

____

____

____

What is your current religion or spiritual orientation?

____

How frequently do you attend church or meet with others who share your spiritual interests?

____

How frequently do you pray, meditate, or read spiritual material?

____

Are you involved in any other religious or spiritual activities (volunteer work, an organized charity, etc.)?

____

Whose deaths have touched you personally?

____

Are you currently experiencing any difficulties or challenges in your spiritual life?

____

____

____

____

PART 4: RECREATION

What are your favorite things to do for fun?

____

____

Are you now involved in any form of regular physical exercise or stretching?

____

Do you follow any particular dietary program? How would you describe your daily eating patterns?

____

What hobbies or activities do you *wish* you could explore or pursue?

____

____

If you were free to go anywhere and do anything you want, what would you do?

____

____

____

____

PART 5: PROGRESS REVIEW

The questions below are intended to help me understand your experience of our work together thus far. We can talk about your responses in person, but I think it is important for you to first have some time and privacy to reflect.

Overall, at this point in time, how satisfied are you with . . .

	Not satisfied			Very satisfied
Progress you have made in therapy.	0	0	0	0
The quality of our relationship.	0	0	0	0
Feeling safe with me.	0	0	0	0
Feeling understood by me.	0	0	0	0
Feeling encouraged by me.	0	0	0	0
Skills that you have learned in therapy.	0	0	0	0
Your feelings about yourself.	0	0	0	0

Please describe your experience of our work together thus far.

____

____

____

____

____

Do you have any questions or suggestions?

____

____

____

____

PART 6: REFLECTIONS

In my experience as a therapist, I have found it valuable to talk with my clients about our mutual experiences in working together when we are nearing the end of our regularly scheduled meetings.

I will prepare a brief personal summary of my experience of you and our work together. I will give my summary to you at our last meeting.

I would appreciate your candid reflections on our work together, and I encourage you to consider themes or issues that we did and did not address. Your reflections may help you to better understand your experience of therapy, and your feedback will help me learn how I might refine my services to future clients. Thank you.

____

____

____

____

____

____

____

____

____

____

____

____

____

____

____

____

____

____

____

____

____

____

____

____

____

APPENDIX D

Breathing Exercises

RELEASE BREATHING

In release breathing, one takes a comfortably deep breath and then—at the very top of the inhalation—one simply releases the air with an open mouth and throat. This may produce the soft sound of an "aahhhhhh," as if one were settling into a tub of water that is at just the right temperature. A release breath may also feel and sound like a sigh of relief.

Pause for a moment. Take in a deep breath. When your lungs feel comfortably full, simply let go of the air and listen to it go. Allow your shoulders to drop as the air leaves your body. Don't force the air out or hold it back. Just let it go. Repeat this slowly two or three times.

Release breaths are good exercises for reducing stress at regular intervals throughout the day.

PAUSE BREATHING

In pause breathing, you insert a brief (and gradually longer) pause between the end of each exhalation and the beginning of the next "in breath." Rapid and shallow breathing results in an excess of oxygen (relative to carbon dioxide) in the blood, and the body and brain react strongly to such changes in blood gases. The old trick of breathing into a paper bag can help (because, after a few breaths, the air in the bag has a lower oxygen ratio than the outside air). One can also breathe into cupped hands for a similar effect. However, pause breathing is generally more effective.

To pause breathe, focus on letting your lungs empty. When it feels like all of the air is out of them, count slowly "one thousand, two thousand, three thousand, four thousand." Do not take in another breath until you reach the second or third count. Try to exhale slowly. It may help to purse your lips while you exhale (as if you were blowing air over a cup of hot coffee or soup). Lip pursing helps to equalize the pressure inside the chest. Continue this exercise as long as necessary, with special emphasis on slow, regular exhalations, each followed by a pause of 2–5 seconds. The calming effect will usually be felt in less than a minute, but it may take another few minutes to relax into trusting in your breathing and well-being. Pause breathing is recommended not just for people who suffer bouts of panic. It is useful for just about anyone as a basic bodily relaxation exercise.

ALTERNATE CONTROL AND SURRENDER BREATHING

This exercise is actually a combination of several basic breathing skills. It can be practiced in several positions, including sitting or standing, but I prefer the form in which one is lying on one's back. Alternate breathing takes a few minutes and it practices the contrast between controlling and letting go of control. The essence of alternate breathing is the alternation between an active and passive attitude toward one's breathing.

Active Phase

During the active phase, I recommend pause breathing. You can perform three to five pause breaths. In each of these, you are in control of how much you exhale and how long you wait before you take in your next breath.

Transition

After your last paused breath, let go of being in control of your breathing. A release breath is a good way of doing this.

Passive Phase

Now simply watch your breathing take care of itself. Feel your abdomen rise gently and then fall. Be aware of the gentle breeze created by the air entering and leaving your nostrils, your sinuses, or your mouth. Simply witness with wonder and appreciation.

Repeat

After perhaps a dozen passive breath cycles, return to the active phase. Repeat the sequence a second and perhaps third time. Relax your need to get anything from the exercise other than the sensations. If you find your mind racing or wandering, consider exploring other forms of meditation.

APPENDIX E

Body Balance Exercises

Find a floor area that is free of objects and where you can practice these exercises without distraction or interruption. If you have concerns about your stability, stand near a wall or a stable piece of furniture that you can easily reach with your hands. Take whatever precautions are necessary to avoid falling. Be gentle with yourself and make yourself comfortable. These exercises can be done in flat shoes, socks, or barefoot.

STANDING CENTER

Stand in a comfortable position with your trunk and head erect, and your hands by your sides. Focus your gaze ahead of you on some object or area that is at eye level. Take a deep release breath and relax. Very slowly and gently begin to lean slightly forward (somewhat like a ski jumper in the middle of a jump, only with much less of an angle). Take about 10 seconds to reach your farthest forward angle. If you lean so far forward that you need to take a step to avoid falling, you have gone too far. As you lean slowly forward, you will feel more pressure on the balls of your feet (just behind the big toe). Spend a couple of seconds near your most forward point of balance. Now reverse the direction of your lean and slowly shift your weight backward. You will pass through your original position and begin to feel more pressure on your heels. If you have to step backward to avoid falling, you have again gone too far. Spend a second at your farthest backward point, then reverse direction and repeat this cycle at least three times.

Take about 10 seconds for each direction, and slowly rock forward and backward. After doing this several times with your eyes open, and if it is safe to do so, consider experimenting with closing your eyes either partially or completely. You may notice two things with your vision reduced: (1) that it is easier to feel the sensations in your soles (and other parts of your body), and (2) that it is a little more difficult to balance.

Finally, with your eyes open or closed (whichever you prefer), allow your slow-motion rocking to come to a halt and let yourself stand comfortably still. Pay special attention to the sensations in the soles of your feet. You may feel three main areas: the balls, the heels, and the outside edges. Perhaps the sensations will remind you of the indentation your foot makes in soft, loose sand. Notice that when you are standing still, your center is still moving, even if ever so slightly. Your weight is distributed between the front and back of your foot and then from side to side, in the area of your arch. If we could hang a tiny plumb line from the middle of your arch, it would trace a gently swaying pattern on the floor as your body continuously compensates for slight movements. Call this middle region your center or base. It is your gravitational home. Invite yourself to stand comfortably relaxed and let your body rock gently through this center. Slowly let yourself settle into a comfortable sense of stillness. Feel it deeply as a familiar and secure base.

ONE-LEG STAND

People with ankle or knee problems should approach this exercise cautiously. (It is frequently used in physical therapy for rehabilitation after injury to these joints, but such therapy should be supervised by a qualified health professional.) Begin by standing in a comfortably relaxed position with your back straight and your head level. Release breathe. Focus your gaze forward at eye level. Your goal is eventually to stand safely balanced on one leg. Approach this goal very slowly, gently, and with a keen awareness of what you feel as you do this. Imagine yourself to be wearing a baseball cap with a string hanging from the center front of the visor. When you are standing on both feet, the string would hang directly between your eyes, in front of your nose, and touch the ground between your feet, probably just in front of your big toes.

With your back remaining straight, begin to slowly shift your weight from one foot to the other in an alternating and very slight sideways rocking motion. Continue this gentle sideways rocking for perhaps 30 seconds and focus on the sensations in your legs and feet. Then, choose which foot you will lift. As you begin to shift your weight to the other foot, your physical sense of center will also shift. The bottom of that imaginary string will slowly begin to shift toward the foot on which you will be standing. Notice the very subtle adjustments you make in your pelvis and hips. Feel a gentle change in the pressure on your weight-bearing leg (particularly in the knee, the ankle, and the sole of that foot). Be aware of the changing feelings in the foot you are about to lift. Notice that you are slowly pushing it off the floor and that the last part to leave the ground is the ball of the foot and the big toe. You may need to touch down several times with that toe before you feel steady and balanced on the other leg. Again notice that your center of balance is dynamic in the sole of your stationary foot. Breathe slowly and notice what else is happening in your upper body during this exercise. As you feel ready, experiment with the differences you feel if you slowly move your elevated leg slightly behind or in front of you. See how long you can balance on one foot before needing to touch the other one on the ground. Experiment with the different feelings produced when you alternate the foot on which you balance.

APPENDIX F

Relaxation

Begin by inviting yourself to gently close your eyes and to center your attention in this moment and in this exercise. Take a comfortably deep release breath, inhaling slowly until your lungs are full, and then gently releasing the air at your own pace, neither rushing nor holding back. Let yourself make the sound of a sigh as you release the air (sigh). Do this several times, slowly, inviting yourself to relax and to let go even more with each breath that you release. Gently letting go of time. Setting aside any worries or plans, and trusting that you can pick them up again when this exercise is finished. Invite yourself to set aside this time as time out from everything else and a special time with yourself and for yourself. Quality time devoted to relaxation and rest. . . . Be gentle with yourself and your way of relaxing. . . . Be aware of the shifts in your attention back and forth between my voice and the music, your thoughts, and your breathing. . . . Simply witness and accept the wandering of your attention. . . . Simply notice and honor the feelings and sensations that flow through you. . . . Inviting yourself to relax more and more deeply as I count slowly from 1 to 10: 1, letting your shoulders drop; 2, allowing the muscles in your jaw to relax; 3, relaxing your forehead; 4, letting the muscles around your eyes relax; 5, breathing slowly; 6, gently moving your fingers; 7, relaxing the muscles around your mouth; 8, letting the muscles in your legs relax; 9, gently stretching your ankles and toes; and 10, allowing yourself to be deeply relaxed.

Respect any requests that your body may now be making for a shift in position, for a gentle stretch, for any movement that would feel more comfortable and comforting. Be gentle with yourself, inviting but not forcing this experience; accepting whatever is happening for you at this moment to be as it should be; trusting in the natural wisdom of your mind and body; and patiently allowing their gentle rhythms to merge and mingle as they find a peaceful balance.

Breathing slowly, and inviting an occasional deep breath and a sigh as you release any tension that you notice in your body (sigh). Gently scanning from head to toe, allowing every muscle to lengthen and stretch, each finding its most comfortable position and its own natural state of rest.

Trusting in your own process of relaxing and honoring both its pauses and progressions, accepting each level while you remain there, and accepting any occasional muscle twitches that signal that you are loosening and letting go.

Become aware of the muscles you use when you swallow and allow them to rest. Witness your breathing: Feel the gentle movement of the air as it enters and leaves your nostrils. Let your breathing take care of itself. Let each breath invite deeply satisfying rest.

Honor your body's requests for movements or changes in position. Notice where your body makes contact with the surface below you—where you are supported—and allow the muscles involved to surrender to the gentle pull of gravity. Sinking more and more into comfort and peace.

Simply witnessing and allowing. Accepting. Inviting. Trusting. Let yourself linger and enjoy, relaxed and at peace. Notice how good it feels. Invite yourself to do this more often—to take time out for yourself, to be with yourself, to pause and to rest, to appreciate the natural wisdom and wonder of your own mind and body.

And now beginning to move your attention toward a slow and gentle emergence from this exercise. Remaining relaxed and at peace as I count backward from 10: 10, returning your attention to where your body is supported; 9, aware of your slow deep breathing; 8, focusing more and more on my voice; 7, noticing the other sounds around you; 6, moving your head slowly from side to side; 5, beginning to open your eyes enough to see some light; 4, blinking gently and focusing on what you can see; 3, noting where you are and what has been happening; 2, breathing a sigh of release as you make the transition from what has been happening to this moment; and 1, beginning to slowly move toward a position that you find comfortable.

Gently, at your pace, beginning to reengage with your world, remaining relaxed and feeling rested. Bring your mind and body back into the flow of this moment and this place.

Relax and return.

APPENDIX G

Mindfulness Meditation

The purpose of this exercise is to practice a gentle witnessing awareness. Select a time and a place where you can be alone without distractions or interruptions for at least 20 minutes. Assume a comfortable sitting position on the floor or in a chair. Unless you need the support of the back of the chair, it is preferable to scoot forward slightly (toward the edge of the seat), so that your primary contact with the chair is on your buttocks and thighs. If you sit on the floor, it may be more comfortable with a cushion underneath you. There are three important points:

1. *Be comfortable*: This is not a pain endurance exercise.
2. *Sit upright*: Your back should be comfortably straight, with your shoulders and ears directly above your hips.
3. *Soft belly*: Your belly should be soft and unrestricted (so that you can breathe comfortably).

Your hands can be folded on your lap, rested on the arms of the chair, folded in a prayerful position, or placed on your abdomen.

Set a timer to signal you after 10–12 minutes (longer, if you prefer).

Begin by taking several slow release breaths. Settle into the exercise. *Slow down.* Allow your eyes to rest on an area of the floor just beneath you. You may feel more comfortable with your eyes lightly closed. If you choose to open your eyes or to lift your gaze, do so in *slow motion.*

Choose a sensation that you feel each time you exhale. It might be the feeling of your shoulders falling very slightly, the feeling of your belly getting smaller, or the feeling of the air moving past the tip of your nose. Choose one of these for a particular session.

Use this sensation as a gentle reference point for your attention. Silently and slowly count each "out breath."

Your attention will stray. Like a small bird in a large tree, your attention will fly from point to point, or it may seem like a river. Imagine that all this is flowing through you—your thoughts, images, sensations, and feelings—like ripples on the surface of a gently moving river. Pretend you are on a bridge over that river. Your reference sensation is that bridge. Looking down, you can watch the flow of your experience. From time to time, something will "hook" you and pull you along with it. Your attention will move downstream. When you realize that you have been hooked, simply go back to the bridge. *Each time you notice this, come back to your reference point*—the sensation you chose. Don't worry about where you left off in your counting. Start over again at "1." It is just like skipping a rope, except you never go past the number "9." When you get to "9," start over again at "1."

Relax. Just pay attention to your reference point. *Be gentle with yourself.* Whatever thoughts or images arise, just watch them and continue breathing slowly.

Again and again, softly return to your outbreaths. Back to sitting upright with a soft belly. Back to counting.

When your timer signals, take a deep release breath. Give yourself credit for investing some quality time in just pausing and witnessing.

APPENDIX H

Mirror Time

The purpose of this exercise is to learn to take a good look at yourself and into yourself. It involves spending 10 minutes in front of a mirror without "doing anything" usual (such as combing your hair, brushing your teeth, applying moisturizers or cosmetics).

Choose a time when you can have privacy. If you prefer to sit, put a chair in front of the mirror. Before you start, set clear intentions for the exercise. Your intentions should be positive or constructive. Your goal is not to "face" some cold, harsh truth. Your goal is to look into your own eyes and connect with yourself in a compassionate way.

If you are concerned about time, set a timer for 8–12 minutes.

Your time in front of the mirror should begin with a few relaxing release breaths. Then look at your face. Look into your own eyes. After about a minute, close your eyes and take another release breath. Be aware of your body. What are you feeling? Where are you feeling it? Release breath. Take your time before proceeding.

Open your eyes again and look at yourself. Your attention may be drawn to many parts of your face and head. Remember to bring your gaze gently back to your own eyes. Experiment with looking at each eye. Do they look the same? Do you feel the same when you look in either eye? (Relax your need to find or feel a difference. Relax your need to understand any difference if you find one.)

Alternate between looking in the mirror and closing your eyes. When your eyes are closed, invite yourself to relax and feel centered. When your eyes are open, simply invite yourself to witness and to feel.

You may feel happy or sad. You may feel mixtures of feelings. You may alternate between noticing features of your face and sensing your insides.

Looking into your own eyes can be a portal for connecting the outside you and the inside you.

If you feel comfortable doing so, experiment with talking out loud to yourself while looking in the mirror. (You may want to record your private conversations for later review.) What do you hear in your voice? Do different feelings have different voices?

At the end of your mirror time, bring the exercise to a close with a release breath and an explicit thought or statement of appreciation. Express gratitude to yourself for taking the time and energy to honor who you are and to refine how you see and feel yourself.

If mirror time feels interesting or promising, consider doing it regularly as part of your self-care. Experiment with different levels of lighting (candlelight can be conducive to a relaxed intimacy).

Remember to emphasize gentleness and self-compassion.

APPENDIX I

Kindly Self-Control

How well do you exercise kindness in setting limits on yourself? This exercise is aimed at refining your ability to set limits and to be compassionate with yourself.

There are two parts to the exercise: (1) giving something up for a day, and (2) being gentle with yourself in the process. The first part teaches skills in impulse control. It is about boundaries. The second part teaches self-compassion. It is about kindness in self-control.

Choose something you can do without for 24 hours. It should be something you enjoy often during an average day. It could be smoking, chewing gum, sweets, soda, radio, television, and so on. Choose only one thing to do without. (Do not give up daily medications, essential food, or water.)

Choose a time to start. Give yourself at least a day to anticipate doing this exercise. Remember that your goal is not just to give something up (to set a limit on yourself). Your goal is to learn to restrain yourself briefly in a compassionate manner. Consider wearing something unusual that day—for example, a special ring or bracelet, or a string around a finger—as a reminder to be kind and mindful.

Pay close and kind attention to what you experience. How do you feel as you prepare for your day of abstention? What are your thoughts? What does it remind you of? How difficult is it? What do you do when an impulse arises? How do you deal with your craving? How do you relate to yourself in the process?

An optional component to the exercise can be added at the end of the first day. In the last 2 hours of the 24, consider whether you want to end the exercise after 1 day as planned or extend it to 48 hours (maximum). Pay attention to how quickly and easily you make this decision. Relax your need to understand all of your reactions. Just focus on learning to watch gently how you deal with limits and how kind you can be with yourself.

APPENDIX J

Self-Comforting Exercise

The purpose of this exercise is to explore and develop your capacities to ask for and receive comfort from yourself. Select a time and a place where you can be alone without distractions or interruptions for at least 20 minutes. Assume a comfortable position sitting or lying down, and allow yourself to relax. Imagine that one part of you wants to be held or comforted in some way. It may be a part of you that is asking for help, for reassurance, for forgiveness, for strength, or for understanding. Then, imagine that there is another part of you that is deeply caring, compassionate, and generous. Perhaps it is the part of you that is called upon when your friends, family or others need your help. Pretend that you can give a different voice to these two parts of yourself: the part that is asking for comfort and the part that is offering comfort. If you find it helpful, you can move your head slightly when you are speaking from each part of you. For example, you can lean your head slightly to the left when you are asking for help, and then lean your head slightly to the right when you are responding to that request from the helping part of you. If you can, you may find this exercise more powerful when you actually speak these voices out loud, but this is not necessary.

Begin with the voice and part of you that is asking for comfort. Use your own words in speaking your request. You might find yourself saying things like, "I feel scared," "I feel lonely," or even "I feel silly doing this." Start out with "I feel" statements. Then pause, shift your head (if you choose to), and allow the comforting part of you to respond. Let the voice of your comforting self sound soothing and reassuring. Perhaps it will sound like the voice of someone who loved you dearly and soothed your pain when you were a child. Your comforting side may begin by saying things like "Yes, darling, I know you are scared. I am here with you." Allow the words to be your own, and be careful not to be impatient or judgmental when you are speaking from your comforting side. That side of you should be infinitely patient and loving. Pause again and allow the "hurting" or "needing" side of you to respond.

Allow a conversation to emerge between these two parts of you. The needing side of you may say anything that comes to mind: "I feel lost," "I want to be held," or "I don't understand." The comforting side of you should be consistently respectful and reassuring. It may feel appropriate to hug yourself or to stroke your hair, your cheek, or your hand. The words "I love you" are always appropriate from your comforting side. Occasionally, your comforting side may offer suggestions or possible solutions to problems, but this is not the main purpose of the exercise. Your primary goal should be to open channels of communication between the parts of you that are distressed and the parts of you that can offer comfort. When you feel ready to finish the exercise, invite each part of you to say something to the other that expresses affection and appreciation.

APPENDIX K

Spiritual Skills Exercises

1. *The sacred art of the pause.* Use some common daily signals to remind you to pause (e.g., a portable timer, the sound of a passing train or ambulance, a glimpse of a child or elder). Take a deep breath and slow down. For even a moment, *be here now.* View all delays (waiting in line, heavy traffic, etc.) as opportunities for mindful pausing.
2. *Witness feeling.* Allow yourself to note and honor the sensations in your body. Be aware of your breathing, and of sounds, sights, smells, being touched (by the wind, by your clothing, by yourself, etc.). Be patient in noticing what you had not been noticing.
3. *Practice compassion and gratefulness.* In the presence of pain or frustration (your own or someone else's), practice compassion. Be sensitive to suffering. When you find yourself judging others, positively or negatively, add the phrase "just like me." Whatever the situation, learn also to appreciate (literally, to find the precious). Be grateful (even without knowing for what or to whom). Out of compassion and gratefulness, practice giving. How and what can you give? Who or what can you forgive? How might you serve?
4. *Trust higher order processes.* Relax your needs to understand, explain, or control all that is happening (in your life and others). Accept the flow, honoring whatever you find sacred (such as love, life, light). Allow yourself to trust in a resonance between your personal ordering processes and higher order ordering processes.
5. Practice meaningful action. From the mobile home of your heart, act from and toward your best intentions.

APPENDIX L

Human Change Processes

A Synopsis

1. Humans are active participants in organizing their experiences of themselves and their worlds. Dynamic and continuous ordering processes construct, maintain, and revise activity patterns.
2. Active ordering processes are primarily tacit and unique to each individual.
3. Those self-organizing processes most vital to life support and individual functioning—what might be called "core ordering processes" (COPs)—are given special protection against changing.
4. COPs organize experiences and activities along interdependent dimensions that include (a) emotionality and valence, (b) reality status, (c) personal identity, and (d) power (control/efficacy/agency).
5. Resistance to change—even desired change—is common, especially when the change is experienced as "too much" or "too quickly." Such resistance reflects basic self-protective processes that serve to maintain the coherence of the living system.
6. Ordering processes always operate in relation to their own contrasts, which are disordering processes. Order and disorder are facets of the same dynamic diamond.
7. The ongoing interaction of ordering and disordering processes creates a simultaneous interplay of both familiar and novel experiences.
8. Novelty is necessary for learning and development. Novelty involves contrast.
9. Familiarity and consistency are essential to life support, systemic coherence, and human well-being.

---

10. The dynamics between familiarity and novelty lie at the heart of human change processes.
11. Disorder is necessary for development.
12. All learning and development involve transitional disruptions or perturbations in systemic functioning. At all levels, development feeds on disruptions and then digests them into familiarity.
13. It is in the context of disorder that a living system exhibits both its greatest rigidity and its greatest variability. When rigidity reigns, stereotyped behavior or frozen passivity are common. Variability may emerge, particularly in a safe relationship that encourages ventures into flexibility. From this flexibility in being and these expressions of variability, more fulfilling and functional activities may emerge and vie for potential selection in the expression of that person's life.
14. When novel experiences—contrasts—are deficient relative to an individual's capacities and developmental needs, stagnation and "hardening of the categories" are likely.
15. When novel experiences greatly exceed the individual's capacities to balance, feelings of being overwhelmed are common. Episodic or chronic disorder and "breakdown" may result.
16. When new experiences are well-timed and suited to the individual's current developmental capacities and edges, developmental "breakthroughs" may emerge and effect whole-system transformations in experiencing.
17. Although disorder may be experienced and expressed in highly patterned processes of human activity, it is diverse, individually unique, and systemic; we advance in our attempts at conceptualization and classification only as we are willing to embrace the limits of symbol systems to capture human uniqueness and the ultimate ineffability of complex system dynamics.
18. Persons can become "trapped" in disorder. Many psychiatric disorders are, in fact, rigidly ordered patterns.
19. Change is a nonlinear process. It is neither continuous nor cumulative. Rather, change processes reflect many small shifts punctuated by occasional sudden leaps and frequent returns to earlier patterns of activity.
20. Change is often experienced in waves or multirhythmic oscillations. Anchors for dimensions of oscillation are often abstract conceptual polarities, such as life–death, right–wrong, good–bad, real–fake, and sacred–profane. Descriptions of experiences of oscillation often include references to opening and closing, expansion and contraction, loosening and tightening, or approach and withdrawal.
21. Change emerges from a shifting matrix of competing possibilities. Old, tenured patterns of activity compete with new and experimental possibilities. Like all other forms of evolution and revolution, this competition is never finished. New patterns, when they gain dominance in the competition, themselves become the "old" and familiar order in contrast with which newer patterns emerge and compete.

22. Ongoing competitions in development are neither "won" nor "lost" in reference to allegedly absolute criteria. Some competitors (i.e., impulses of activity) are selected to assume temporary positions in the "driver's seat" of the body. The old patterns remain as contenders, and they may "win" occasional episodes of ascendancy in future situations. Old habits are not eliminated completely, but they can be effectively displaced by new ones.
23. Selection processes always include human agency. What "decides" the ongoing competition among activity patterns is a complex dynamic system that emerges out of and expresses a human will.
24. Selection processes must mature into retention processes if a chosen activity is to become an influential pattern in ongoing self-organization. A change—to effect a change that makes an enduring and therefore significant difference—must be actively practiced.
25. Successful (adaptive) change is facilitated by a rhythmic orchestration of exploratory, selective, and perpetuating activities (i.e., experiments in living, evaluative choices regarding which experiments are "working," and action patterns that serve to perpetuate and elaborate valued experiences).
26. Self-relationships, which emerge in social and symbolic relationships, powerfully influence life quality and resilience under stress. Awareness, acceptance, and celebration are common quests in self-relating.
27. Interpersonal relationships involving strong emotions are powerful contexts for psychological development. Safe and loving intimacy is an expression of trust, which lies at the core of optimal contexts for development.
28. Symbol systems including language and the arts may offer valuable structure and welcome stimulation in personal development.
29. Conscious practices, both spiritually and secularly pursued, are central to qualities and directions of life experiencing. Intention and action are key (even when the goal is stillness).
30. Psychotherapy should reflect an appreciation for the history and motivational power of personal realities, the role of interpersonal, symbolic, and self-relational processes in the maintenance and change of personal realities; and the complex existential agency and responsibility of the socially embedded individual.
31. Love is basic to life. What is basic to life is basic to psychotherapy. Spiritual and wisdom traditions that embrace these insights may be precious sources of comfort, companionship, and direction in the complex processes of lifespan personal development.

APPENDIX M

Recommendations for Therapist Self-Care

1. *Be gentle with yourself; honor your own process.* Professional responsibilities and life demands will press on you to push yourself too hard and to be impatient with yourself and your limitations. Again and again, learn to relax, to find a comfortable pace, and to forgive yourself.
2. *Get adequate rest.* Learn to take brief naps. If you have trouble sleeping, do everything you can to create time and space that will allow you to rest well when you do rest. If possible, develop work schedules and styles that allow more time for rest between sessions.
3. *Make yourself comfortable.* At work and at home, indulge yourself in comfortable clothing, furniture, decorations, and music. Give yourself things that add comfort to your life. Let yourself enjoy.
4. *Move your body often.* Between and in sessions, perform gentle stretches of your lower back, your shoulders, your neck, your feet, and your hands. Avoid motionless positions that reduce blood circulation. Go for walks. Dance. Spend at least 30 seconds every day with your head below your heart. Develop a comfortable exercise or movement routine that is suited to your personal abilities and enjoyments.
5. *Develop a ritual of transition for leaving work at the office.* Even though you are likely to carry your clients' struggles with you after work, learn to formalize a transition from your professional to your personal life (a walk, a prayer, a brief period of meditation, etc.).
6. *Receive regular professional massages.* Find a licensed massage therapist with whom you are comfortable. Receive regular massages of the form you

prefer (neck and shoulder, hand, scalp, facial, foot, whole body). Learn to massage your own face (where emotions are most often expressed) both during and between sessions. Allow yourself to be touched, and enjoy the process.

7. *Cherish your friendships and intimacy with family.* Call them, send notes, buy flowers, invite laughter, and allow tears. Again and again, say some of the most important words in any language: "I love you," "Please," "Thank you," "I am sorry," "I forgive you."
8. *Cultive your commitment to helping; honor the privilege of our profession.* Despite the changing winds of public policy and professional demands, remember to appreciate the precious intentions at the heart of helping. Take pride in serving human development. Encourage others to do so.
9. *Ask for and accept comfort, help, and counsel.* Find teachers or counselors whom you can talk to and trust. Give yourself permission to be cared for and counseled. Do not expect to be finished with your personal therapy. If you cannot find a therapist, create an imaginary one and have regular sessions.
10. *Create a support network among your colleagues.* Offer to be there for them, and ask them to be there for you. Hug each other, if only over the phone. Kind words mean a lot.
11. *Enjoy yourself.* Play. Adopt a pet. Visit parks where there are children, families, and elders. Whistle, sing, dance, giggle, kiss, and smile into others' eyes. Practice peace with everyone, beginning with yourself.
12. *Follow your heart and embrace your spiritual seeking.* Find people, practices, and communities that serve your needs for meaning, belonging, and encouragement. Keep the faith; share it when you can.

APPENDIX N

Recommendations for Constructive Practice

1. *Prepare for each session in private reflection.* Even if only for a few seconds, take the time to nurture a sense of your own center and your intention to serve another developing being.
2. *Honor the complexity and uniqueness of each client.* Do not presume to know them. Let them be themselves, and invite them to share as much of their uniqueness as they are ready to do so.
3. *Give yourself and your client permission not to know and not to fully understand.* Life is much more than figuring things out; effective therapy does not require complete understanding or definitive explanations.
4. *Let clients set the pace, and honor their process.* Some clients will want to move very quickly; others will not want to move at all. Pushing often results in pushing back or digging in. Expansions and contractions tend to alternate. Recognize and respect the importance of timing.
5. *Encourage (but do not force) emotional expression.* Allow your clients to feel, and to feel freely, but do not convey the message that they must be emotionally expressive if they are to make progress or win your respect or caring. When feelings emerge, invite elaborations and explorations. Seek to understand beyond familiar words and summary labels. Locate felt emotions in bodily sensations.
6. *Allow and invite yourself to feel emotional in the process of counseling.* Let your heart lead your helping. Open yourself to feeling. Learn your patterns around pain. Cultivate compassion, loving kindness, balance, and trust. Recognize that a primary responsibility of your role as a professional

helper is to maintain a spirit of centeredness (balance) large enough to accommodate the combined energies of your client and yourself. *You will be challenged* in your balancing abilities, particularly if you allow yourself to be emotionally alive to your interactions with clients. When you are overwhelmed (e.g., by intense emotions, whether your client's or your own), take a moment to breathe deeply and to refocus on your intentions to help the person you are serving.

7. *Trust that your clients can endure their pain and be strengthened by the process.* You cannot take their pain away, although you might often wish that you could. But you can hold a steady course of confidence in their capacities.
8. *Emphasize safety and offer as much structure as your client needs.* Use routines, rhythms, and rituals to create a sense of order and familiarity. Give your clients freedom to create their own path, yet be ready with suggestions and illustrations when they request direction or structure.
9. *Affirm and encourage experimentation and exploration.* Invite clients to experiment with safe and socially responsible excursions into new patterns of experiencing—especially new patterns of action, interpretation, explanation, or meaning making. Affirm the processes and feelings involved; express genuine respect for the challenges of changing and offer generous encouragement of your clients' active engagement with those challenges.
10. *Teach compassion, forgiveness, and self-care.* Help your clients develop compassion for themselves and others. Encourage forgiveness. Teach self-care: Set a good example.

REFERENCES

Abram, D. (1996). *The spell of the sensuous*. New York: Pantheon.

Ackerman, D. (1990). *A natural history of the senses*. New York: Random House.

Arbib, M. A., & Hesse, M. B. (1986). *The construction of reality*. Cambridge, UK: Cambridge University Press.

Ainsworth, M. D. S. (1979). Infant–mother attachment. *American Psychologist, 34*, 932–937.

Alford, B. A., & Beck, A. T. (1997). *The integrative power of cognitive therapy*. New York: Guilford Press.

Almaas, A. H. (1988). *The pearl beyond price: Integration of personality into being: An object relations approach*. Berkeley, CA: Diamond Books.

Anderson, B. (1980). *Stretching*. Bolinas, CA: Shelter.

Anderson, W. T. (1990). *Reality isn't what it used to be*. San Francisco: Harper & Row.

Anderson, W. T. (Ed.). (1995). *The truth about the truth: De-confusing and re-constructing the postmodern world*. New York: Putnam.

Anderson, W. T. (1997). *The future of the self: Inventing the postmodern person*. New York: Tarcher & Putnam.

Anderson, W. T. (2003). *The next Enlightenment*. New York: St. Martin's.

Angus, L. (1996). Metaphor and the transformation of meaning in psychotherapy. In J. Mio & A. Katz (Eds.), *Metaphor: Pragmatics and applications*. Hillsdale, NJ: Erlbaum.

Angus, L., & Hardtke, K. (1994). Narrative processes in psychotherapy. *Canadian Psychology, 35*, 190–203.

Antonovsky, A. (1979). *Health, stress and coping*. San Francisco: Jossey-Bass.

Arciero, G. (1999). *Constructive coherence: Emotionality, identity, and narrative processes in psychotherapy*. Unpublished manuscript, Rome, Italy.

Arciero, G., Gaetano, P., Maselli, P., & Gentili, N. (2003). Identity, personality, and emotional regulation. *Constructivism in the Human Sciences, 8*, 7–18.

Arciero, G., & Guidano, V. F. (2000). Experience, explanation, and the quest for coherence. In R. A. Neimeyer & J. D. Raskin (Eds.), *Constructions of disor-*

der: Meaning-making perspectives for psychotherapy (pp. 91–118). Washington, DC: American Psychological Association.

Aron, E., & Aron, A. (1987). The influence of inner state on self-reported long-term happiness. *Journal of Humanistic Psychology, 27*, 248–270.

Atkinson, L., & Zucker, K. J. (Eds.). (1997). *Attachment and psychopathology.* New York: Guilford Press.

Austin, J. H. (1998). *Zen and the brain.* Cambridge, MA: MIT Press.

Baars, B. J. (1997). *In the theater of consciousness.* Oxford, UK: Oxford University Press.

Badiner, A. H., & Grey, A. (2002). *Zig zag Zen: Buddhism and psychedelics.* San Francisco: Chronicle Books.

Bailey, K. G., Wood, H. E., & Nava, G. R. (1992). What do clients want?: Role of psychological kinship in professional helping. *Journal of Psychotherapy Integration*, 2, 125–147.

Bakal, D. A. (1999). *Minding the body: Clinical uses of somatic awareness.* New York: Guilford Press.

Bakhtin, M. M. (1975). *The dialogic imagination.* Austin: University of Texas Press.

Bakhtin, M. M. (1986). *Speech genres and other late essays.* Austin: University of Texas Press.

Baldwin, C. (1990). *Life's companion: Journal writing as a spiritual quest.* New York: Bantam.

Ballou, M., & Brown, L. S. (Eds.). (2002). *Rethinking mental health and disorder: Feminist perspectives.* New York: Guilford Press.

Baltes, P. B., & Staudinger, U. M. (2000). Wisdom: A metaheuristic (pragmatic) to orchestrate mind and virtue toward excellence. *American Psychologist, 55*, 122–136.

Bandura, A. (1969). *Principles of behavior modification.* New York: Holt, Rinehart & Winston.

Bandura, A. (1977). Self-efficacy: Toward a unifying theory of behavioral change. *Psychological Review, 84*, 191–215.

Bandura, A. (1982). The psychology of chance encounters in life paths. *American Psychologist, 37*, 747–755.

Bandura, A. (1986). *Social foundations of thought and action: A social cognitive theory.* Englewood Cliffs, NJ: Prentice-Hall.

Bandura, A. (1997). *Self-efficacy: The exercise of control.* New York: Freeman.

Baringholtz, S. (1998). Constructive psychotherapy and the therapist: Some considerations. *Constructivism in the Human Sciences, 3*, 83–92.

Barnard, K. E., & Brazelton, T. B. (Eds.). (1990). *Touch: The foundation of experience.* Madison, CT: International Universities Press.

Barrett, L. F., & Russell, J. A. (1999). The structure of current affect: Controversies and emerging consensus. *Current Directions in Psychological Science, 8*, 10–14.

Barrett, W. (1958). *Irrational man: A study in existential philosophy.* New York: Doubleday.

Barrett, W. (1967). *The illusion of technique.* New York: Doubleday.

Bartlett, F. C. (1932). *Remembering.* Cambridge, UK: Cambridge University Press.

Bartley, W. W. (1984). *The retreat to commitment* (2nd ed.). La Salle, IL: Open Court. (Original published in 1962)

Batchelor, S. (1994). *The awakening of the West: The encounter of Buddhism and Western culture*. Berkeley, CA: Parallax Press.

Batchelor, S. (1997). *Buddhism without beliefs: A contemporary guide to awakening*. New York: Riverhead Books.

Bateson, G. (1972). *Steps to an ecology of mind*. New York: Ballantine.

Bateson, G. (1979). *Mind and nature: A necessary unity*. New York: Bantam.

Bateson, P., & Martin, P. (2000). *Design for a life*. New York: Touchstone.

Baumeister, R. F. (1991). *Meanings of life*. New York: Guilford Press.

Baumeister, R. F. (1994). The crystalization of discontent in the process of major life change. In T. F. Heatherton & J. L. Weinberger (Eds.), *Can personality change?* (pp. 281–297). Washington, DC: American Psychological Association.

Bechara, A., Damasio, H., Tranel, D., & Damasio, A. R. (1997). Deciding advantageous before knowing the advantageous strategy. *Science, 275*, 1293–1295.

Beck, A. T. (1976). *Cognitive therapy and the emotional disorders*. New York: International Universities Press.

Beck, A. T., Rush, A. J., Shaw, B. F., & Emery, G. (1979). *Cognitive therapy of depression*. New York: Guilford Press.

Beck, D. E., & Cowan, C. C. (1996). *Spiral dynamics*. Oxford, UK: Blackwell.

Beck, J. S. (1995). *Cognitive therapy: Basics and beyond*. New York: Guilford Press.

Becker, E. (1973). *The denial of death*. New York: Free Press.

Beiser, M. (1974). Components and correlates of mental well-being. *Journal of Health and Social Behavior, 15*, 320–327.

Belenky, M. F., Clinchy, B. McV., Goldberger, N. R., & Tarule, J. M. (1986). *Women's ways of knowing: The development of self, voice, and mind*. New York: Basic Books.

Benthal, J., & Polhemus, T. (Eds.). (1975). *The body as a medium of expression*. New York: Dutton.

Berger, P. L. (1967). *The sacred canopy: Elements of a sociological theory of religion*. New York: Anchor.

Berger, P. L., & Luckman, T. (1966). *The social construction of reality: A treatise in the sociology of knowledge*. Garden City, NY: Anchor.

Bergner, R. M. (1997). What is psychopathology? And so what? *Clinical Psychology: Science and Practice, 4*, 235–248.

Berlin, I. (1976). *Vico and Herder: Two studies in the history of ideas*. New York: Viking Press.

Berman, M. (1981). *The reenchantment of the world*. New York: Bantam.

Berman, M. (1989). *Coming to our senses: Body and spirit in the hidden history of the West*. New York: Bantam.

Bermúdez, J. L., Marcel, A., & Eilan, N. (Eds.). (1995). *The body and the self*. Cambridge, MA: MIT Press.

Bernstein, R. J. (1983). *Beyond objectivism and relativism: Science, hermeneutics, and praxis*. Philadelphia: University of Pennsylvania Press.

Beskow, J., & Palm, A. (1998). The mirror technique. *Constructivism in the Human Sciences, 3*, 20–22.

Bloom, H. (2000). *Global brain*. New York: Wiley.

Bloor, D. (1976). *Knowledge and social imagery*. Chicago: University of Chicago Press.

Blumenthal, A. L. (1975). A reappraisal of Wilhelm Wundt. *American Psychologist, 30*, 1081–1088.

Blumenthal, A. L. (1980). Wilhelm Wundt and early American psychology: A clash of cultures. In R. Rieber & K. Salzinger (Eds.), *Psychology: Theoretical–historical perspectives* (pp. 25–42). New York: Academic Press.

Blumenthal, A. L. (1985). Wilhelm Wundt: Psychology as the propaedeutic science. In C. Buxton (Ed.), *Points of view of the history of modern psychology* (pp. 19–49). New York: Academic Press.

Bohart, A. C., & Greenberg, L. S. (1997). *Empathy reconsidered: New directions in psychotherapy.* Washington, DC: American Psychological Association.

Bohart, A. C., & Tallman, K. (1999). *How clients make therapy work: The process of active self-healing.* Washington, DC: American Psychological Association.

Bohm, D. (1985). *Unfolding meaning: A weekend of dialogue.* London: Routledge.

Bohm, D. (1996). *On dialogue.* London: Routledge.

Boorstein, S. (1996). *Don't just do something, sit there.* New York: HarperCollins.

Bowman, T. (1994). Using poetry, fiction, and essays to help people face shattered dreams. *Journal of Poetry Therapy, 8*, 81–89.

Bowker, G. C., & Starr, S. L. (1999). *Sorting things out: Classification and its consequences.* Cambridge, MA: MIT Press.

Bowlby, J. (1969). *Attachment and loss: Vol. I. Attachment.* New York: Basic Books.

Bowlby, J. (1973). *Attachment and loss: Vol. II. Separation: Anxiety and anger.* New York: Basic Books.

Bowlby, J. (1979). *The making and breaking of affectional bonds.* London: Tavistock.

Bowlby, J. (1980). *Attachment and loss: Vol. III. Loss: Sadness and depression.* London: Hogarth Press.

Bowlby, J. (1985). The role of childhood experience in cognitive disturbance. In M. J. Mahoney & A. Freeman (Eds.), *Cognition and psychotherapy* (pp. 181–199). New York: Plenum Press.

Bowlby, J. (1988). *A secure base: Parent–child attachment and healthy human development.* New York: Basic Books.

Bowlby, J. (1990). *Charles Darwin: A new life.* New York: Norton.

Brand, A. G. (1980). *Therapy in writing: A psycho-educational enterprise.* Lexington, MA: Heath.

Brent, S. B. (1978). Prigogine's model for self-organization in nonequilibrium systems: Its relevance for developmental psychology. *Human Development, 21*, 374–387.

Bretherton, I. (1995). A communication perspective on attachment relationships and internal working models. In E. Waters, B. E. Vaughn, G. Posada, & K. Kondo-Ikemura (Eds.), *Caregiving, cultural, and cognitive perspectives on secure-base behavior and working models* (pp. 310–329). Chicago: Monographs of the Society for Research in Child Development (University of Chicago Press).

Brown, L. B. (1994). *The human side of prayer: The psychology of praying.* Birmingham, AL: Religious Education Press.

Brown, W. S. (Ed.). (2000). *Understanding wisdom: Sources, science, and society.* Radnor, PA: Templeton Foundation.

Brower, A. M., & Nurius P. S. (1993). *Social cognition and individual change: Current theory and counseling guidelines*. Newbury Park, CA: Sage.
Bruner, J. (1979). *On knowing: Essays for the left hand*. Cambridge, MA: Harvard University Press.
Bruner, J. (1986). *Actual minds, possible worlds*. Cambridge, MA: Harvard University Press.
Bruner, J. (1990). *Acts of meaning*. Cambridge, MA: Harvard University Press.
Bruner, J. (1994). The view from the heart's eye: A commentary. In P. M. Niedenthal & S. Kitayama (Eds.), *The heart's eye: Emotional influences in perception and attention* (pp. 269–286). New York: Academic Press.
Bruner, J. (2002). *Making stories: Law, literature, life*. New York: Farrar, Straus & Giroux.
Bruner, J., & Kalmar, D. A. (1998). Narrative and metanarrative in the construction of the self. In M. Ferrari & R. J. Sternberg (Eds.), *Self-awareness: Its nature and development* (pp. 308–331). New York: Guilford Press.
Brussat, F., & Brussat, M. A. (1996). *Spiritual literacy: Reading the sacred in everyday life*. New York: Scribner's.
Buber, M. (1958). *I and thou*. New York: Scribner's.
Bucci, W. (1997). *Psychoanalysis and cognitive science: A multiple code theory*. New York: Guilford Press.
Bugental, J. F. T. (1965). *The search for authenticity*. New York: Holt, Rinehart & Winston.
Bugental, J. F. T. (1978). *Psychotherapy and process: The fundamentals of an existential–humanistic approach*. Reading, MA: Addison-Wesley.
Bugental, J. F. T. (1981). *The search for authenticity*. New York: Irvington.
Bugental, J. F. T. (1987). *The art of the psychotherapist*. New York: Norton.
Camus, A. (1955). *The myth of Sisyphus*. New York: Random House.
Capra, F. (1996). *The web of life*. New York: Anchor.
Caputi, A. (1988). *Pirandello and the crisis of modern consciousness*. Urbana: University of Illinois Press.
Caputo, J. D. (1987). *Radical hermeneutics: Repetition, deconstruction, and the hermeneutic project*. Bloomington: Indiana University Press.
Carlin, G. (1997). *Brain droppings*. New York: Hyperion.
Carlsen, M. B. (1988). *Meaning-making: Therapeutic processes in adult development*. New York: Norton.
Carlsen, M. B. (1995). Meaning-making and creative aging. In R. A. Neimeyer & M. J. Mahoney (Eds.), *Constructivism in psychotherapy* (pp. 127–153). Washington, DC: American Psychological Association.
Carlson, J., & Sperry, L. (1998). Adlerian psychotherapy as a constructivist psychotherapy. In M. F. Hoyt (Ed.), *The handbook of constructive therapies* (pp. 68–82). San Francisco: Jossey-Bass.
Caro, I. (Ed.). (1993). *Psicoterapia e investigación de procesos*. Valencia, Spain: Promolibro.
Caro, I. (1994). *La práctica de la terapia lingüística de evaluación*. Salamanca, Spain: Amaru Ediciones.
Caro, I. (Ed.). (1997). *Manual de psicoterapias cognitivas*. Barcelona, Spain: Paidós.
Caro, I., & Read, C. S. (Eds.). (2002). *General semantics in psychotherapy: Selected*

wrings on methods aiding therapy. Brooklyn, NY: Institute of General Semantics.

Carstensen, L. L., Pasupathi, M., Mayr, U., & Nesselrode, J. R. (2000). Emotional experience in everyday life across the adult life span. *Journal of Personality and Social Psychology, 79*, 644–655.

Cassidy, J., & Mohr, J. J. (2001). Unsolvable fear, trauma, and psychopathology: Theory, research, and clinical considerations related to disorganized attachment across the life span. *Clinical Psychology: Science and Practice, 8*, 275–298.

Cassidy, J., & Shaver, P. R. (Eds.). (1999). *Handbook of attachment: Theory, research, and clinical applications*. New York: Guilford Press.

Cassileth, B. R. (1998). *The alternative medicine handbook*. New York: Norton.

Cervone, D., & Shoda, Y. (Eds.). (1999). *The coherence of personality: Social-cognitive bases of consistency, variability, and organization*. New York: Guilford Press.

Chamberlain, L. L., & Bütz, M. R. (Eds.). (1998). *Clinical chaos*. New York: Brunner/Mazel.

Chodorow, J. (1991). *Dance therapy and depth psychology: The moving imagination*. New York: Routledge.

Chödrön, P. (1997). *When things fall apart: Heart advice for difficult times*. Boston: Shambhala.

Combs, A. (1996). *The radiance of being: Complexity, chaos, and the evolution of consciousness*. St. Paul, MN: Paragon House.

Crosby, A. W. (1997). *The measure of reality: Quantification and western society, 1250–1600*. Oxford, UK: Oxford University Press.

Csordas, T. J. (Ed.). (1994). *Embodiment and experience: The existential ground of culture and self*. Cambridge, UK: Cambridge University Press.

Cushman, P. (1995). *Constructing the self, constructing America: A cultural history of psychotherapy*. Reading, MA: Addison-Wesley.

Cytowic, R. E. (1998). *The man who tasted shapes*. Cambridge, MA: MIT Press.

Daloz, L. A. (1999). *Mentor: Guiding the journey of adult learners*. San Francisco: Jossey-Bass.

Damasio, A. (1995). *Descartes' error*. New York: Harcourt Brace.

Damasio, A. (1999). *The feeling of what happens: Body and emotion in the making of consciousness*. New York: Harcourt Brace.

Davis, D., & Hollon, S. D. (1999). Reframing resistance and noncompliance in cognitive therapy. *Journal of Psychotherapy Integration, 9*, 33–55.

Davis, P. J., & Hersh, R. (1986). *Descartes' dream: The world according to mathematics*. Boston, MA: Houghton Mifflin.

Davisson, A. (1978). George Kelly and the American mind (or why has he been obscure for so long in the U.S.A. and whence the new interest?). In F. Fransella (Ed.), *Personal construct psychology 1977* (pp. 25–33). London: Academic Press.

DeAngelis, T. (2001). APA has lead role in revising classification system. *Monitor on Psychology, 32*(2), 54–56.

Debats, D. L. (1999). Sources of meaning: An investigation of significant commitments in life. *Journal of Humanistic Psychology, 39*, 30–57.

Dell, P. F. (1982a). Beyond homeostatsis: Toward a concept of coherence. *Family Process*, *21*, 21–41.

Dell, P. F. (1982b). In search of truth: On the way to clinical epistemology. *Family Process*, *21*, 407–414.

Dell, P. F., & Goolishian, H. A. (1981). Order through fluctuation: An evolutionary epistemology for human systems. *Australian Journal of Family Therapy, 2*, 175–184.

de Rivera, J., & Sarbin, T. R. (Eds.). (1998). *Believed-in imaginings: The narrative construction of reality.* Washington, DC: American Psychological Association.

de Shazer, S. (1994). *Words were originally magic*. New York: Norton.

Diener, E. (2000). Subjective well-being: The science of happiness and a proposal for a national index. *American Psychologist*, *55*, 34–43.

Diener, E., & Larsen, R. J. (1993). The experience of emotional well-being. In M. Lewis & J. M. Haviland (Eds.), *Handbook of emotions* (pp. 405–415). New York: Guilford Press.

Doherty, W. J. (1995). *Soul searching: Why psychotherapy must promote moral responsibility.* New York: Basic Books.

Dollinger, S. J. (1986). The need for meaning following disaster: Attributions and emotional upset. *Personality and Social Psychology Bulletin*, *12,* 300–310.

Dowd, E. T. (1999). Why don't people change? What stops them from changing?: An integrative commentary on the special issue on resistance. *Journal of Psychotherapy Integration*, *9*, 119–131.

Drechsler, A. (1998). *The weightlifting encyclopedia*. Flushing, NY: A Is A Communications.

Duncan, B. L., Hubble, M. A., Miller, S. D., & Coleman, S. T. (1998). Escaping the lost world of impossibility: Honoring clients' language, motivation, and theories of change. In M. F. Hoyt (Ed.), *The handbook of constructive therapies* (pp. 293–313). San Francisco: Jossey-Bass.

Durant, W. (1926). *The story of philosophy.* Garden City, NY: Garden City Publishing.

Durant, W., & Durant, A. (1935–1975). *The story of civilization* (11 vols.). New York: Simon & Schuster.

Eagle, M. (1999). Why don't people change?: A psychoanalytic perspective. *Journal of Psychotherapy Integration*, *9*, 3–32.

Ecker, B., & Hulley, L. (2000). The order in clinical "disorder": Symptom coherence in depth-oriented brief psychotherapy. In R. A. Neimeyer & J. D. Raskin (Eds.), *Constructions of disorder: Meaning-making frameworks for psychotherapy* (pp. 63–89). Washington, DC: American Psychological Association.

Efran, J., Lukens, M. D., & Lukens, R. J. (1990). *Language, structure, and change.* New York: Norton.

Elliott, D. M., & Guy, J. D. (1993). Mental health professionals versus non-mental-health professionals: Childhood trauma and adult functioning. *Professional Psychology: Research and Practice, 24,* 83–90.

Ellis, A. (1962). *Reason and emotion in psychotherapy.* New York: Stuart.

Ellis, A. (1998). How rational emotive behavior therapy belongs in the constructivist camp. In M. F. Hoyt (Ed.), *The handbook of constructive therapies* (pp. 83–99). San Francisco: Jossey-Bass.

Emmett, G. J. (1998). *The process of ritual: A twenty-year survey of literature.* Unpublished master's thesis, University of North Texas, Denton.

Emmons, R. A. (1999). *The psychology of ultimate concerns: Motivation and spirituality in personality.* New York: Guilford Press.

Epstein, M. (1995). *Thoughts without a thinker: Psychotherapy from a Buddhist perspective.* New York: Basic Books.

Epstein, S. (1973). The self-concept revisited: Or a theory of a theory. *American Psychologist, 28,* 404–416.

Epstein, S. (1993). Emotion and self theory. In M. Lewis & J. M. Haviland (Eds.), *Handbook of emotions* (pp. 313–326). New York: Guilford Press.

Epstein, S. (1998). *Constructive thinking: The key to emotional intelligence.* London: Praeger.

Faidley, A. J., & Leitner, L. M. (1993). *Assessing experience in psychotherapy: Personal construct alternatives.* Westport, CT: Praeger.

Ferreira, R. F., & Nabuco, C. (Eds.). (1998). *Psicoterapia e constructivismo: Considerações teóricas e práticas.* São Paulo: Artes Médicas.

Feixas, G. (1990a). Personal construct theory and systemic therapies. *Journal of Marital and Family Therapy, 16,* 1–20.

Feixas, G. (1990b). Approaching the individual, approaching the system. *Journal of Family Psychology, 4,* 4–35.

Feixas, G. (1995). Personal constructs in systemic practice. In R. A. Neimeyer & M. J. Mahoney (Eds.), *Constructivism in psychotherapy* (pp. 305–337). Washington, DC: American Psychological Association.

Feixas, G., Procter, H. G., & Neimeyer, G. J. (1993). Convergent lines of assessment: Systemic and constructivist contributions. In G. J. Neimeyer (Ed.), *Constructivist assessment: A casebook* (pp. 143–178). London: Sage.

Feldman-Barrett, L., & Russell, J. A. (1999). The structure of current affect: Controversies and emerging consensus. *Current Directions in Psychological Science, 8,* 10–14.

Ferrari, M., & Sternberg, R. J. (1998). *Self-awareness: Its nature and development.* New York: Guilford Press.

Fischer, C. T. (1980). Phenomenology and psychological assessment: Representational description. *Journal of Phenomenological Psychology, 11,* 79–105.

Fischer, C. T. (Ed.). (2002). Approaches to humanistic psychological assessment. *The Humanistic Psychologist, 30*(Issues 1–3).

Fischer, R. (1987). On fact and fiction—the structures of stories that the brain tells to itself about itself. *Journal of Social and Biological Structures, 10,* 343–351.

Flack, W. F., & Laird, J. D. (Eds.). (1998). *Emotions in psychopathology.* Oxford, UK: Oxford University Press.

Fogel, A. (1993). *Developing through relationships: Origins of communication, self, and culture.* Chicago: University of Chicago Press.

Fogel, D. O. (1978). Learned helplessness and learned restlessness. *Psychotherapy, 15,* 39–47.

Follette, W. C. (1996). Introduction to the Special Section on the development of theoretically coherent alternatives to the DSM system. *Journal of Consulting and Clinical Psychology, 64,* 1117–1119.

Ford, D. H. (1987). *Humans as self-constructing living systems: A developmental perspective on behavior and personality.* Hillsdale, NJ: Erlbaum.

Ford, D. H., & Urban, H. B. (1998). *Contemporary models of psychotherapy: A comparative analysis* (2nd ed.). New York: Wiley.

Fortun, M., & Bernstein, H. J. (1998). *Muddling through: Pursuing science and truths in the 21st century.* Washington, DC: Counterpoint.

Fosha, D. (2000). *The transforming power of affect: A model of accelerated change.* New York: Basic Books.

Fosha, D. (2001). Trauma reveals the roots of resilience. *Constructivism in the Human Sciences, 6,* 7–15.

Foster, D., & Arvay, M. J. (2003). Wilber's all-quadrant model: Implications for constructive postmodern counseling research and practice. *Constructivism in the Human Sciences, 8,* 159–172.

Foucault, M. (1965). *Madness and civilization: A history of insanity in the age of reason* (R. Howard, trans.). New York: Random House.

Foucault, M. (1970). *The order of things: An archeology of the human sciences.* New York: Random House.

Foulkes, D. (1985). *Dreaming: A cognitive-psychological analysis.* Hillsdale, NJ: Erlbaum.

Foulkes, D. (1999). *Children's dreaming and the development of consciousness.* Cambridge, MA: Harvard University Press.

Frank, J. D. (1973). *Persuasion and healing* (2nd ed.). Baltimore: Johns Hopkins University Press.

Frankl, V. E. (1959). *Man's search for meaning: An introduction to logotherapy.* New York: Washington Square Press.

Frankl, V. E. (1985). Logos, paradox, and the search for meaning. In M. J. Mahoney & A. Freeman (Eds.), *Cognition and psychotherapy* (pp. 259–275). New York: Plenum Press.

Franklin, C., & Nurius, P. S. (1998). *Constructivism in practice: Methods and challenges.* Milwaukee, WI: Families International.

Freedland, R. L., & Bertenthal, B. I. (1994). Developmental changes in interlimb coordination: Transition to hands-and-knees crawling. *Psychological Science, 5,* 26–32.

Freeman, W. (1995). *Societies of brains.* Hillsdale, NJ: Erlbaum.

French, M. (1985). *Beyond power: On women, men, and morals.* New York: Summit Books.

Friedman, L., & Moon, S. (Eds.). (1997). *Being bodies: Buddhist women on the paradox of embodiment.* Boston: Shambhala.

Friedman, S. (Ed.). (1993). *The new language of change: Constructive collaboration in psychotherapy.* New York: Guilford Press.

Freud, S. (1988). *My three mothers and other passions.* New York: New York University Press.

Freud, S. (2003). The opposite is also true: A backwards look at attachment. *Constructivism in the Human Sciences, 8,* 37–46.

Fromm, E. (1956). *The art of loving.* New York: Harper.

Fuller, S. (2000). Science studies through the looking glass: An intellectual itinerary. In U. Segerstråle (Ed.), *Beyond the science wars: The missing discourse about science and society* (pp. 185–217). Albany, NY: SUNY Press.

Gallagher, S., & Shear, J. (Eds.). (1999). *Models of the self*. Bowling Green, OH: Imprint Academic.

Gallese, V. (1995). The "shared manifold" hypothesis: From mirror neurons to empathy. In E. Thompson (Ed.), *Between ourselves* (pp. 33–50). Charlottesville, VA: Imprint Academic.

Gallop, J. (1988). *Thinking through the body*. New York: Columbia University Press.

Garvey, J. (Ed.). (1985). *Modern spirituality: An anthology*. Springfield, IL: Templegate.

Gavin, J. (1988). *Body moves: The psychology of exercise*. Harrisburg, PA: Stackpole.

Geertz, C. (2000). *Available light: Anthropological reflections on philosophical topics*. Princeton, NJ: Princeton University Press.

Geller, J. D., & Spector, P. D. (Eds.). (1987). *Psychotherapy: Portraits in fiction*. Northvale, NJ: Aronson.

Gendlin, E. T. (1996). *Focusing-oriented psychotherapy: A manual of the experiential method*. New York: Guilford Press.

Gergen, K. J. (1991). *The saturated self*. New York: Basic Books.

Gergen, K. J. (1994). *Realities and relationships: Soundings in social construction*. Cambridge, MA: Harvard University Press.

Gergen, K. J. (1999). *An invitation to social construction*. London: Sage.

Gergen, K. J. (2000). The coming of creative confluence in therapeutic practice. *Psychotherapy, 37*, 364–369.

Gibson, E. J. (1988). Exploratory behavior in the development of perceiving, acting, and the acquiring of knowledge. *Annual Review of Psychology, 39*, 1–41.

Gilbert, P., & Bailey, K. G. (Eds.). (2000). *Genes on the couch: Explorations in evolutionary psychotherapy*. Philadelphia: Taylor & Francis.

Gillham, N. W. (2001). *A life of Sir Francis Galton*. Oxford, UK: Oxford University Press.

Gilligan, S. (1997). *The courage to love: Principles and practices of self-relations psychotherapy*. New York: Norton.

Glazer, S. (Ed.). (1999). *The heart of learning: Spirituality in education*. New York: Tarcher.

Gleick, J. (1987). *Chaos: Making a new science*. New York: Viking Press.

Goldberg, N. (1986). *Writing down the bones: Freeing the writer within*. Boston: Shambhala.

Goldberger, N., Tarule, J., Clinchy, B., & Belenky, M. (Eds.). (1996). *Knowledge, difference, and power: Essays inspired by* Women's Ways of Knowing. New York: Basic Books.

Goldfried, M. R. (1995). *From cognitive-behavior therapy to psychotherapy integration*. New York: Plenum Press.

Goleman, D. (1988). *The meditative mind: The varieties of meditative experience*. Los Angeles: J. P. Tarcher.

Goleman, D. (1995). *Emotional intelligence*. New York: Bantam.

Gonçalves, M., & Gonçalves, O. F. (1998). Political functions of the concept of identity. *Constructivism in the Human Sciences, 3*, 129–151.

Gonçalves, O. F. (1994). Cognitive narrative psychotherapy: The hermeneutic construction of alternatives. *Journal of Cognitive Psychotherapy: An International Quarterly, 8*, 105–125.

Gonçalves, O. F. (1995). Hermeneutics, constructivism, and cognitive-behavioral therapies: From the object to the project. In R. A. Neimeyer & M. J. Mahoney (Eds.), *Constructivism in psychotherapy* (pp. 195–230). Washington, DC: American Psychological Association.

Gonçalves, O. F., Korman, Y., & Angus, L. (2000). Constructing psychopathology from a cognitive narrative perspective. In R. A. Neimeyer & J. D. Raskin (Eds.), *Constructions of disorder: Meaning-making frameworks for psychotherapy* (pp. 265–284). Washington, DC: American Psychological Association.

Gonçalves, O. F., & Machado, P. P. (1999). Cognitive narrative psychotherapy: Research foundations. *Journal of Clinical Psychology, 55*, 1179–1191.

Gould, S. J. (2000). Deconstructing the "science wars" by reconstructing an old mold. *Science, 287*, 253–261.

Graci, G. M., O'Rourke, N., & Mahoney, M. J. (2003). Personal meanings of spirituality. *Constructivism in the Human Sciences, 8*, 47–56.

Greenberg, L. S. (2002). *Emotion-focused psychotherapy.* Washington, DC: American Psychological Association.

Greenberg, L. S., & Paivio, S. C. (1997). *Working with emotions in psychotherapy.* New York: Guilford Press.

Greenberg, L. S., & Pascual-Leone, J. (1995). A dialectical constructivist approach to experiential change. In R. A. Neimeyer & M. J. Mahoney (Eds.), *Constructivism in psychotherapy* (pp. 169–191). Washington, DC: American Psychological Association.

Greenberg, L. S., Watson, J. C., & Lietaer, G. (1998). *Handbook of experiential psychotherapy.* New York: Guilford Press.

Greenberger, D., & Padesky, C. A. (1995). *Mind over mood: Change how you feel by changing the way you think*. New York: Guilford Press.

Greene, B. (1999). *The elegant universe: Superstrings, hidden dimensions, and the quest for the ultimate theory.* New York: Random House.

Greher, M. R., & Mahoney, M. J. (2001). Behavioral and self-report measures of attention. *Constructivism in the Human Sciences*, 6, 87–93.

Griffith, J. L., & Griffith, M. E. (1994). *The body speaks: Therapeutic dialogues for mind–body problems*. New York: Basic Books.

Grof, S. (1975). *Realms of the human unconscious*. New York: Viking.

Grof, S., & Grof, C. (Eds.). (1989). *Spiritual emergency: When personal transformation becomes a crisis*. Los Angeles: Tarcher.

Guidano, V. F. (1987). *Complexity of the self: A developmental approach to psychopathology and therapy.* New York: Guilford Press.

Guidano, V. F. (1991). *The self in process: Toward a post-rationalist cognitive therapy.* New York: Guilford Press.

Guidano, V. F. (1995a). Constructive psychotherapy: A theoretical framework. In R. A. Neimeyer & M. J. Mahoney (Eds.), *Constructivism in psychotherapy* (pp. 93–108). Washington, DC: American Psychological Association.

Guidano, V. F. (1995b). Self-observation in constructivist psychotherapy. In R. A. Neimeyer & M. J. Mahoney (Eds.), *Constructivism in psychotherapy* (pp. 155–168). Washington, DC: American Psychological Association.

Guy, J. D. (1987). *The personal life of the psychotherapist*. New York: Wiley.

Haken, H. (1984). *The science of structure synergetics*. New York: Van Nostrand Reinhold.

Haken, H. (1996). *Principles of brain functioning*. New York: Springer.

Hanna, T. (1970). *Bodies in revolt: A primer in somatic thinking*. New York: Holt, Rinehart & Winston.

Harding, D. E. (1961). *On having no head: Zen and the rediscovery of the obvious*. London: Penguin.

Hargens, S. (2001). Intersubjective musings: A response to Christian de Quincey's "The promise of Integralism." *Journal of Consciousness Studies*, *8*(12), 35–78.

Harner, M. (1982). *The way of the shaman*. New York: Bantam.

Harre, R. (1991). *Physical being: A theory for corporeal psychology*. Oxford, UK: Blackwell.

Haruki, Y., Homma, I., Umezawa, A., & Masaoka, Y. (Eds.). (2001). *Respiration and emotion*. New York: Springer.

Haruki, Y., Ishii, Y., & Suzuki, M. (Eds.). (1996). *Comparative and psychological study on meditation*. Delft, the Netherlands: Eburon.

Haviland, J. M., & Kahlbaugh, P. (1993). Emotion and identity. In M. Lewis & J. M. Haviland (Eds.), *Handbook of emotions* (pp. 327–339). New York: Guilford Press.

Hayek, F. A. (1952). *The sensory order*. Chicago: University of Chicago Press.

Hayek, F. A. (1964). The theory of complex phenomena. In M. Bunge (Ed.), *The critical approach to science and philosophy: Essays in honor of K. R. Popper*. New York: Free Press.

Hayes, A. M. (1996). Dynamic systems theory as a paradigm for studying the process of change in psychotherapy for depression. *Constructivism in the Human Sciences*, *1*(1), 9–12.

Hays, K. F. (1999). *Working it out: Using exercise in psychotherapy*. Washington, DC: American Psychological Association.

Heatherton, T. F., & Weinberger, J. L. (Eds.). (1994). *Can personality change?* Washington, DC: American Psychological Association.

Heidrich, S. M., Forsthoff, C. A., & Ward, S. E. (1994). Psychological adjustments in adults with cancer: The self as a mediator. *Health Psychology*, *13*, 346–353.

Hermans, H. J. M., & Hermans-Jansen, E. (1995). *Self-narratives: The construction of meaning in psychotherapy*. New York: Guilford Press.

Hill, C. E. (1996). *Working with dreams in psychotherapy*. New York: Guilford Press.

Hoffman, I. Z. (1998). *Ritual and spontaneity in the psychoanalytic process: A dialectical-constructivist view*. Hillsdale, NJ: Analytic Press.

Horwitz, A. V. (2002). *Creating mental illness*. Chicago: University of Chicago Press.

Hoshmand, L. T. (1993). The personal narrative in the communal construction of self and life issues. In G. J. Neimeyer (Ed.), *Constructivist assessment: A casebook* (pp. 179–205). London: Sage.

Hoyt, M. F. (Ed.). (1994). *Constructive therapies: Volume 1*. New York: Guilford Press.

Hoyt, M. F. (Ed.). (1996). *Constructive therapies: Volume 2*. New York: Guilford Press.

Hoyt, M. F. (Ed.). (1998). *The handbook of constructive therapies*. San Francisco: Jossey-Bass.

Hoyt, M. F. (2000). *Some stories are better than others*. New York: Brunner/Mazel.

Hubble, M. A., Duncan, B. L., & Miller, S. D. (Eds.). (1999). *The heart and soul of change: What works in therapy.* Washington, DC: American Psychological Association.

Hunt, H. T. (1995). *On the nature of consciousness: Cognitive, phenomenological, and transpersonal perspectives.* New Haven, CT: Yale University Press.

Huxley, A. (1944). *The perennial philosophy.* New York: Harper & Row.

Ishai, A. (2002). Streams of consciousness. *Journal of Cognitive Neuroscience, 14,* 832–833.

Ivey, A. E. (1986). *Developmental therapy.* San Francisco: Jossey-Bass.

Ivey, A. E., & Gonçalves, O. F. (1988). Developmental therapy: Integrating development processes into clinical practice. *Journal of Counseling and Development, 66,* 406–413.

James, W. (1890). *Principles of psychology* (2 vols.). New York: Harper, Holt.

James, W. (1897). *The will to believe.* London: Longman, Green.

James, W. (1902). *The varieties of religious experience.* New York: New American Library.

Jankowicz, A. D. (1987). Whatever became of George Kelly?: Applications and implications. *American Psychologist, 42,* 481–487.

Johnson, D. H. (1994). *Body, spirit, and democracy.* Berkeley, CA: North Atlantic Books.

Johnson, M. (1987). *The body in the mind: The bodily basis of meaning, imagination, and reason.* Chicago: University of Chicago Press.

Joyce-Moniz, L. (1985). Epistemological therapy and constructivism. In M. J. Mahoney & A. Freeman (Eds.), *Cognition and psychotherapy* (pp. 143–179). New York: Plenum Press.

Kabat-Zinn, J. (1990). *Full catastrophe living.* New York: Dell.

Kabat-Zinn, J. (1994). *Wherever you go, there you are: Mindfulness meditation in everyday life.* New York: Hyperion.

Kahn, M. (1991). *Between therapist and client: The new relationship.* New York: Freeman.

Kant, I. (1929). *The critique of pure reason* (N. K. Smith, Trans.). New York: Macmillan. (Original published in 1781)

Kapleau, R. P. (1980). *The three pillars of Zen* (25th anniversary ed.). New York: Anchor Doubleday.

Karen, R. (1998). *Becoming attached.* Oxford, UK: Oxford University Press.

Kauffman, S. A. (1993). *The origins of order: Self-organization and selection in evolution.* Oxford, UK: Oxford University Press.

Kauffman, S. A. (1995). *At home in the universe.* Oxford: Oxford University Press.

Kaufmann, W. (1974). *Nietzsche: Philosopher, psychologist, antichrist.* Princeton, NJ: Princeton University Press.

Kazantzakis, N. (1960). *The saviors of god: Spiritual exercises.* New York: Simon & Schuster.

Kazantzis, N., Deane, F. P., & Ronan, K. R. (2000). Homework assignments in cognitive and behavioral therapy: A meta-analysis. *Clinical Psychology: Science and Practice, 7,* 189–202.

Keats, P. A. (2003). Constructing masks of the self in therapy. *Constructivism in the Human Sciences, 8,* 103–122.

Kegan, R. (1982). *The evolving self.* Cambridge, MA: Harvard University Press.

Kegan, R. (1994). *In over our heads: The mental demands of modern life*. Cambridge, MA: Harvard University Press.

Kegan, R., & Lahey, L. L. (2001). *How the way we talk can change the way we work*. San Francisco: Jossey-Bass.

Keller, E. F. (1983). *A feeling for the organism: The life and work of Barbara McClintock*. New York: Freeman.

Keller, E. F. (1985). *Reflections on gender and science*. New Haven, CT: Yale University Press.

Kelly, G. A. (1955). *The psychology of personal constructs*. New York: Norton.

Kelly, G. A. (1969a). In whom confide: On whom depend for what? In B. Maher (Ed.), *Clinical psychology and personality: The selected papers of George Kelly* (pp. 189–206). New York: Wiley.

Kelly, G. A. (1969b). Ontological accelerations. In B. Maher (Ed.), *Clinical psychology and personality: The selected papers of George Kelly* (pp. 7–45). New York: Wiley.

Kelly, G. A. (1969c). Personal construct theory and the psychotherapeutic interview. In B. Maher (Ed.), *Clinical psychology and personality: The selected papers of George Kelly* (pp. 224–264). New York: Wiley.

Kelly, G. A. (1969d). The psychotherapeutic relationship. In B. Maher (Ed.), *Clinical psychology and personality: The selected papers of George Kelly* (pp. 216–223). New York: Wiley.

Kelly, G. A. (1973). Fixed-role therapy. In R.-R. M. Jurjevich (Ed.), *Direct psychotherapy: 28 American originals* (pp. 394–422). Coral Gables, FL: University of Miami Press.

Kelso, J. A. S. (1995). *Dynamic patterns: The self-organization of brain and behavior.* Cambridge, MA: MIT Press.

Kenny, V., & Delmonte, M. (1986). Meditation as viewed through personal construct theory. *Journal of Contemporary Psychotherapy, 16*, 4–22.

Kernberg, O. F. (1975). *Borderline conditions and pathological narcissism*. New York: Jason Aronson.

Kernberg, O. F. (1976). *Object relations theory and clinical psychoanalysis*. New York: Jason Aronson.

Kernberg, O. F. (1995). *Internal world and external reality: Object relations theory applied*. New York: Jason Aronson.

Kierkegaard, S. (1938). *Purity of heart is to will one thing* (D. V. Steere, Trans.). New York: Harper & Row.

Kirsch, I. (1999). *How expectancies shape experience*. Washington, DC: American Psychological Association.

Kitayama, S., & Markus, H. R. (Eds.). (1994). *Emotion and culture: Empirical studies and mutual influences*. Washington, DC: American Psychological Association.

Klinger, E. (1971). *The structure and functions of fantasy.* New York: Wiley.

Knaster, M. (1996). *Discovering the body's wisdom*. New York: Bantam.

Knorr-Cetina, K. (1999). *Epistemic cultures: How the sciences make knowledge*. Cambridge, MA: Harvard University Press.

Koestler, A. (1978). *Janus: A summing up*. London: Hutchinson.

Kohut, H. (1971). *The analysis of the self*. New York: International Universities Press.

Kohut, H. (1977). *The restoration of the self.* New York: International University Press.

Kokoszka, A. (1999). Information metabolism as a model of human experiences. *International Journal of Neuroscience, 97,* 169–178.

Kono, T. (2001). *Olympic style weightlifting.* Aiea, HI: Hawaii Kono Company.

Kopp, S. B. (1972). *If you meet the Buddha on the road, kill him!* New York: Bantam.

Kornfield, J. (1993). *A path with heart: A guide through the perils and promises of spiritual life.* New York: Bantam.

Kornfield, J. (2000). *After the ecstasy, the laundry.* New York: Bantam.

Korzybski, A. (1937). *General semantics.* Englewood, NJ: Institute of General Semantics.

Kovel, J. (1991). *History and spirit: An inquiry into the philosophy of liberation.* Boston: Beacon.

Krippner, S. (1994). Humanistic psychology and chaos theory: The third revolution and the third force. *Journal of Humanistic Psychology, 34,* 48–61.

Kris, A. O. (1996). *Free association: Method and process* (rev. ed.). Hillsdale, NJ: Analytic Press.

Kuhn, T. S. (1962). *The structure of scientific revolutions.* Chicago: University of Chicago Press.

Kuhn, T. S. (1977). *The essential tension.* Chicago: University of Chicago Press.

Kuhn, T. S. (2000). *The road since structure.* Chicago: University of Chicago Press.

Kühnlein, I. (1999). Psychotherapy as a process of transformation: Analysis of posttherapeutic autobiographic narrations. *Psychotherapy Research, 9,* 274–288.

Kurtz, R. (1986). *Hakomi therapy.* Boulder, CO: Hakomi Institute.

Kurtz, R. (1990). *Body-centered psychotherapy: The Hakomi method.* Mendocino, CA: LifeRhythm.

Kwee, M. G. T., & Holdstock, T. L. (Eds.). (1996). *Western and Buddhist psychology: Clinical perspectives.* Delft, the Netherlands: Eburon.

LaBerge, S. (1985). *Lucid dreaming.* New York: Ballantine.

LaBerge, S., & Kahan, T. (1994). Lucid dreaming as metacognition: Implications for cognitive science. *Consciousness and Cognition, 3,* 246–264.

Lakoff, G. (1987). *Women, fire, and dangerous things: What categories reveal about the mind.* Chicago: University of Chicago Press.

Lakoff, G., & Johnson, M. (1980). *Metaphors we live by.* Chicago: University of Chicago Press.

Lakoff, G., & Johnson, M. (1999). *Philosophy in the flesh: The embodied mind and its challenge to Western thought.* New York: Basic Books.

Lakoff, G., & Núñez, R. E. (2000). *Where mathematics comes from: How the embodied mind brings mathematics into being.* New York: Basic Books.

Lambert, M. J. (1989). The individual therapist's contribution to psychotherapy process and outcome. *Clinical Psychology Review, 9,* 469–485.

Lamiell, J. T. (1987). *The psychology of personality: An epistemological approach.* New York: Columbia University Press.

Lash, J. (1990). *The seeker's handbook: The complete guide to spiritual pathfinding.* New York: Harmony Books.

Leder, D. (1990). *The absent body.* Chicago: University of Chicago Press.

Leder, D. (1997). *Spiritual passages: Embracing life's sacred journey.* New York: Tarcher/Putnam.

Lee, J. (1994). *Writing from the body.* New York: St. Martin's Press.

Leitner, L. M. (1995). Optimal therapeutic distance: A therapist's experience of personal construct psychotherapy. In R. A. Neimeyer & M. J. Mahoney (Eds.), *Constructivism in psychotherapy* (pp. 357–370). Washington, DC: American Psychological Association.

Leitner, L. M., & Faidley, A. J. (1999). Creativity in experiential personal construct psychotherapy. *Journal of Constructivist Psychology, 12*, 273–286.

Leonard, G. (1995). *The Tao of practice.* Mill Valley, CA: Integral Tranformation Practices.

Leonard, G., & Murphy, G. (1995). *The life we are given.* New York: Tarcher/Putnam.

Lesser, E. (1999). *The new American spirituality.* New York: Random House.

Levin, D. M. (1985). *The body's recollection of being: Phenomenological psychology and the deconstruction of nihilism.* London: Routledge & Kegan Paul.

Levin, D. M. (1988). *The opening of vision: Nihilism and the postmodern situation.* New York: Routledge.

Levine, S. (1979). *A gradual awakening.* Garden City, NY: Anchor.

Levine, S., & Levine, O. (1997). *To love and be loved: The difficult yoga of relationships.* Boulder, CO: Sounds True.

Lewis, M. (1992). *Shame: The exposed self.* New York: Free Press.

Lewis, M. (1997). *Altering fate: Why the past does not predict the future.* New York: Guilford Press.

Lewis, M., & Haviland, J. M. (Eds.). (1993). *Handbook of emotions.* New York: Guilford Press.

Lewis, M. D., & Granic, I. (Eds.). (2000). *Emotion, development, and self-organization: Dynamic systems approaches to emotional development.* Cambridge, UK: Cambridge University Press.

Livesley, W. J., Schroeder, M. L., Jackson, D. N., & Jang, K. L. (1994). Categorical distinctions in the study of personality disorder: Implications for classification. *Journal of Abnormal Psychology, 103.* 6–17.

Loder, J. E. (1981). *The transforming moment: Understanding convictional experiences.* New York: Harper & Row.

Lowen, W. (1982). *Dichotomies of the mind.* New York: Wiley.

Luborsky, L., Barber, J., & Digeur, L. (1992). The meanings of narratives told during psychotherapy: The fruits of a new observational unit. *Psychotherapy Research, 2*, 277–291.

Luhmann, N. (2002). *Theories of distinction: Redescribing the descriptions of modernity.* Stanford, CA: Stanford University Press.

Lutz, T. (1999). *Crying: The natural and cultural history of tears.* New York: Norton.

Lyddon, W. J. (1993). Contrast, contradiction, and change in psychotherapy. *Psychotherapy, 30*, 383–390.

Lyddon, W. J. (1995). Forms and facets of constructivist psychology. In R. A. Neimeyer & M. J. Mahoney (Eds.), *Constructivism in psychotherapy* (pp. 69–92). Washington, DC: American Psychological Association.

Lyddon, W. J., & Alford, D. J. (1993). Constructivist assessment: A developmental–epistemic perspective. In G. J. Neimeyer (Ed.), *Constructivist assessment: A casebook* (pp. 31–57). London: Sage.

Magai, C., & McFadden, S. H. (1995). *The role of emotions in social and personality development.* New York: Plenum Press.

Magee, B. (1983). *The philosophy of Schopenhauer.* Oxford, UK: Oxford University Press.

Magee, B. (1997). *Confessions of a philosopher.* New York: Random House.

Maher, B. (Ed.). (1969). *Clinical psychology and personality: The selected papers of George Kelly.* New York: Wiley.

Mahler, M. (1968). *On human symbiosis and the vicissitudes of individuation.* New York: International Universities Press.

Mahler, M., Pine, F., & Bergman, A. (1975). *The psychological birth of the infant.* New York: Basic Books.

Mahoney, M. J. (1974). *Cognition and behavior modification.* Cambridge, MA: Ballinger.

Mahoney, M. J. (1979). *Self-change: Strategies for solving personal problems.* New York: Norton.

Mahoney, M. J. (1983). *Stream of consciousness: A therapeutic application.* Keystone Heights, FL: PsychoEducational Resources.

Mahoney, M. J. (1988). Cognitive metatheory: II. Implications for psychotherapy. *International Journal of Personal Construct Psychology, 1,* 299–315.

Mahoney, M. J. (1991). *Human change processes.* New York: Basic Books.

Mahoney, M. J. (Ed.). (1995a). *Cognitive and constructive psychotherapies: Theory, research, and practice.* New York: Springer.

Mahoney, M. J. (1995b). Continuing evolution of the cognitive sciences and psychotherapies. In R. A. Neimeyer & M. J. Mahoney (Eds.), *Constructivism in psychotherapy* (pp. 39–67). Washington, DC: American Psychological Association.

Mahoney, M. J. (1996). Authentic presence and compassionate wisdom: The art of Jim Bugental. *Journal of Humanistic Psychology, 36,* 58–66.

Mahoney, M. J. (1997a). Brief moments and enduring effects: Reflections on time and timing in psychotherapy. In W. J. Matthews & J. Edgette (Eds.), *Current thinking and research in brief therapy: Solutions, strategies, narratives* (pp. 25–38). New York: Brunner/Mazel.

Mahoney, M. J. (1997b). Psychotherapists' personal problems and self-care patterns. *Professional Psychology: Research and Practice, 28,* 14–16.

Mahoney, M. J. (1999). Vittorio F. Guidano: 1944–1999. *Constructivism in the Human Sciences, 4,* 5–11.

Mahoney, M. J. (2000a). Behaviorism, cognitivism, and constructivism: Reflections on persons and patterns in my intellectual development. In M. R. Goldfried (Ed.), *How therapists change* (pp. 183–200). Washington, DC: American Psychological Association.

Mahoney, M. J. (2000b). A constructive view of disorder and development. In R. A. Neimeyer & J. D. Raskin (Eds.), *Constructions of disorder: Meaning-making frameworks for psychotherapy* (pp. 43–62). Washington, DC: American Psychological Association.

Mahoney, M. J. (2003). *Pilgrim in process: Collected poems*. Plainfield, IL: Kinder Path Press.

Mahoney, M. J. (in press-a). Minding science: Constructivism and the discourse of inquiry. *Cognitive Therapy and Research*.

Mahoney, M. J. (in press-b). *Scientist as subject: The psychological imperative*. Clinton Corners, NY: Eliot Werner. (Original published in 1976)

Mahoney, M. J., & Fernandez-Alvarez, H. (1998). La vida personal del psicoterapeuta/The personal life of the psychotherapist. *Avances en Psicología Clínica Latinoamericana, 16*, 9–22.

Mahoney, M. J., & Graci, G. M. (1999). The meanings and correlates of spirituality: Suggestions from an exploratory survey of experts. *Death Studies, 23*, 521–528.

Mahoney, M. J., & Mahoney, S. M. (2001). Living within essential tensions: Dialectics and future development. In K. J. Schneider, J. F. T. Bugental & J. F. Pierson (Eds.), *The handbook of humanistic psychology* (pp. 659–665). Thousand Oaks, CA: Sage.

Mahoney, M. J., & Marquis, A. (2002). Integral constructivism and dynamic systems in psychotherapy processes. *Psychoanalytic Inquiry, 22*, 794–813.

Mahoney, M. J., & Moes, A. J. (1997). Complexity and psychotherapy: Promising dialogues and practical issues. In F. Masterpasqua & P. A. Perna (Eds.), *The psychological meaning of chaos: Self-organization in human development and psychotherapy* (pp. 177–198). Washington, DC: American Psychological Association.

Mahoney, M. J., & Weimer, W. B. (1994). Friedrich A. Hayek 1899–1992. *American Psychologist, 49*, 63.

Mahrer, A. R. (1983). *Experiential psychotherapy: Basic practices*. New York: Brunner/Mazel.

Mancuso, J. C. (2001). Claiming Giambattista Vico as a narrativist/constructivist. Karl Jaspers Forum, Target Article 33; *http://www.douglashospital.qc.ca/fdg/kjf/33–taman.htm*

Mancuso, J. C., & Shaw, M. L. (1988). *Cognition and personal structure*. New York: Praeger.

Mangione, C. (1978). *Children of Sanchez* [cassette]. Los Angeles: A & M Records.

Margulis, L. (1998). *Symbiotic planet: A new look at evolution*. New York: Basic Books.

Margulis, L., & Sagan, D. (1995). *What is life?* New York: Simon & Schuster.

Markus, H., & Nurius, P. (1986). Possible selves. *American Psychologist, 41*, 954–969.

Marlatt, G. A. (Ed.). (1998). *Harm reduction: Pragmatic strategies for managing high-risk behaviors*. New York: Guilford Press.

Marrone, R. (1990). *Body of knowledge: An introduction to body/mind psychology*. Albany, NY: SUNY Press.

Marquis, A. (2002). *Comparing eclectic, Adlerian, and integral intake instruments*. Unpublished doctoral dissertation, University of North Texas, Denton.

Martin, J. (1994). *The construction and understanding of psychotherapeutic change: Conversations, memories, and theories*. New York: Teachers College Press.

Maslow, A. (1968). *Toward a psychology of being* (2nd ed.). New York: Van Nostrand Reinhold.

Maslow, A. (1971). *The farther reaches of human nature.* New York: Penguin.

Masterpasqua, F., & Perna, P. A. (Eds.). (1997). *The psychological meaning of chaos: Translating theory into practice.* Washington, DC: American Psychological Association.

Maturana, H. R. (1975). The organization of the living: A theory of the living organization. *International Journal of Man–Machine Studies, 7,* 313–332.

Maturana, H. R., & Varela, F. J. (1980). *Autopoiesis and cognition: The realization of the living.* Boston: Reidel.

Maturana, H. R., & Varela, F. J. (1987). *The tree of knowledge: The biological roots of human understanding.* Boston: Shambhala.

May, R. (1969). *Love and will.* New York: Norton.

Mayeroff, M. (1971). *On caring.* New York: Harper & Row.

Mazzotta, G. (1999). *The new map of the world: The poetic philosophy of Giambattista Vico.* Princeton, NJ: Princeton University Press.

McAdams, D. P. (1993). *The stories we live by: Personal myths and the making of the self.* New York: Guilford Press.

McAdams, D. P. (1994). Can personality change?: Levels of stability and growth in personality across the life span. In T. F. Heatherton & J. L. Weinberger (Eds.), *Can personality change?* (pp. 299–313). Washington, DC: American Psychological Association.

McCullough, M. E., Pargament, K. I., & Thoresen, C. E. (Eds.). (1999). *Forgiveness: Theory, research, and practice.* New York: Guilford Press.

Melville, S. W. (1986). *Philosophy beside itself: On deconstruction and modernism.* Minneapolis: University of Minnesota Press.

Merleau-Ponty, M. (1942). *The structure of behavior.* Boston: Beacon.

Merleau-Ponty, M. (1962). *Phenomenology of perception* (C. Smith, Trans.). London: Routledge & Kegan Paul.

Merton, T. (1968). *Zen and the birds of appetite.* New York: New Directions.

Messer, S. B., Sass, L. A., & Woolfolk, R. L. (Eds.). (1988). *Hermeneutics and psychological theory: Interpretive perspectives on personality, psychotherapy, and psychopathology.* New Brunswick, NJ: Rutgers University Press.

Mikulas, W. L. (2002). *The integrative helper: Convergence of eastern and western traditions.* Pacific Grove, CA: Brooks/Cole.

Miller, W. R. (Ed.). (1999). *Integrating spirituality into treatment: Resources for practitioners.* Washington, DC: American Psychological Association.

Miller, W. R., & C'deBaca, J. (1994). Quantum change: Toward a psychology of transformation. In T. F. Heatherton & J. L. Weinberger (Eds.), *Can personality change?* (pp. 253–280). Washington, DC: American Psychological Association.

Miller, W. R., & C'de Baca, J. (2001). *Quantum change: When epiphanies and sudden insights transform ordinary lives.* New York: Guilford Press.

Minton, S. C. (1989). *Body and self: Partners in movement.* Champaign, IL: Human Kinetics Books.

Mischel, W. (1980). George Kelly's anticipation of psychology. In M. J. Mahoney (Ed.), *Psychotherapy process: Current issues and future directions* (pp. 85–87). New York: Plenum Press.

Mitchell, S. A. (1988). *Relational concepts in psychoanalysis: An integration*. Cambridge, MA: Harvard University Press.

Mitchell, S. A. (1997). *Influence and autonomy in psychoanalysis*. Hillsdale, NJ: Analytic Press.

Mitchell, S. A., & Black, M. J. (1995). *Freud and beyond: A history of modern psychoanalytic thought*. New York: Basic Books.

Montagu, A. (1978). *Touching: The human significance of the skin* (2nd ed.). New York: Harper & Row.

Moore, R. (2000). *The creation of reality in psychoanalysis: A view of the contributions of Donald Spence, Roy Schafer, Robert Stolorow, Irwin Z. Hoffman, and beyond*. Hillsdale, NJ: Analytic Press.

Moreno, J. (1946). *Psychodrama* (Vol. 1). New York: Beacon House.

Moreno, J. (1959). *Psychodrama* (Vol. 2). New York: Beacon House.

Moreno, J. (1962). *Psychodrama* (Vol. 3). New York: Beacon House.

Muller, W. (1992). *Legacy of the heart: The spiritual advantages of a painful childhood*. New York: Simon & Schuster.

Murphy, M. (1992). *The future of the body: Explorations into the further evolution of human nature*. Los Angeles: Tarcher.

Murphy, M., & Donovan, S. (1997). *The physical and psychological effects of meditation: A review of contemporary research with a comprehensive bibliography 1931–1996*. Sausalito, CA: Institute of Noetic Sciences.

Nachmanovitch, S. (1990). *Free play: Improvisation in life and art*. New York: Tarcher.

Nash, S. A., & Merkert, J. (Eds.). (1985). *Naum Gabo: Sixty years of constructivism*. Munich: Prestl-Verlag.

Natsoulas, T. (1996–1997). The stream of consciousness: XIII. Bodily self-awareness and Aron Gurwitsch's margin. In K. S. Pope & J. L. Singer (Eds.), *Imagination cognition and personality: Consciousness in theory, research, and clinical practice* (pp. 281–300). New York: Baywood.

Neimeyer, G. J. (Ed.). (1993). *Constructivist assessment: A casebook*. London: Sage.

Neimeyer, R. A. (1985). *The development of personal construct psychology*. Lincoln: University of Nebraska Press.

Neimeyer, R. A. (1995a). Client-generated narratives in psychotherapy. In R. A. Neimeyer & M. J. Mahoney (Eds.), *Constructivism in psychotherapy* (pp. 231–246). Washington, DC: American Psychological Association.

Neimeyer, R. A. (1995b). Constructivist psychotherapies: Features, foundations, and future directions. In R. A. Neimeyer & M. J. Mahoney (Eds.), *Constructivism in psychotherapy* (pp. 11–38). Washington, DC: American Psychological Association.

Neimeyer, R. A., & Mahoney, M. J. (Eds.). (1995). *Constructivism in psychotherapy*. Washington, DC: American Psychological Association.

Neimeyer, R. A., & Neimeyer, G. J. (Eds.). (1987). *Personal construct therapy casebook*. New York: Springer.

Neimeyer, R. A., & Raskin, J. D. (2000). *Constructions of disorder: Meaning-making frameworks for psychotherapy*. Washington, DC: American Psychological Association.

Nepo, M. (2000). *The book of awakening*. Berkeley, CA: Canari Press.

Niedenthal, P. M., & Kitayama, S. (Eds.). (1994). *The heart's eye: Emotional influences in perception and attention*. New York: Academic Press.

Nietzsche, F. (1996). *Human, all too human* (R. J. Hollingdale, Trans.). London: Cambridge University Press. (Original published in 1878)

Nisbett, R. E., & Wilson, T. D. (1977). Telling more than we can know: Verbal reports on mental processes. *Psychological Review, 84*, 231–259.

Norcross, J. C., & Goldfried, M. R. (Eds.). (1992). *Handbook of psychotherapy integration*. New York: Basic Books.

Norcross, J. C., Santrock, J. W., Campbell, L. F., Smith, T. S., Sommer, R., & Zuckerman, E. L. (2003). *Authoritative guide to self-help resources in mental health* (rev. ed.). New York: Guilford Press.

Nørrestranders, T. (1998). *The user illusion: Cutting consciousness down to size*. New York: Penguin.

Norris, K. (1998). *Amazing grace: A vocabulary of faith*. New York: Riverhead Books.

Nuland, S. B. (1997). *The wisdom of the body*. New York: Knopf.

Núñez, R., & Freeman, W. J. (Eds.). (1999). *Reclaiming cognition: The primacy of action, intention and emotion*. Tucson, AZ: Imprint Academic.

Oberst, U. E. (1998). Alfred Adler's individual psychology in the context of constructivism. *Constructivism in the Human Sciences, 3*, 153–176.

O'Donahue, J. (1997). *Anam cara: A book of Celtic wisdom*. New York: HarperCollins.

O'Donahue, J. (1998). *Eternal echoes: Exploring our hunger to belong*. London: Bantam.

Oldfather, P., West, J., White, J., & Wilmarth, J. (1999). *Learning through children's eyes: Social constructivism and the desire to learn*. Washington, DC: American Psychological Association.

Omer, H., & Alon, N. (1997). *Constructing therapeutic narratives*. Northvale, NJ: Jason Aronson.

Orlinsky, D., Ambühl, H., Rønnestad, M. H., Davis, J., Gerin, P., Davis, M., et al. (1999). Development of psychotherapists: Concepts, questions, and methods of a collaborative international study. *Psychotherapy Research, 9*, 127–153.

Orlinsky, D. E., Grawe, K., & Parks, B. (1994). Process and outcome in psychotherapy—noch einmal. In A. E. Bergin & S. L. Garfield (Eds.), *Handbook of psychotherapy and behavior change* (4th ed., pp. 270–376). New York: Wiley.

Orlinsky, D. E., & Howard, K. I. (1975). *Varieties of psychotherapeutic experience*. New York: Teachers College Press.

Orlinsky, D., Rønnestad, M. H., Ambühl, H., Willutzki, U., Botermans, J.-F., Cierpka, M., et al. (1999). Psychotherapists' assessments of their development at different career levels. *Psychotherapy, 36*, 203–215.

Oyama, S. (2000). *Evolution's eye: A systems view of the biology-culture divide*. Durham, NC: Duke University Press.

Padesky, C. A., & Greenberger, D. (1995). Clinician's guide to *Mind over Mood*. New York: Guilford Press.

Pagels, H. (1988). *The dreams of reason: The computer and the rise of the sciences of complexity*. New York: Simon & Schuster.

Palmer, P. J. (1998). *The courage to teach: Exploring the inner landscape of a teacher's life*. San Francisco: Jossey-Bass.

Palmer, R. E. (1969). *Hermeneutics: Interpretation theory in Schleiermacher, Dilthey, Heidegger, and Gadamer.* Evanston, IL: Northwestern University Press.

Palombo, S. (1999). *The emergent ego: Complexity and co-evolution in the psychoanalytic process*. Madison, CT: International Universities Press.

Panksepp, J. (1998). *Affective neuroscience: The foundations of human and animal emotions*. New York: Oxford University Press.

Pargament, K. I. (1997). *The psychology of religion and coping: Theory, research, practice*. New York: Guilford Press.

Partridge, E. (1983). *Origins: A short etymological dictionary of modern English*. New York: Greenwich House.

Pattee, H. H. (1973). *Hierarchy theory: The challenge of complex systems*. New York: George Braziller.

Peele, S. (1985). *The nature of addiction*. Lexington, MA: Heath.

Peele, S. (1999). *Diseasing of America*. San Francisco: Jossey-Bass.

Pennebaker, J. W. (1990). *Opening up: The healing power of expressing emotions*. New York: Guilford Press.

Pennebaker, J. W. (Ed.). (1995). *Emotion, disclosure, and health*. Washington, DC: American Psychological Association.

Pennebaker, J. W. (1997). Writing about emotional experiences as a therapeutic process. *Psychological Science*, *8*, 162–166.

Pera, M. (1994). *The discourses of science*. Chicago: University of Chicago Press.

Person, E. S. (1995). *By force of fantasy: How we make our lives*. New York: Basic Books.

Pervin, L. A. (1994). Personality stability, personality change, and the question of process. In T. F. Heatherton & J. L. Weinberger (Eds.), *Can personality change?* (pp. 315–330). Washington, DC: American Psychological Association.

Pessoa, F. (1974). *Selected poems* (2nd ed.). New York: Penguin.

Pessoa, F. (1991). *The book of disquiet*. New York: Pantheon.

Petitot, J., Varela, F. J., Pachoud, B., & Roy, J.-M. (Eds.). (1999). *Naturalizing phenomenology: Issues in contemporary phenomenology and cognitive science*. Stanford, CA: Stanford University Press.

Philippot, P., & Rimé, B. (1998). Social and cognitive processing in emotion: A heuristic for psychopathology. In W. F. Flack & J. D. Laird (Eds.), *Emotions in psychopathology* (pp. 114–129). Oxford, UK: Oxford University Press.

Piaget, J. (1926). *The language and thought of the child*. New York: Harcourt Brace.

Piaget, J. (1970). *Psychology and epistemology: Towards a theory of knowledge*. New York: Viking.

Piaget, J. (1981). *Intelligence and affectivity: Their relationship during child development*. Palo Alto, CA: Annual Reviews.

Piaget, J. (1987a). *Possibility and necessity: Vol. 1. The role of possibility in cognitive development* (H. Feider, Trans.). Minneapolis: University of Minnesota Press.

Piaget, J. (1987b). *Possibility and necessity: Vol. 2. The role of necessity in cognitive development* (H. Feider, Trans.). Minneapolis: University of Minnesota Press.

Piaget, J., & Inhelder, B. (1963). *The psychology of the child.* New York: Basic Books.

Polanyi, M. (1958). *Personal knowledge: Towards a post-critical philosophy.* Chicago: University of Chicago Press.

Polanyi, M. (1966). *The tacit dimension.* New York: Doubleday.

Polkinghorne, D. E. (1988). *Narrative knowing and the human sciences.* New York: SUNY Press.

Pompa, L. (1975). *Vico: A study of the "New Science."* Cambridge, UK: Cambridge University Press.

Pope, K. S., & Singer, J. L. (1978). *The stream of consciousness: Scientific investigations into the flow of human experience.* New York: Plenum Press.

Prigogine, I. (1980). *From being to becoming: Time and complexity in the physical sciences.* San Francisco: Freeman.

Prigogine, I., & Stengers, I. (1984). *Order out of chaos: Man's new dialogue with nature.* New York: Bantam.

Prochaska, J. O., & Prochaska, J. M. (1999). Why don't continents move? Why don't people change? *Journal of Psychotherapy Integration, 9,* 83–102.

Quintana, S. M. (1993). Toward an expanded and updated conceptualization of termination: Implications for short-term, individual psychotherapy. *Professional Psychology: Research and Practice, 24,* 426–432.

Radeke, J. T., & Mahoney, M. J. (2000). Comparing the personal lives of psychotherapists and research psychologists. *Professional Psychology: Research and Practice, 31,* 82–84.

Rainer, T. (1978). *The new diary.* New York: Tarcher.

Ram Dass. (1970). *The only dance there is.* Garden City, NY: Anchor.

Ram Dass. (1971). *Be here now.* San Cristobal, NM: Lama Foundation.

Ram Dass & Gorman, P. (1985). *How can I help?: Stories and reflections on service.* New York: Knopf.

Raskin, J. D. (2001). On relativism in constructivist psychology. *Journal of Constructivist Psychology, 14,* 285–313.

Raskin, J. D., & Bridges, S. K. (2002). *Studies in meaning: Exploring constructivist psychology.* Albany, NY: Pace University Press.

Rea, B. D. (2001). Finding our balance: The investigation and clinical application of intuition. *Psychotherapy, 38,* 97–106.

Reber, A. S. (1993). *Implicit learning and tacit knowledge: An essay on the cognitive unconscious.* Oxford, UK: Oxford University Press.

Reid, T. (1999). A cultural perspective on resistance. *Journal of Psychotherapy Integration, 9,* 57–81.

Rennie, D. L. (1994). Storytelling in psychotherapy: The client's subjective experience. *Psychotherapy, 31,* 234–243.

Rice, L. N., & Greenberg, L. S. (1984). *Patterns of change.* New York: Guilford Press.

Rimé, B. (1995). Mental rumination, social sharing, and the recovery from emotional exposure. In J. W. Pennebaker (Ed.), *Emotion, disclosure, and health* (pp. 271–291). Washington, DC: American Psychological Association.

Robertson, R., & Combs, A. (Eds.). (1995). *Chaos theory and psychology in the life sciences*. Mahwah, NJ: Erlbaum.

Rogers, C. R. (1957). The necessary and sufficient conditions of therapeutic personality change. *Journal of Consulting Psychology, 21*, 95–103.

Rogers, C. R. (1961). *On becoming a person*. Boston: Houghton Mifflin.

Rogers, C. R. (1980). *A way of being*. Boston: Houghton Mifflin.

Ronen, T. (1997). *Cognitive developmental therapy with children*. Chichester, UK: Wiley.

Ronen, T. (1999). *Cognitive constructive therapy with children*. New York: Jason Aronson.

Ronen, T. (2003). *Cognitive-constructivist psychotherapy with children and adolescents*. New York: Kluwer Academic/Plenum.

Roof, W. C. (1993). *A generation of seekers: The spiritual journeys of the baby boom generation*. San Francisco: Harper.

Rosen, H., & Kuehlwein, K. T. (Eds.). (1996). *Constructing realities: Meaning-making perspectives for psychotherapists*. San Francisco: Jossey-Bass.

Rosenbaum, M. (Ed.). (1990). *Learned resourcefulness: On coping skills, self-control, and adaptive behavior*. New York: Springer.

Rosenbaum, M. (1998). Opening versus closing strategies in controlling one's responses to experience. In M. Kofta, G. Weary, & G. Sedek (Eds.), *Personal control in action: Cognitive and motivational mechanisms*. New York: Plenum Press.

Rosenberg, M. (1979). *Conceiving the self*. New York: Basic Books.

Roth, G. (1997). *Sweat your prayers: Movement as spiritual practice*. New York: Penguin.

Russell, B. (1945). *A history of western philosophy*. New York: Simon & Schuster.

Russell, P. (1992). *Waking up in time: Finding inner peace in times of accelerating change*. Novato, CA: Origin Press.

Rychlak, J. F. (2003). *The human image in postmodern America*. Washington, DC: American Psychological Association.

Safran, J. D., & Muran, J. C. (2000). *Negotiating the therapeutic alliance: A relational treatment guide*. New York: Guilford Press.

Salovey, P., Rothman, A. J., Detweiler, J. B., & Steward, W. T. (2000). Emotional states and physical health. *American Psychologist, 55*, 110–121.

Salkovskis, P. M. (Ed.). (1996). *Frontiers of cognitive therapy*. New York: Guilford Press.

Sampson, E. E. (1993). Identity politics: Challenges to psychology's understanding. *American Psychologist, 48*, 1219–1230.

Sarbin, T. R., & Keen, E. (1998). Sanity and madness: Conventional and unconventional narratives of emotional life. In W. F. Flack & J. D. Laird (Eds.), *Emotions in psychopathology* (pp. 130–142). Oxford, UK: Oxford University Press.

Sass, L. A. (1992). *Madness and modernism: Insanity in the light of modern art, literature, and thought*. New York: Basic Books.

Scarr, S. (1985). Constructing psychology: Making facts and fables for our times. *American Psychologist, 40*, 499–512.

Schafer, R. (1992). *Retelling a life*. New York: Basic Books.

Schaie, K. W., & Lawton, M. P. (Eds.). (1997). *Annual review of gerontology and geriatrics: Focus on emotion and adult development*. New York: Springer.

Schiepek, G., Eckert, H., & Weihrauch, S. (2003). Critical fluctations and clinical change: Data-based assessment in dynamic systems. *Constructivism in the Human Sciences, 8*, 57–82.

Schopenhauer, A. (1932). *The wisdom of life and other essays*. New York: Walter J. Black.

Schore, A. N. (1994). *Affect regulation and the origin of the self*. Hillsdale, NJ: Erlbaum.

Schwartz, B. (2000). Self-determination: The tyranny of freedom. *American Psychologist, 55*, 79–88.

Schwartz, J. M., & Begley, S. (2002). *The mind and the brain: Neuroplasticity and the power of mental force*. New York: HarperCollins.

Schwartz, R. S. (1993). Managing closeness in psychotherapy. *Psychotherapy, 30*, 601–607.

Schwartz, T. (1995). *What really matters: Searching for wisdom in America*. New York: Bantam.

Scott, G. A. (Ed.). (2002). *Does Socrates have a method?: Rethinking the* Elenchus *in Plato's dialogues and beyond*. University Park, PA: Pennsylvania State University Press.

Segal, L. (1986). *The dream of reality: Heinz von Foerster's constructivism*. New York: Norton.

Segal, Z. V., Williams, J. M. G., & Teasdale, J. D. (2002). *Mindfulness-based cognitive therapy for depression*. New York: Guilford Press.

Segerstråle, U. (Ed.). (2000). *Beyond the science wars: The missing discourse about science and society*. Albany, NY: SUNY Press.

Selby, C. B., & Mahoney, M. J. (2002). Psychological and physiological correlates of self-complexity and authenticity. *Constructivism in the Human Sciences, 7*, 39–52.

Seligman, M. E. P., & Csikszentmihalyi, M. (2000). Positive psychology: An introduction. *American Psychologist, 55*, 5–14.

Sewell, K. W. (1995). Personal construct therapy and the relation between cognition and affect. In M. J. Mahoney (Ed.), *Cognitive and constructive psychotherapies: Theory, research, and practice* (pp. 121–138). New York: Springer.

Sewell, K. W. (1997). Posttraumatic stress: Towards a constructivist model of psychotherapy. In R. A. Neimeyer & G. J. Neimeyer (Eds.), *Advances in personal construct psychology* (Vol. IV, pp. 207–235). Greenwich, CT: JAI Press.

Sewell, K. W. (1998). Embodiment, sexuality, and self-understanding: Constructivist elaborations of theatrical acting. *Constructivism in the Human Sciences, 3*, 56–69.

Sexton, A. T. L., & Griffin, B. L. (Eds.). (1997). *Constructivist thinking in counseling practice, research, and training*. New York: Teachers College Press.

Shafranske, E. P. (Ed.). (1996). *Religion and the clinical practice of psychology*. Washington, DC: American Psychological Association.

Shepherd, L. J. (1993). *Lifting the veil: The feminine face of science*. Boston: Shambhala.

Sherrington, C. S. (1906). *The integrative action of the nervous system* (Silliman Lectures). New Haven, CT: Yale University Press.

Shevrin, H., Bond, J. A., Brakel, L. A. W., Hertel, R. K., & Williams, W. J. (1996).

Conscious and unconscious processes: Psychodynamic, cognitive, and neurophysiological convergences. New York: Guilford Press.

Siegler, R. S. (1994). Cognitive variability: A key to understanding cognitive development. *Current Directions in Psychological Science*, *3*, 1–5.

Simon, L. (1998). *Genuine reality: A life of William James*. New York: Harcourt Brace.

Simpson, J. A., & Rholes, W. S. (Eds.). (1997). *Attachment theory and close relationships*. New York: Guilford Press.

Skovholt, T. M., & Rønnestad, M. H. (1992). *The evolving professional self: Stages and themes in therapist and counselor development*. New York: Wiley.

Sluzki, C. E. (1992). Transformations: A blueprint for narrative changes in therapy. *Family Process*, *31*, 217–230.

Sluzki, C. E. (1998). Strange attractors and the transformation of narratives in family therapy. In M. F. Hoyt (Ed.), *The handbook of constructive therapies* (pp. 159–179). San Francisco: Jossey-Bass.

Smith, B. H. (1988). *Contingencies of value*. Cambridge, MA: Harvard University Press.

Smith, C., & Nylund, D. (1997). *Narrative therapies with children and adolescents*. New York: Guilford Press.

Smith, E. W. L., Clance, P. R., & Imes, S. (Eds.). (1998). *Touch in psychotherapy: Theory, research, and practice*. New York: Guilford Press.

Smith, H. (1958). *The religions of man*. New York: Harper & Row.

Smith, H. (1998). Foreword. In P. Cousineau, *The art of pilgrimage: The seeker's guide to making travel sacred* (pp. xi–xiv). York Beach, ME: Conari Press.

Smith, H. (2000). *Cleansing the doors of perception*. New York: Tarcher.

Smith, S. G. (1988). *The concept of the spiritual: An essay in first philosophy*. Philadelphia: University of Pennsylvania Press.

Snyder, C. R. (Ed.). (1999). *Coping: The psychology of what works*. Oxford, UK: Oxford University Press.

Snyder, C. R., & Ingram, R. E. (Eds.). (2000). *Handbook of psychological change*. New York: Wiley.

Snyder, C. R., & Lopez, S. J. (Eds.). (2001). *Handbook of positive psychology*. Oxford, UK: Oxford University Press.

Snyder, C. R., McDermott, D., Cook, W., & Rapoff, M. A. (1997). *Hope for the journey: Helping children through good times and bad*. Boulder, CO: Westview Press.

Sokal, A., & Bricmont, J.(1998). *Postmodern intellectuals' abuse of science*. New York: Picador Books.

Soldz, S., & McCullough, L. (1999). *Reconciling empirical knowledge and clinical experience: The art and science of psychotherapy*. Washington, DC: American Psychological Association.

Solomon, J., & George, C. (Eds.). (1999). *Attachment disorganization*. New York: Guilford Press.

Sorabji, R. (2000). *Emotion and peace of mind: From Stoic agitation to Christian temptation*. Oxford, UK: Oxford University Press.

Spence, D. P. (1982). *Narrative truth and historical truth: Meaning and interpretation in psychoanalysis*. New York: Norton.

Spence, D. P. (1987). *The Freudian metaphor: Toward paradigm change in psychoanalysis*. New York: Norton.

Sperry, R. W. (1988). Psychology's mentalist paradigm and the religion/science tension. *American Psychologist, 43*, 607–613.

Sroufe, L. A. (1979). The coherence of individual development: Early care, attachment, and subsequent developmental issues. *American Psychologist, 34*, 834–841.

Steindl-Rast, B. D. (1983). *A listening heart: The spirituality of sacred sensuousness*. New York: Crossroad.

Steindl-Rast, B. D. (1984). *Gratefulness, the heart of prayer.* Ramsey, NJ: Paulist Press.

Stern, D. B. (1983). Unformulated experience. *Contemporary Psychoanalysis, 19*, 71–99.

Stern, D. N. (1985). *The interpersonal world of the infant.* New York: Basic Books.

Stewart, A. E., & Berry, J. R. (1991). Origins of George Kelly's constructivism in the work of Korzybski and Moreno. *International Journal of Personal Construct Psychology, 4*, 121–136.

Stolorow, R. D., & Atwood, G. E. (1992). *Contexts of being: The intersubjective foundations of psychological life*. Hillsdale, NJ: Analytic Press.

Stolorow, R. D., & Atwood, G. E., & Orange, D. M. (2002). *Worlds of experience: Interweaving philosophical and clinical dimensions in psychoanalysis*. New York: Basic Books.

Stone, H., & Winkelman, S. (1985). *Embracing our selves: Voice dialogue manual.* Marina del Rey, CA: DeVorss.

Strauch, I., & Meier, B. (1996). *In search of dreams: Results of experimental dream research*. Albany, NY: SUNY Press.

Taubes, G. (1999). String theorists find a rosetta stone. *Science, 285*, 512–517.

Taylor, E. (1996). *William James on consciousness beyond the margin*. Princeton, NJ: Princeton University Press.

Taylor, E. (1999). *Shadow culture: Psychology and spirituality in America*. Washington, DC: Counterpoint.

Taylor, J. (1992). *Where people fly and water runs uphill.* New York: Warner Books.

Taylor, K. (1995). *The ethics of caring: Honoring the web of life in our professional healing relationships*. Boston: Shambhala.

Tellegen, A., Watson, D., & Clark, L. A. (1999). On the dimensional and hierarchical structure of affect. *Psychological Science, 10*, 297–303.

Thakker, J., Ward, T., & Strongman, K. T. (1999). Mental disorder and cross-cultural psychology: A constructivist perspective. *Clinical Psychology Review, 19*, 843–874.

Thelen, E. (1992). Development as a dynamic system. *Current Directions in Psychological Science, 1*, 189–193.

Thelen, E., & Smith, L. B. (1994). *A dynamic systems approach to the development of cognition and action*. Cambridge, MA: MIT Press.

Thompson, E. (Ed.). (2001). *Between ourselves: Second-person issues in the study of consciousness*. Charlottesville, VA: Imprint Academic.

Thompson, M. G., Thompson, L., & Gallagher-Thompson, D. (1995). Linear and non-linear changes in mood between psychotherapy sessions: Implications for treatment outcome and relapse risk. *Psychotherapy Research*, *5*, 327–336.

Thompson, W. I. (1996). *Coming into being*. New York: St. Martin's Press.

Tillich, P. (1952). *The courage to be*. New Haven, CT: Yale University Press.

Tobias, S. (1997). *Faces of feminism*. New York: HarperCollins.

Ueland, B. (1987). *If you want to write: A book about art, independence and spirit* (2nd ed.). St. Paul, MN: Graywolf Press.

U. S. Olympic Committee Strength and Conditioning Staff. (1999). Is Olympic-style weightlifting important for sport performance? *Olympic Coach*, *9*(4), 14–15.

Vaihinger, H. (1924). *The philosophy of "as if."* Berlin: Reuther & Reichard. (Original published in 1911)

Van Geert, P. (1998). A dynamic systems model of basic developmental mechanisms: Piaget, Vygotsky and beyond. *Psychological Review*, *105*, 634–677.

Van Geert, P. (2000). The dynamics of general developmental mechanisms: From Piaget to Vygotsky to dynamic systems models. *Current Directions in Psychological Science*, *9*, 64–68.

Van Maanen, M. (1990). *Researching lived experience*. New York: SUNY Press.

Van Raalte, J. L., & Brewer, B. W. (Eds.). (1996). *Exploring sport and exercise psychology*. Washington, DC: American Psychological Association.

Van Zuuren, F. J., Schoutrop, M. J. A., Lange, A., Louis, C. M., & Slegers, J. E. M. (1999). Effective and ineffective ways of writing about traumatic experiences: A qualitative study. *Psychotherapy Research*, *9*, 363–380.

Varela, F. J. (1979). *Principles of biological autonomy*. New York: Elsevier/North Holland.

Varela, F. J. (1986). *The science and technology of cognition: Emergent directions*. Florence: Hopeful Monster.

Varela, F. J. (1999). *Ethical know-how: Action, wisdom, and cognition*. Stanford, CA: Stanford University Press.

Varela, F. J., & Shear, J. (Eds.). (1999). *The view from within: First-person approaches to the study of consciousness*. Bowling Green, OH: Imprint Academic.

Varela, F. J., & Singer, W. (1987). Neuronal dynamics in the visual corticothalamic pathway revealed through binocular rivalry. *Experimental Brain Research*, *66*, 10–20.

Varela, F. J., Thompson, E., & Rosch, E. (1991). *The embodied mind: Cognitive science and human experience*. Cambridge, MA: MIT Press.

Vaughan, F. (1979). *Awakening intuition*. New York: Anchor.

Vaughan, F. (1986). *The inward arc*. Boston: Shambhala.

Vaughan, F. (1995). *Shadows of the sacred: Seeing through spiritual illusions*. Wheaton, IL: Quest Books.

Velmans, M. (Ed.). (2000). *Investigating phenomenal consciousness: New methodologies and maps*. Amsterdam: Benjamins.

Verene, D. P. (1971). *Vico's science of imagination*. Ithaca, NY: Cornell University Press.

Vico, G. (1988). *On the most ancient wisdom of the Italians* (L. M. Palmer, Trans.). Ithaca, NY: Cornell University Press. (Original published in 1710)

Vico, G. (1948). *The new science* (T. G. Bergin & M. H. Fisch, Trans.). Ithaca, NY: Cornell University Press. (Original published in 1725)

Volk, T. (1995). *Metapatterns: Across space, time, and mind.* New York: Columbia University Press.

von Foerster, H. (1984). On constructing a reality. In P. Watzlawick (Ed.), *The invented reality* (pp. 41–61). New York: Norton.

von Glasersfeld, E. (1984). An introduction to radical constructivism. In P. Watzlawick (Ed.), *The invented reality* (pp. 18–40). New York: Norton.

Wachtel, P. L. (Ed.). (1982). *Resistance: Psychodynamic and behavioral approaches.* New York: Plenum Press.

Wachtel, P. L. (1987). *Action and insight.* New York: Guilford Press.

Wachtel, P. L. (1999). Resistance as a problem for practice and theory. *Journal of Psychotherapy Integration, 9,* 103–117.

Wade, J. (1996). *Changes of mind: A holonomic theory of the evolution of consciousness.* Albany, NY: SUNY Press.

Walker, B. E., Costigan, J., Viney, L. L., & Warren, W. G. (Eds.). (1996). *Personal construct theory: A psychology for the future.* Melbourne: APS Imprint Books.

Walsh, F. (1999). *Spiritual resources in family therapy.* New York: Guilford Press.

Walsh, M. W., Cushman, S., & Mahoney, M. J. (2003). *Dancing and well-being.* Unpublished manuscript.

Walsh, R. N. (1976). Reflections on psychotherapy. *Journal of Transpersonal Psychology, 8,* 100–111.

Walsh, R. N. (1990). *The spirit of shamanism.* Los Angeles: Tarcher.

Walsh, R. N. (1999). *Essential spirituality.* New York: Wiley.

Walsh, R. N., & Vaughan, F. (Eds.). (1980). *Beyond ego: Transpersonal dimensions in psychology.* Los Angeles: Tarcher.

Walsh, R. N., & Vaughan, F. (Eds.). (1993). *Paths beyond ego: The transpersonal vision.* Los Angeles: Tarcher Perigree.

Washington, P. (1993). *Madame Blavatsky's baboon.* New York: Schocken.

Watkins, M. (1986). *Invisible guests: The development of imaginal dialogues.* New York: Analytic Press.

Watts, A. (1963). *The two hands of God: The myths of polarity.* New York: Macmillan.

Watts, A. (1966). *The book: On the taboo against knowing who you are.* New York: Random House.

Watzlawick, P. (Ed.). (1984). *The invented reality: Contributions to constructivism.* New York: Norton.

Watzlawick, P., & Hoyt, M. F. (1998). Constructing therapeutic realities: A conversation with Paul Watzlawick. In M. F. Hoyt (Ed.), *The handbook of constructive therapies* (pp. 183–197). San Francisco: Jossey-Bass.

Weidong, W., Sasaki, Y., & Haruki, Y. (Eds.). (2000). *Bodywork and psychotherapy in the East.* Delft, the Netherlands: Eburon.

Weil, A. (1972). *The natural mind.* Boston: Houghton Mifflin.

Weil, A. (1983). *Health and healing.* Boston: Houghton Mifflin.

Weimer, W. B. (1977). A conceptual framework for cognitive psychology: Motor theories of mind. In R. Shaw & J. Bransford (Eds.), *Perceiving, acting, and knowing* (pp. 267–311). Hillsdale, NJ: Erlbaum.

Weimer, W. B. (1979). *Notes on the methodology of scientific research*. Hillsdale, NJ: Erlbaum.

Weimer, W. B. (1980). Psychotherapy and philosophy of science: Examples of a two-way street in search of traffic. In M. J. Mahoney (Ed.), *Psychotherapy process: Current issues and future directions* (pp. 369–393). New York: Plenum Press.

Weimer, W. B. (1982). Hayek's approach to the problems of complex phenomena: An introduction to the theoretical psychology of *The Sensory Order.* In W. B. Weimer & D. S. Palermo (Eds.), *Cognition and the symbolic processes* (Vol. 2, pp. 267–311). Hillsdale, NJ: Erlbaum.

Weimer, W. B. (1987). Spontaneously ordered complex phenomena and the unity of the moral sciences. In G. Radnitzky (Ed.), *Centripetal forces in the universe* (pp. 257–296). New York: Paragon House.

Wendell, S. (1996). *The rejected body: Feminist philosophical reflections on disability.* New York: Routledge.

Werner, H. (1948). *The comparative psychology of mental development*. New York: Science Editions.

West, B. J., & Schlesinger, M. (1990). The noise in natural phenomena. *American Scientist*, *78*, 40–45.

Wheeler, G. (2000*). Beyond individualism: Toward a new understanding of self, relationship, and experience*. Hillsdale, NJ: Analytic Press.

White, M., & Epston, D. (1990). *Narrative means to therapeutic ends*. New York: Norton.

Wiener, D. J. (Ed.). (1999). *Beyond talk therapy: Using movement and expressive techniques in clinical practice*. Washington, DC: American Psychological Association.

Wilber, K. (1998). *The marriage of sense and soul: Integrating science and religion*. New York: Random House.

Wilber, K. (1999). *Collected works* (4 vols.). Boston: Shambhala.

Williams, A. M., Diehl, N. H., & Mahoney, M. J. (2002). Mirror-time: Empirical findings and implications for a constructivist psychotherapeutic technique. *Journal of Constructivist Psychology, 15*, 21–39.

Williamson, C. (1975). *The changer and the changed* [CD]. Oakland, CA: Olivia Records.

Woodcock, A., & Davis, M. (1978). *Catastrophe theory.* New York: Avon.

Woodruff, P. (2001). *Reverence: Renewing a forgotten virtue*. London: Oxford University Press.

Wright, B. A. (1991). Labeling: The need for greater person–environment individuation. In C. R. Snyder & D. R. Forsyth (Eds.), *Handbook of social and clinical psychology.* New York: Pergamon.

Wundt, W. (1912). *An introduction to psychology.* New York: Macmillan.

Zimmerman, J., & McCandless, J. (1998). *Flesh and spirit: The mystery of intimate relationship*. Ojai, CA: Bramble Books.

INDEX

Abreaction, 148
Absolute relativism, 218
Activity
  assessment, 43
  behaviorism principle, 76
  collaboration role in, 19–21
  constructivism theme, 5, 6, 32
  in problem solving, 76, 77
Adler, Alfred, 4, 7, 85, 215
Aerobic exercise
  individualized program, 119
  and pain, 119
"Affirmation," 21–23
  case illustration, 22, 23
  and hope, 23
  reinforcement distinction, 21
Agency
  and affirmation, 22, 23
  in change process, 19–21
  therapeutic collaboration role in, 19–21
Aggressive challenge, and change, 27
Alexander technique, 116
Altered states of consciousness, 143
"Alternate control and surrender breathing," 61, 243
Anaerobic exercise
  individualized program, 119
  and pain, 119
Anxiety, and exercise, 119
Arrival myth, 165, 166
"As if" philosophy, 4, 135, 215
"As if" role playing, 131–135
Asklepios, 197
Assessment, 38–56
  constructivist themes in, 42–44
  at intake interview, 52, 53
  intervention link, 53, 54
  pathology focus of, 41
  and personal meanings, 40
  of problems and patterns, 44–48, 53
  of processes, 44–48
  quantitative method limitations, 39
Attachment relationships, and emotionality, 181
Attunement, 52–56

Balance exercises (*see* Body balance exercises)
Balance metaphor
  in constructive psychotherapy, 29
  and range of movement exercises, 116
Bandura, Albert, 4, 5, 7, 80
Bartlett, Frederic, 216
Bateson, Gregory, 4, 6, 177
Behavioral techniques, 73–87
  activity importance in, 76, 77
  consequences importance, 78, 79
  consistency in application of, 80, 81
  in problem solving, 76–81
  "successive approximation" in, 79, 80
Bibliotherapy, 91, 105
Bodhisattva phenomenon, 210*n*12
Body balance exercises, 62–66, 244–246
  rationale, 62
  techniques, 62–66, 244–246
Body work (*see* Embodiment exercises)

Boundary issues, and therapeutic touch, 124, 125
Breathing exercises, 59–62, 105, 242, 243
  and meditation, 111, 112
  and panic episodes, 60
  rationale, 59, 60
  techniques, 60–62, 242, 243
Bruner, Jerome, 4, 6, 7, 107
Buddhism, 3, 108, 212, 213
Bugental, James, 4, 6, 144

Car screaming exercise, 126
Caring, 14–18
  as heart of psychotherapy, 14–18
  progressive challenge compatibility, 27, 28
  role of "presence" in, 15, 16
Catharsis, 148
Caulkins, Mary Whiton, 4, 7, 215
Centering, 57–72
  body balance exercises, 62–66, 116
  breathing exercises, 58–62
  entry meditation function, 68, 69
  individual differences in response to, 59
  main purpose of, 69
  mindfulness meditation function, 163
  and process change, 58
  range of movement exercises in, 116, 117
  and relaxation, 66–69
  and ritual, 58, 59
  as streaming antidote, 143
Challenges, in change process, 26–28
  aggressive versus progressive 27
  caring compatibility, 27, 28
Change process, 1–3, 170–192, 257–259
  case illustrations, 170–172, 175, 176, 183–187
  challenge in, 26–28
  collaboration and action in, 19–21
  complexity of, 9, 10
  constructive psychotherapy principles, 36, 37
  constructivism role in, 2, 3
  and core ordering processes, 50, 51
  courage in, 181, 182
  and emotionality, 180, 181
  "opening and closing" metaphor, 24–26
  and personal revolutions, 177–180, 190*n*8
  relational context of, 2
  resistance to, 173–177
  synopsis, 257–259
  therapist's "comforting and challenging" in, 26–28
  therapist's creativity in, 181–187
  types of, 177
Chaos theory
  and constructivism, 10
  and dreaming, 137
Character sketch role play, 132
Classical conditioning, 77
Classification, 40, 41
Client-therapist relationship (*see* Therapeutic relationship)
Cognitive restructuring, 81–85
  and meditation, 83, 162
  perspective-taking function, 162
  situational reaction reinterpretation, 82, 83
  stages in teaching of, 82
Collaboration, 19–21
  in active change process, 19–21
  definition, 19, 20
  essential dimensions, 20
Collective voice, power of, 127
"Comforting and challenges" approach, 26–28
"Coming home" meditation, 69, 70
Compassion, 14–18
  as heart of psychotherapy, 14–18
  role of "presence" in, 15, 16
Complexity theory
  and constructivism, 10
  and dreaming, 137
Confidentiality
  as sacred responsibility, 210*n*14
  in therapists' personal therapy, 199, 200, 210*n*14
Consciousness, and constructivism, 221–223
Consent form, 53, 226–229
Consequences
  and behavioral techniques, 78, 79
  time course factor, 79, 80
Consistency
  behavioral reinforcement importance, 80, 81
  in habit development, 71, 72
Constructivism, 1–12, 211–225
  and assessment, 42–44
  basic themes, 4–9
  in change processes, 1–3, 9–12
  and consciousness, 221–223
  essence of, 3–9
  history and current relevance, 211–225
  and the "science wars," 217–221

Coordination, in therapeutic collaboration, 20, 21
Coordination of movement, 117
Core ordering processes, 48–52
in change process, 50, 51
definition, 49
perceptual constancy in, 48
and resistance to change, 176, 177
spiritual skills link, 161
themes in, 49, 50
therapeutic risks, 47, 48, 131
Courage, in change process, 181, 182
Creativity, of therapist, 182–187
Crying, 127
Cultural studies, 218, 219

Daily notes, in problem solving evaluation, 75, 76
Damapada, 213
Dance
as metaphor, 122
and well-being, 121, 122
Daydreaming, 135, 136
Delayed-onset muscle soreness, 119
Depersonalization, 178
Depression
individualized exercise program, 119
perspective-taking effect on, 162
Derealization, 178
Developmental processes
assessment, 44
complexity of, 9, 10
constructivism theme, 8, 9, 33, 34
Diagnostic and Statistical Manual of Mental Disorders, 40, 41
Diagnostics, 38–42
pathology emphasis of, 41
quantitative method limitations, 39, 40
Dialectics
constructivism theme, 33, 34
in "opening and closing" process, 26
in science, 220, 221
Dialogue, in therapeutic collaboration, 20, 21
Diary writing, 90
Disorder, and constructivism, 10, 11
Drama, 130–135
Dramatic change (*see* Personal revolutions)
Dream-image dictionaries, 139
Dreams, 135–140
alternate identity in, 138
biologic evolutionary processes in, 137
and boundary fuzziness, 137, 138
fantasy distinction, 136
function of, 136, 137
interpretation of, 139, 140
journaling of, 140
and process-level change, 51
three-stage model of work in, 139, 140
Dynamic systems theory
and constructivism, 10
and dreaming, 137

Embodiment exercises, 113–128
range of movement methods, 116, 117
rationale, 113–115
resistance techniques, 117–120
rhythm techniques, 120–122
touch dimension, 122–125
voice dimension, 125–128
Emotion-focused psychotherapy, 181
Emotions
and change, 180, 181
constructive view of, 6
in "opening and closing" process, 25, 26
relaxation and centering effect on, 68
Enactment sketch role play, 132
"Entry meditation," 68, 69
Epistemotion, 51
Ethics
and constructivism, 217, 218
therapeutic touch, 124, 125
Evolutionary factors
and dreams, 137
in transformational change, 179, 180
"Exaptations," 139,
Exercise (*see* Resistance exercises)
Exercise machines, 118
Externalization
in narrative reconstruction, 102
and problem identification, 74, 75

Fantasy, 135–140
Fees, 228
Feldenkrais method, 116
Feminist theory, 218, 219
First interview, 52, 53
First-order change, 177
"Fixed-role therapy, 132–134
Frankl, Viktor, 4, 6, 161
Free association
measures of, 141
versus streaming, 142
Free weight training, 118
Functional fictions principle, 215

Gergen, Kenneth, 4, 7
"Gestalting" a dream, 138
"Grand unifying theory," 222
Guidano, Vittorio, 4, 6, 7, 84, 101, 109, 177

Habits
centering function, 71, 72
and change, 173
Haken, Hermann, 4, 6
Harding, Sandra, 4, 7
Hayek, Friedrich, 4, 6, 49, 50, 86, 216
Heisenberg principle, 75, 141
Hellerwork, 116
Heraclitus, 4, 100, 108, 212, 213
Holism, 114
"Home" concept, 69, 70
Homework assignments
and affirmation, 23
change process importance, 19
Hope, 21–23
and affirmation, 21–23
therapist as guardian of, 196, 197
"Hope from hell" paradox, 196, 197
"Hot" therapeutic moments, 20, 21
Hyperventilation, and breathing exercises, 59–61
"Hypnogogic" processes, 137
Hypochondriasis, 114, 115

Identity (*see also* Self-relationship)
assessment, 43, 44
constructivism theme, 6, 7, 32, 33
in dreams, 139
spiritual skills link, 161
Imagery, in relaxation exercises, 67
Individual differences, and treatment response, 59
Informed consent
form for, 53, 226–229
and streaming, 143
Initial interview, 52, 53
Instrumental conditioning, 77
Intake interview, 52, 53
Intermittent reinforcement, 80, 81
Internalization
in narrative reconstruction, 102
and problem identification, 74, 75
International Classification of Diseases, 40, 41
Internet, 70
Intersubjectivity, 54, 55
Introspection training, 83, 140
Isometric exercise, 117

James, William, 4, 6, 7, 80, 140, 141, 143, 152, 153, 161, 215
Journal writing
and dream work, 140
in pattern-level work, 90–92

Kant, Immanuel, 4, 10, 135, 214, 215
Keller, Evelinn Fox, 4, 7
Kelly, George A., 4, 7, 50, 74, 104, 132, 216, 217
Kindly self-control, 253
Knorr-Cetina, Karin, 4, 7

Languaging, 80, 97
Lao Tzu, 3, 108, 212, 213
Laughing meditation, 127
Laughter, healing potential, 127
Life collage, 98
Life Companion (Baldwin), 90
Life-review exercises, 95–100
format, 96
purpose of, 95, 96
Life story method, 96, 97
Lifespan development, constructivism theme, 8, 9
Lucid dreaming, 138

Massage
benefits, 122
and professional boundaries, 124, 125
Maturana, Humberto, 4, 7, 80
Meaning making
narrative reconstruction function, 100, 101
in stories, 7, 8
Measurement, 38–42
and individual differences, 39, 40
pathology focus of, 41
and personal meanings, 40
quantitative method limitations, 39
Meditation, 110–113, 249, 250
and breathing exercises, 59–62, 111, 112
centering function of, 69
and cognitive therapy, 83
and embodiment exercises, 113–115
and posture, 111
in process-level work, 46, 47
and relapse prevention, 83
relaxation distinction, 111, 112
"streaming" distinction, 141, 142
Mind-body dualism, 114

Mindfulness meditation, 112, 113, 247, 248
basic goal of, 112
cognitive therapy integration, 162
and perspective-taking, 162
in relapse prevention, 83, 162, 163
technique, 112, 113, 247, 248
"Miracle question," 85
Mirror time, 154–161, 251, 252
case example, 154–156
dialectical balance in, 158, 159
protocol, 156, 157, 251, 252
self-relationship effect, 154–161
therapist coaching in, 158, 159
trespasso exercise in, 159, 160
Morality, and constructivism, 217, 218
"Moses complex," 199
Movement meditation, 115 (*see also* Embodiment exercises)
Music
centering function of, 71
and rhythm exercises, 120, 121
Musical memories method, 97, 98, 120
Myth of arrival, 165, 166

Narrative reconstruction, 100–104
and dreams, 140
meaning making function, 100, 101
nonlinear course of, 101
polarization of problems in, 101, 102
"possible selves" in, 102, 103
turning points exercise, 103
"Narrative turn," 100
Necker cube, 109, 110
Negative reinforcement, 78–80
Negative thoughts, meditation effect on, 162
"Negative triad," 82
The New Diary (Rainer), 90

Object relations, 54
Objectivity, 55
Olympic weightlifting, 118, 119
"One-leg stand" exercise, 64–66, 245, 246
adaptation for athletes, 65, 66
metaphors in, 65
technique, 64, 65, 245, 246
"Opening and closing" metaphor, 24–26
and change process, 25
dynamics, 25
thinking and feeling experience of, 25, 26
Operant conditioning, 77
Order dimension
assessment, 43
in constructivism, 6, 32
and "opening and closing" metaphor, 24–26
and routines, 71
Origins pilgrimage, 98–100
"Out breath" counting, 112

Pain, and physical exercise, 119
Panic episodes, breathing exercises, 60
"Parallel processes," 112

Pattern-level work, 88–107
bibliotherapy, 91
life-review exercises in, 95–100
narrative reconstruction in, 100–104
personal journaling method, 90–95
"unsent letter" exercise in, 92–95
Patterns, 44–48
assessment, 44–48
definition, 45, 46
essence of, 89
"Pause breathing," 60, 61, 242, 243
Pavlovian conditioning, 77
Perceptual constancy, 48, 49
Persona, 90
Personal construct theory, 216, 217
Personal Experience Report, 75, 230–241
and body awareness, 115
dreams in, 138
rating scale structure of, 75
Personal identity (*see* Identity)
Personal journaling, 90–92
Personal revolutions, 177–180, 190*n*8 (*see also* Quantum change)
and attachment to therapist, 179
case illustrations, 183–187
courage role in, 181, 182
evolutionary aspects, 179, 180
phenomenology of, 109, 178, 179
and therapist's creativity, 181–187
Personality, emotionality interactions, 180
Personality change, 178, 190*n*8
Pets, 70
Physical exercise (*see* Resistance exercise)
Piaget, Jean, 4, 6, 8, 51, 216
Places, as source of stability, 70, 72
Poetry, functions of, 108, 109
"Positive" psychology
affirmation role in, 23
constructivism link, 14
Positive reinforcement, 78–80

"Possible selves," 102, 103
Postmodernism, 218
"Postural sway," 64
Posture
  alignment techniques, 116, 117
  balance in, 116, 117
  and meditation, 111
Power, in core ordering process, 50
"Power walk," 120, 129*n*16
"Praxis," 19
"Presence"
  definition, 15, 16
  therapeutic relationship factor, 15, 16
Problem-solving level, 73–87, 105
  behavioral techniques, 76–81
  cognitive restructuring, 81–85
  evaluation methods, 75, 76
  phases of, 74
  solution-focused approach, 85
Problems, 44–48
  assessment of, 44–48
  definition, 45
  function of, 174
Process-level work, 108–129
  "as if" role playing in, 131–135
  and core ordering processes change, 51, 131
  embodiment exercises role, 113–128
  fantasy and dreams in, 135–140
  and meditation, 110–113
  poetry relationship, 109
  risks, 47, 48, 131
  role playing in, 131–135
  and streaming, 46, 51, 140–149
  techniques, 46, 47, 51, 110–113
Processes, 44–48
  assessment, 44–48
  and change, 51, 58
  definition, 46
  therapeutic techniques, 46, 47
Professional boundaries, and touch, 124, 125
Progressive challenge
  versus aggressive challenge, 27
  caring compatibility, 27, 28
  therapeutic relationship link, 27, 28
Progressive muscle relaxation, 66–69
  centering function of, 66–69
  individual differences in response to, 59
Psychodrama, 131, 132
Psychological tests, 141
Psychotropic medication, and diagnosis, 41
Punishment
  and behavioral methods, 78, 79
  time course factor, 79

Qi Gong, 115
"Quantophilia," 39
Quantum change, 109, 128, 177–180, 190*n*8

Range of movement, 116, 117
  balance metaphor, 116
  and postural alignment techniques, 116, 117
Rating scales, 75, 76
Rational-emotive therapy, 81
Rationalism, and neglect of body, 114
Reading, as centering exercise, 70
Reinforcement techniques
  consistency in, 80, 81
  principles, 78–80
Relapse prevention, 83, 162
Relationship theme
  assessment, 44
  and centering, 69, 70
  in constructivism, 7, 8, 33
Relativism, 218
Relaxation exercises, 66–69, 105, 247, 248
  centering function of, 66–69
  individual differences in response to, 59
  main purpose of, 69
  meditation distinction, 111, 112
  techniques, 67–69, 247, 248
"Release breathing," 61, 62, 242
Repressed memories, and streaming, 148
Resistance exercises, 117–120
  forms of, 117–119
  individualized programs, 119
  and pain, 119
Resistance to change, 173–177
  case illustration, 174, 175
  definition, 173, 174
"Reversing consequences gradient"
  practical implications, 45
  principle of, 79
Reward
  and behavioral methods, 78, 79
  time course factor, 79
Rhythm exercises, 120–122
Rituals
  centering techniques link, 58, 71, 72
  in constructive psychotherapy, 36

Role playing, 131–135
"as if" method, 131–133
benefits, 134, 135
Rolfing, 116
Routines, order function of, 71, 72
Rychlak, Joseph, 4, 7

Scaffolding, and spirituality, 164
Schedules of reinforcement, 80, 81
Schopenhauer, Arthur, 4, 10, 13, 214, 215
Science, 217–221
constructivism in, 217–221
dialectical model, 220, 221
social studies of, 218–220
SCIENCE acronym, 74
"Science wars," 217–221
Second-order change, 177
Secure base, and change, 173
Self-care, therapists, 205, 206, 260, 261
Self-comforting exercise, 254, 255
Self-compassion, 153, 154
Self-control 253
Self-efficacy
constructivism emphasis on, 5, 6
learning of, 80
Self-help books
function, 70
limitations, 166
Self psychology, 54
Self-regulation, behavioral principles, 79
Self-relationship, 152–169
assessment, 43, 44
in constructivism, 6, 7, 32, 33
and core ordering process, 50
and mirror time, 154–161
self-esteem distinction, 153
and spiritual skills, 161–167
transformational change effects on, 180
Self-report measures, 141
Sense of self (*see* Self-relationship)
Sensory deprivation experiences, 148
Sexual abuse survivors, touch ethics, 125
Shaping technique, 79, 80
Slow-motion walking, 66
Social studies of science, 218–220
Social-symbolic relatedness
assessment, 44
centering function, 69, 70
in constructivism, 7, 8, 33
Socratic method, 83
"The Sokal hoax," 219
"Solution-focused" approach, 85
Sound exchange exercise, 126
Spiritual skills, 161–168, 169n14, 256
basic themes, 164, 165
exercises, 256
morale restoration, 163, 164
path to happiness misconception, 165, 166
scaffolding effect, 164
in therapists, 206, 207
"Standing center" exercises, 62–64, 244, 245
metaphor of, 63, 64
technique, 62, 63, 116, 244, 245
Stationary meditation, 113
"Stimulus control," 76, 77
Stories, in meaning making, 7, 8, 33
Stream of consciousness reporting, 140–149
abreaction and catharsis in, 148
case illustration, 144–147
developmental acceleration effect, 142
disorganizing effects, 142, 143
free association distinction, 142, 143
meditation distinction, 141, 142
in process-level work, 46, 51, 140–149
and repressed memories, 148, 149
therapeutic relationship effects of, 149
three-stage therapist response, 151*n*28
video of, 151*n*28
working alliance importance in, 143
Strength training, 117–119
advantages and disadvantages, 118
individualized programs, 119
and pain, 119
Structure, as root of constructivism, 80
Subjectivity, objectivity polarity, 55
"Successive approximation," 79, 80
"Superconscious," 49
Supportive relationships, 70
Symbolic processes, in constructivism, 7, 8, 33

Tacit dimension, in core ordering processes, 49
Tai Chi, 115
Taoism, 3, 108, 212
Teleonomy, 20, 30*n*11
Termination, 187–190
clinical illustration, 187, 188
"transitional objects" in, 187
Thelen, Esther, 4, 8
Therapeutic relationship
affirmation as basic dimension, 21
collaboration in, 19–21
"presence" role in, 15, 16

Therapeutic relationship *(cont.)*
  progressive challenge link, 27, 28
  streaming effects on, 149
Therapeutic writing, 90–95, 105
Therapists, 193–210
  constructive psychotherapy challenges, 207–209
  creativity in change process, 181–187
  negative stereotypes, 197–199
  personal life of, 197–204
  personal therapy of, 199–204
  as protectors of hope, 23, 196
  psychological development, 206, 207
  self-care, 205, 206, 260, 261
  spiritual development, 206, 207
  vicarious suffering, 195–197
"Three R's" mnemonic, 115
Touch, 122–125
  benefits of, 122
  case illustration, 122, 123
  and professional boundaries, 124, 125
Transference, and transformational change, 179
Transformational change (*see* Personal revolutions)
"Transpersonal" option, 160, 169*n*10
"Transitional objects," and termination, 187
Trauma memories, and streaming, 148, 149
Trespasso exercise, 159, 160, 169*n*9
Turning points exercise, 103
"TV" mnemonic, 115

"Unconscious," and core ordering processes, 49
Unsent letter exercise, 92–95

Vaihinger, Hans, 4, 135, 214, 215
Values, and constructivism, 218
Varela, Francisco, 4, 7
Vicarious learning, 78, 80
Vicarious suffering, therapists, 195–197
Vico, Giambattista, 4, 135, 214, 215
Vipassana meditation, 112
Vocal intonation, 125, 126
Voice, 125–128
  intonation importance, 125–127
  and play, 127
  in process-level work, 125–128
Vowel movements exercise, 126

Walking, 120
Watzlawick, Paul, 4, 7, 217
Weight training, 117–119
  advantages and disadvantages, 118
  individualized programs, 119
Word association, 141
"Wounded healer" stereotype, 197–199